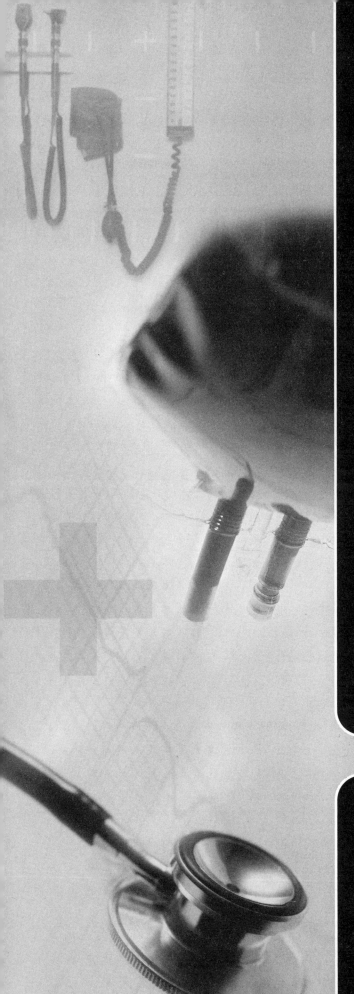

AMERICAN
ASSOCIATION
of CRITICAL-CARE
NURSES

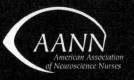

AANN
American Association
of Neuroscience Nurses

AACN-AANN
Protocols for Practice

Monitoring
Technologies
in Critically Ill
Neuroscience Patients

Edited by
Linda R. Littlejohns, RN, MSN, CCRN, CNRN
Vice President of Clinical Development
Integra NeuroSciences
San Diego, California

Mary Kay Bader, RN, MSN, CCRN, CNRN, CCNS
Neuroscience/Critical Care Clinical Nurse Specialist
Mission Hospital
Mission Viejo, California

D1211598

JONES AND BARTLETT PUBLISHERS
Sudbury, Massachusetts
BOSTON   TORONTO   LONDON   SINGAPORE

World Headquarters
Jones and Bartlett Publishers
40 Tall Pine Drive
Sudbury, MA 01776
978-443-5000
info@jbpub.com
www.jbpub.com

Jones and Bartlett Publishers Canada
6339 Ormindale Way
Mississauga, Ontario L5V 1J2
Canada

Jones and Bartlett Publishers International
Barb House, Barb Mews
London W6 7PA
United Kingdom

Jones and Bartlett's books and products are available through most bookstores and online booksellers. To contact Jones and Bartlett Publishers directly, call 800-832-0034, fax 978-443-8000, or visit our website www.jbpub.com.

Substantial discounts on bulk quantities of Jones and Bartlett's publications are available to corporations, professional associations, and other qualified organizations. For details and specific discount information, contact the special sales department at Jones and Bartlett via the above contact information or send an email to specialsales@jbpub.com.

The authors, editor, and publisher have made every effort to provide accurate information. However, they are not responsible for errors, omissions, or for any outcomes related to the use of the contents of this book and take no responsibility for the use of the products and procedures described. Treatments and side effects described in this book may not be applicable to all people; likewise, some people may require a dose or experience a side effect that is not described herein. Drugs and medical devices are discussed that may have limited availability controlled by the Food and Drug Administration (FDA) for use only in a research study or clinical trial. Research, clinical practice, and government regulations often change the accepted standard in this field. When consideration is being given to use of any drug in the clinical setting, the health care provider or reader is responsible for determining FDA status of the drug, reading the package insert, and reviewing prescribing information for the most up-to-date recommendations on dose, precautions, and contraindications, and determining the appropriate usage for the product. This is especially important in the case of drugs that are new or seldom used.

Production Credits
Executive Editor: Kevin Sullivan
Acquisitions Editor: Emily Ekle
Acquisitions Editor: Amy Sibley
Editorial Assistant: Patricia Donnelly
Production Director: Amy Rose
Associate Production Editor: Wendy Swanson
Associate Marketing Manager: Ilana Goddess
Manufacturing and Inventory Control Supervisor: Amy Bacus
Composition: Shepherd, Inc.
Cover Design: Timothy Dziewit
Cover Image: © Photos.com
Printing and Binding: Courier Stoughton
Cover Printing: Courier Stoughton

Library of Congress Cataloging-in-Publication Data

AACN-AANN protocols for practice : monitoring technologies in critically ill neuroscience patients/edited by Linda R. Littlejohns, Mary Kay Bader.
    p. ; cm.
  Includes bibliographical references.
  ISBN-13: 978-0-7637-4156-3 (pbk. : alk. paper)
  ISBN-10: 0-7637-4156-6 (pbk. : alk. paper) 1. Neurological nursing. 2. Patient monitoring. 3. Nursing care plans.
I. Littlejohns, Linda R. II. Bader, Mary Kay. III. American Association of Critical-Care Nurses. IV. American Association of Neuroscience Nurses. V. Title: Protocols for practice.
  [DNLM: 1. Nervous System Diseases—nursing—Practice Guideline. 2. Critical Care—methods—Practice Guideline. 3. Monitoring, Physiologic—methods—Practice Guideline. WY 160.5 A111 2008]

RC350.5.A117 2008
616.8'04231—dc22

                    2007049764

6048

Printed in the United States of America
12 11 10 09 08   10 9 8 7 6 5 4 3 2 1

Dedication

We dedicate this book to Deborah J. Webb, RN, MSN, for her commitment to the practice of neuroscience and critical care nursing. We miss her expertise.

Contents

About the Protocols

Recognizing that clinical practice must continually evolve to keep up with current science, busy bedside clinicians and advanced practice nurses asked the American Association of Critical-Care Nurses for help in using available research to change acute and critical care practice. They asked for studies to be translated into a format in which findings were demystified and their strength evaluated. They would use this tool to advocate for necessary changes in practice because such changes were based on the latest evidence and because they carried the weight of the association's credibility and influence.

In 1994 the American Association of Critical-Care Nurses began developing research-based practice protocols as one of several responses to this request. AACN's Protocols for Practice are designed to provide clinicians at the point of care with the latest patient care research findings in a format that is easy to understand and integrate into clinical practice. The protocols outline the latest thinking on how to best provide care when using technology and in specific patient care situations. Experts in each topic area develop a concise list of recommendations that are appropriate to incorporate into practice routines for patients with a particular situation or device. Recommendations are based on a comprehensive review of the science related to the situation or technology and include only those that are based on research and/or expert consensus positions.

PROTOCOL STRUCTURE

Clinical recommendations represent the core of each protocol. Recommendations are organized in a logical order, usually chronologically, starting with the time before a device is used or an occurrence begins and continuing until after the device is discontinued or the occurrence ends. Recommendations address the following:

Selection of Patients: Including indications, contraindications, and special considerations for use, such as age, physiologic status, and intermittent or continuous monitoring. Depending on the device or procedure, a clinical decision-making algorithm may be provided.

Application of Device and Initial Use: Where appropriate, important considerations during device or procedure application, such as patient preparation, preapplication calibration, and preparation of application site.

Ongoing Monitoring: Important considerations for maintaining the patient during the procedure or for monitoring the device, such as monitoring frequency and clinical factors influencing accuracy and positioning.

Prevention of Complications: Key strategies for prevention or early identification of complications, such as infection, skin breakdown, pain, or discomfort.

Quality Control: Requirements to maintain accuracy of the device under circumstances of normal use.

Recommendation Level: Each recommendation is rated according to the level of information available to support the statement. A scale ranging from I to VI represents progressively stronger levels of scientific basis for the recommendation. Ratings are defined as:

I   Manufacturer's recommendation only

II   Theory-based. No research data to support recommendations; recommendations from expert consensus groups may exist

III   Laboratory data only, no clinical data to support recommendations

IV   Limited clinical studies to support recommendations

V   Clinical studies in more than 1 or 2 different populations and situations to support recommendations

VI   Clinical studies in a variety of patient populations and situations to support recommendations

Along with clinical recommendations, each protocol includes these elements:

- **Case Study:** One or more brief case studies describing a common patient care situation related to the protocol topic
- **General Description:** General description of the device or patient care situation addressed by the protocol
- **Accuracy:** For medical devices, a general description of the accuracy of the device, including precision and bias, with range of accuracy given when variation exists between models and/or manufacturers
- **Competency:** Specific skill or knowledge verification that is important in determining a nurse's competency
- **Ethical Considerations:** Ethical implications or considerations related to the device or patient care situation
- **Occupational Hazards:** Hazards that may be associated with a device or patient care situation, such as electrical safety or exposure to blood-borne pathogens
- **Future Research:** Suggested areas of future research needed to strengthen the research basis of practice related to the protocol content. This may include key points of research methodology important for clinical studies in this category, such as dependent variables to be measured or confounding variables to be considered
- **Annotated Bibliography:** Summary of important aspects of key studies on the topic
- **Suggested Readings:** Resources for additional information on the protocol topic

USING THE PROTOCOLS

The protocols are designed to guide care in a variety of acute and critical care settings, including intensive care, progressive care, and medical-surgical units. Selected topics may also be appropriate for long-term and home care. Clinicians should select those elements that apply to their practice setting.

The protocols are not intended to be used as a step-by-step procedure or comprehensive education resource alone. For this reason, each protocol includes additional informa-

tion sources. Where available and appropriate, protocols include other essential information such as details about the proper application of devices or patient management algorithms. Clinicians may consider first using a protocol to assess the topic's current status in their practice. From this baseline assessment, they can evaluate the merits of changing current practice drawing from the protocol's evaluation of evidence that would support a change in practice.

Protocols will be valuable adjuncts in nursing education because they succinctly summarize the state of the science on a specific topic and identify areas for future research. Nursing students are often exposed to wide variation in practice in equally varied clinical settings. Protocols help to identify whether a variation is based on science.

Experienced researchers will find the protocols useful in identifying areas of inquiry. The evidence supporting each action in a protocol is rated according to its level of scientific information. Lower level ratings indicate there is insufficient research to support a strong scientific base. Users with limited expertise in research methods will find that the protocols accurately summarize the research base using a user-friendly, concise approach with minimal jargon. They have been reviewed for scientific merit, readability, and clinical usefulness as of the time of publication.

AACN PRACTICE ALERTS

Recognizing that clinical practice is ever evolving, the American Association of Critical-Care Nurses issues practice alerts as a real-time complement to the protocols. Practice alerts are succinct dynamic directives supported by authoritative evidence to ensure excellence in practice and a safe and humane work environment. The alerts address nursing and multidisciplinary activities of importance to acutely and critically ill patients and environments in order to close the gap between research and practice, provide guidance in changing practice, standardize practice, and identify and inform about advances and new trends in the science. Practice alerts are posted at www.aacn.org.

Acknowledgments

We would like to thank the nurses and physicians in the surgical intensive care unit at Mission Hospital, Mission Viejo, California, for their commitment to keeping an open mind and their incredible spirit of discovery, which has expanded our knowledge and understanding of the complex physiologic processes inside the cranial vault. Their pursuit of knowledge has provided the foundation for the development and implementation of technology in neuroscience critical care.

We would like to thank the leadership at the American Association of Critical-Care Nurses and the American Association of Neuroscience Nurses for their trust in allowing us to explore this topic and expand our collective knowledge in neuroscience critical care, and to the AACN and AANN national office staff, especially Laura Baerenklau, Anne Costello, Ellen French, Diane Simmons, and Teresa A. Wavra.

We would also like to thank our employers—Mission Hospital and Integra NeuroSciences—for allowing us the time and energy to develop this book. Lastly, we would like to acknowledge the extraordinary contributors and reviewers who provided the evidence-based knowledge and clinical applications to create and refine these protocols. Thanks to Donna St. John, REEGT, lab supervisor, and Colleen Bynum, REEGT, neurodiagnostic center, Albert Einstein Healthcare Network, for assistance in developing illustrations for Chapter 6. Our hope is that the knowledge and information in these protocols will enable nurses at the bedside to apply technology in their quest to choose the appropriate interventions to manage our complex critically ill neuroscience patients.

Contributors

Richard Arbour, RN, MSN, CCRN, CNRN, FAAN
Critical Care Clinical Nurse Specialist
Albert Einstein Medical Center
Philadelphia, Pennsylvania

Mary Kay Bader, RN, MSN, CCRN, CNRN, CCNS
Neuroscience/Critical Care Clinical Nurse Specialist
Mission Hospital
Mission Viejo, California

Patricia A. Blissitt, RN, PhD, CCRN, CNRN, CCM, APRN, BC
Neuroscience Clinical Nurse Specialist
Harborview Medical Center
Seattle, Washington

Catherine Kirkness, RN, PhD
Research Associate Professor
Biobehavioral Nursing and Health System
University of Washington
Seattle, Washington

Barbara "Bobbi" Leeper, RN, MN, CCRN
Clinical Nurse Specialist
Cardiovascular Services
Baylor University Medical Center
Dallas, Texas

Rose Lewis, RN, MSN, ACNP
Long-Term Ventilated Patient Outcomes Manager
Neurosciences
University of Virginia Health System
Charlottesville, Virginia

Linda R. Littlejohns, RN, MSN, CCRN, CNRN
Vice President of Clinical Development
Integra NeuroSciences
San Diego, California

Darlene Lovasik, RN, MN, CCRN, CNRN
Advanced Practice Nurse
UPMC Presbyterian, University of Pittsburgh Medical Center
Pittsburgh, Pennsylvania

Lori Madden, RN, MS, CCRN, CNRN, ACNP-C
Nurse Practitioner
Department of Neurological Surgery
University of California, Davis
Sacramento, California

Dea Mahanes, RN, MSN, CCRN, CNRN, CCNS
Clinical Nurse Specialist
Nerancy Neuroscience ICU
University of Virginia Health System
Charlottesville, Virginia

Karen March, RN, MN, CCRN, CNRN
Director of Clinical Development
Integra LifeSciences
Sammamish, Washington

Reviewers

Suzanne M. Burns, RN, MSN, RRT, ACNP, CCRN, FAAN, FCCM, FAANP
Professor of Nursing and APN 2, Medical ICU
Director of Professional Nursing Staff Organization
    Clinical Research Program
University of Virginia
Charlottesville, Virginia
Ventilatory Management

Elizabeth Crago, RN, MSN, APN
Research Associate
University of Pittsburgh School of Nursing
Pittsburgh, Pennsylvania
Cerebral Blood Flow Monitoring

Laura M. Criddle, RN, MS, CCRN, CCNS, APRN, CFRN
Clinical Nurse Specialist
Organ Health and Science University
Scappoose, Oregon
Brain Oxygen Monitoring

Janice L. Hinkle, RN, PhD, CNRN
Acute Stroke Program
Nuffield Department of Clinical Medicine
Level 7, John Radcliffe Hospital Headington, Oxford,
    United Kingdom
Cerebral Blood Flow Monitoring

Norma D. McNair, RN, MSN, CCRN, CNRN, APRN-BC
Neuroscience Clinical Nurse Specialist
UCLA Medical Center
Los Angeles, California
Cerebrospinal Drainage Systems

Susan T. McNamara, RNC, MSN, CPNP
Children's Hospital Boston
Braintree, Massachusetts
Electroencephalograph-Derived Monitoring

DaiWai M. Olson, RN, PhD
Staff Nurse, Neurocritical Care Unit
Research Associate, Department of Neurology/
    Division of Medicine
Duke University
Durham, North Carolina
Electroencephalograph-Derived Monitoring

Virginia Prendergast, RN, MSN, CNRN, NP-C
Nurse Practitioner
Division of Neurological Surgery
Barrow Neurological Institute
St. Joseph's Hospital
Phoenix, Arizona
Intracranial Pressure Management

Janice M. Powers, RN, MSN, CCRN, CCNS, CNRN, CWCN, FCCM
Director, Clinical Nurse Specialists
Critical Care Clinical Nurse Specialist
St. Vincent Hospital,
Indianapolis, Indiana
Ventilatory Management

Jeannette Richardson, RN, MS, CNRN
ICU Clinical Nurse Specialist
Portland VA Medical Center
Portland, Oregon
Electroencephalograph-Derived Monitoring

Angela Starkweather, PhD, ACNP, CCRN, CNRN
Assistant Professor
Intercollegiate College of Nursing
Washington State University
Spokane, Washington
Cerebrospinal Drainage Systems

Michelle VanDemark, RN, MSN, CNRN
Neuroscience Clinical Nurse Specialist
Sanford USD Medical Center
Sioux Falls, South Dakota
Intracranial Pressure Management

Deborah J. Webb, RN, MSN, CNRN†
Neuroscience Clinical Nurse Specialist
Harborview Medical Center
Seattle, Washington
Intracranial Pressure Management
Cerebrospinal Drainage Systems
†Died June 14, 2007

Eileen Maloney Wilensky, MSN, APRN, BC
Director, Clinical Research Division
Director, CRNP/PA Program
Department of Neurosurgery
University of Pennsylvania
Philadelphia, Pennsylvania
Cerebral Blood Flow Monitoring

Susan C. Yeager, RN, MSN, CCRN, ACNP
Neuroscience Nurse Practitioner
Riverside Methodist Hospital
Columbus, Ohio
Ventilatory Management
Cerebral Blood Flow Monitoring

Ventilatory Management

Dea Mahanes, RN, MSN, CCRN, CNRN, CCNS
and Rose Lewis, RN, MSN, ACNP

CASE STUDY 1: AIRWAY PROTECTION

Mr H., a 33-year-old man, was injured in a motorcycle crash. He was wearing a helmet at the time of the crash and was thrown approximately 20 feet after the initial impact. Mr H. sustained a traumatic brain injury with bifrontal contusions and a small traumatic subarachnoid hemorrhage (SAH); a complete trauma work-up revealed no other injuries. Twenty-four hours after admission to the neuroscience intensive care unit (ICU), Mr H. underwent a bifrontal decompressive craniectomy to treat refractory elevated intracranial pressure (ICP). On hospital day 3, Mr H. remained heavily sedated due to intermittent elevated ICP and required vasopressors to maintain adequate cerebral perfusion pressure (CPP). On hospital day 4, his ICP began to stabilize and sedation and vasopressors were weaned. On hospital day 6, he was localizing to painful stimuli and opening his eyes spontaneously, but was agitated and not following any commands. Also on day 6, Mr H. successfully passed an hour-long spontaneous breathing trial on continuous positive airway pressure (CPAP) of 5 cm H_2O. He coughed spontaneously and was being suctioned every 4 hours for thick yellow sputum. The ICU team was faced with the decision of whether to extubate Mr H., and decided to remove the endotracheal tube. Mr H. was able to productively cough and protect his airway. Due to his decreased mental status, inability to follow commands, and impaired gag, he was unable to successfully pass a swallow evaluation, and tube feedings were used to maintain nutrition. Mr H. was transferred to the acute care area on hospital day 7. On hospital day 10, a percutaneous endoscopic gastrostomy tube was placed for nutrition. He continued to slowly improve neurologically and was discharged to a rehabilitation facility on hospital day 12.

CASE STUDY 2: NEUROMUSCULAR WEAKNESS

Mr J., a 52-year-old man, first experienced tingling in his feet 2 days prior to hospital admission. He experienced increasing weakness and came to the emergency department when he was no longer able to walk unassisted. Mr J. was admitted to the neurology unit with a diagnosis of Guillain-Barré syndrome (GBS). Orders were placed for serial monitoring (every 6 hours) of bedside pulmonary function parameters (see Table 1-1): forced vital capacity (FVC), maximal inspiratory pressure (MIP), and maximal expiratory pressure (MEP). On admission, his FVC was 2.1 L (28 mL/kg, ideal body weight 75 kg), MIP –36 cm H_2O, and MEP 52 cm H_2O. About 4 hours later, the nurse noted that Mr J. was speaking only in single words or short phrases, and had difficulty lifting his head. The nurse collaborated with the respiratory therapist to obtain a new set of respiratory parameters; FVC was 1.2 L (16 mL/kg), MIP –28 cm H_2O, and MEP 42 cm H_2O. Due to the decline in FVC, decreasing MIP, and rapid disease progression, Mr J. was moved to the ICU and electively intubated. Plasma exchange was initiated. Mr J. continued to decline; by the 7th day of hospitalization he was unable to move anything except for his eyes. Because weaning from mechanical ventilation was likely to be prolonged, a tracheostomy was performed on hospital day 8. Plasma exchange treatment continued for a total of 5 sessions. A communication system was established using an eye gaze board and yes/no responses. The interdisciplinary team optimized supportive care, involving Mr J. and his family in care planning. Careful attention was given to pain management, nutrition, and psychological support. The head of Mr J.'s bed was kept elevated 30° to 45° to decrease the risk of ventilator-associated pneumonia.

Table 1-1   Bedside Pulmonary Function Parameters Used in the Management of Patients with Neuromuscular Disease

Parameter	Description	Comments
FVC	Measures the maximum volume of air that can be forcefully expired in 1 breath after a maximal inspiration.	Threshold forced vital capacity (FVC) for weaning in the general patient population is ≥ 15 mL/kg.
MIP	Measures the pressure generated by maximal inhalation against a closed system. Maximal inspiratory pressure (MIP) is an indicator of inspiratory muscle strength.	Also called negative inspiratory force (NIF) or negative inspiratory pressure (NIP). Threshold MIP for weaning is ≤ -20 cm H_2O in the general patient population.
MEP	Measures the pressure generated by forced exhalation against a closed system. Maximal expiratory pressure (MEP) is primarily an indicator of expiratory muscle strength.	Also called positive expiratory force (PEF) or positive expiratory pressure (PEP). Threshold MEP for weaning is ≥ 30 cm H_2O in the general patient population.

Source: Adapted from: Burns SM. Weaning from mechanical ventilation, Appendix 3B: traditional weaning indices. In Burns SM (ed). *AACN Protocols for Practice: Care of Mechanically Ventilated Patients*, 2nd ed. Sudbury, MA: Jones and Bartlett; 2007:97–154.

Mechanical and pharmacological strategies were used to prevent venous thromboembolism. A schedule was created to provide periods of activity alternating with periods of rest, and to allow for uninterrupted sleep at night. Mr J.'s skeletal and respiratory muscle strength gradually improved, and ventilator weaning was initiated on hospital day 17, when his FVC was 550 mL (a little more than 7 mL/kg, a level found to be consistent with readiness to begin weaning in a small study; Other References: 24). Mr J. was weaned using pressure support, which was gradually reduced as tolerated by the patient. Signs of intolerance were clearly established: tachypnea (respiratory rate ≥ 30 for more than 5 minutes), oxygen saturation <92%, change in blood pressure or heart rate of $\geq 20\%$ from baseline, or the use of respiratory accessory muscles. Mr J. was returned to full ventilatory support (pressure support adequate to maintain respiratory rate ≤ 20 breaths/minute) at night to promote rest. By hospital day 27, Mr J. no longer required mechanical ventilation, was able to cough up secretions through his tracheostomy, and only required tracheal suctioning every 4 to 6 hours. He was transferred to the acute care floor, and moved to a rehabilitation center a few days later. His tracheostomy was removed at the rehabilitation center once he demonstrated the ability to clear his own airway. After 5 weeks of rehabilitation, Mr J. returned home. During his visit to the ICU 10 months later, Mr J. reported that he was back at work with no notable deficits except for occasional fatigue and slightly decreased facial strength.

GENERAL DESCRIPTION

As these 2 case studies illustrate, intubation and mechanical ventilation are treatment strategies for critically ill neuroscience patients who present with a variety of indications. While most patients require mechanical ventilation because of oxygenation problems and have underlying lung pathology, critically ill neuroscience patients often have normal lungs. Lack of adequate airway protection is frequently the cause for intubation. Loss of airway protection may be due to decreased mental status or bulbar impairment. Decreased

mental status can be a direct consequence of neuronal injury or can result from the secondary effects of increased pressure within the cranial vault due to trauma, stroke, infection, or other pathologies. Patients with cranial nerve deficits (commonly seen with brainstem or cerebellar lesions) may be unable to swallow or cough effectively, leading to aspiration of oral secretions. Neuromuscular diseases often affect the oropharyngeal muscles, causing decreased secretion clearance and loss of airway protection.

Neuroscience patients also may require mechanical ventilation because of inspiratory or expiratory muscle weakness. Neuromuscular diseases and spinal cord injury affect the function of the muscles of respiration, often leading to hypoventilation and atelectasis. Development of neuromuscular respiratory weakness is frequently insidious and standard parameters (eg, arterial blood gases) may not reflect the need for ventilation until respiratory failure is imminent. Respiratory muscle weakness may develop due to an acute neuromuscular disease such as GBS or exacerbation of a chronic neuromuscular disease such as myasthenia gravis (MG). GBS causes progressive muscle weakness due to demyelination of the peripheral nerves. Weakness typically starts in the lower extremities and ascends, with approximately 20% to 30% of individuals requiring mechanical ventilation (Other References: 23, 42, 94). Treatment consists of plasma exchange or intravenous immunoglobulin, and supportive care. Most patients recover, but hospitalization is often prolonged (Other References: 46). MG is an autoimmune disease of the neuromuscular junction; a decrease in neuromuscular impulse transmission causes muscle weakness that may include the muscles of respiration. Patients with MG experience periodic exacerbations, which sometimes necessitate mechanical ventilation (*myasthenic crisis*). These episodes are typically treated with plasma exchange or intravenous immunoglobulin (Other References: 61). Patients with cervical or thoracic spinal cord injury can also develop neuromuscular respiratory failure, with the degree of respiratory involvement dependent on the level of cord impairment.

Patients with complete injuries above C3 do not initiate respirations due to loss of diaphragmatic innervation and require ventilation to survive. Complete spinal cord injuries below this level cause paralysis of the accessory respiratory muscles to varying degrees, and cough strength is also diminished. Airway management and secretion clearance in patients with spinal cord injuries is further complicated by the need for spine stabilization devices such as cervical collars, halo vests, and other braces.

Other patients require intubation and mechanical ventilation for treatment of their primary neurological problem. Neurological conditions affecting the brainstem may directly impact respiratory drive, causing abnormal breathing patterns or even apnea. Patients with inadequate gas exchange due to abnormal respiratory pattern will require mechanical ventilation. As mentioned previously, lesions in this area also frequently cause bulbar dysfunction resulting in loss of airway protection and the need for intubation. Pathologies such as traumatic brain injury, hydrocephalus, neuro-infectious processes, stroke, aneurysmal SAH, and postcraniotomy cerebral edema may cause increased ICP and impact mental status. Management of elevated ICP often includes the use of sedative medications, necessitating placement of an artificial airway and mechanical ventilation. Although routine hyperventilation is no longer recommended in the care of neurological patients, hyperventilation is sometimes used for short periods to control elevated ICP while other interventions are taking place. Recently, the use of devices that measure cerebral oxygenation (brain tissue oxygen monitoring) has become widespread. The data obtained from these devices emphasize the impact of respiratory management on preventing cerebral ischemia. Arterial levels of both oxygen and carbon dioxide have a marked impact on cerebral hemodynamics and perfusion.

Finally, neuroscience patients may require mechanical ventilation for concomitant lung injury or underlying chronic cardiac or pulmonary disease. For example, patients with central nervous system (CNS) trauma also may have thoracic trauma such as rib fracture, pneumothorax, hemothorax, and pulmonary contusions, or may have facial trauma that produces airway compromise. Aspiration prior to intubation is common in patients with decreased mental status and can result in pneumonia. Neurogenic pulmonary edema (NPE) may develop in patients with significant CNS dysfunction, and compromises oxygenation. Cardiogenic pulmonary edema also occurs, especially in patients receiving hyperdynamic therapy for the treatment of cerebral vasospasm or CPP augmentation due to elevated ICP. While these therapies are necessary for management of the primary neurological condition, they can complicate pulmonary care, especially in patients with pre-existing cardiac or pulmonary disease.

Research into specific weaning strategies for patients with neurological illness or injury is very limited. In fact, most studies of mechanical ventilation and weaning either

---

Table 1-2 Weaning Readiness Criteria

Neurological process stable or improving

Sao_2 >92% on Fio_2 <0.50

PEEP <6 cm H_2O

Minute ventilation <12 L/min

Hemodynamically stable (no dysrhythmias, heart rate <120)

If monitored, ICP stable without aggressive intervention

Sao_2, arterial oxygen saturation; Fio_2, fraction of inspired oxygen; PEEP, positive end-expiratory pressure; ICP, intracranial pressure

---

Table 1-3 Intolerance Criteria

Respiration rate >30 breaths per minute for >5 minutes

Sao_2 <92% (unless concomitant respiratory disease)

Change in heart rate or blood pressure of <20% from baseline

Accessory muscle use

Sao_2, arterial oxygen saturation

---

include only very small numbers of neuroscience patients or exclude them completely. In the absence of sufficient research that specifically addresses neuroscience patients, clinicians combine the available evidence on ventilator weaning with an understanding of the pathophysiology of neurological disease or injury to determine best practice. Evidence-based guidelines for weaning patients from mechanical ventilation advocate the use of spontaneous breathing protocols using CPAP or T-piece as the preferred mode (Other References: 74). In comparison, a trial by Esteban and colleagues suggests that the use of pressure support as a weaning modality is equivalent to the use of T-piece (Other References: 38). Pressure support weaning is often used for those patients who do not tolerate CPAP trials. The use of weaning protocols decreases practice variation, assures aggressive testing of readiness, and is associated with decreased ventilation duration (Other References: 36, 65). Weaning protocols should include distinct readiness criteria for initiating trials, the method and duration of weaning trials (typically CPAP or T-piece for between 30 minutes and 2 hours), and intolerance criteria for stopping trials (Other References: 19). Patients should be evaluated daily for weaning readiness (Table 1-2), and trials should be initiated as soon as readiness criteria are met. Intolerance criteria (Table 1-3) indicate the need to stop a weaning trial and return the patient to full ventilatory support. In addition to weaning protocols, the algorithmic management of sedation and the use of protocols to wean sedative infusions have resulted in shorter duration of mechanical ventilation and shorter ICU and hospital length of stay (Other References: 14, 66). In summary, a comprehensive, interdisciplinary approach, which includes a systematic plan that decreases variability in care, weaning assessment, weaning trials, and weaning off of sedative infusions is the objective (Other References: 19).

Though extubation is the final goal, often neuroscience patients can be weaned (ie, able to sustain spontaneous breathing) but still require an artificial airway for airway protection. Readiness for extubation must be evaluated separately from the ability to wean from mechanical ventilation. Patients with decreased mental status pose a particular challenge. Frequently these patients can be successfully extubated, provided they have a strong cough and minimal secretions. For patients with neuromuscular disease, the approach to weaning and extubation varies based on the disease process. Some patients, including those with GBS or high cervical spinal cord injury, may benefit from early tracheostomy to improve comfort and facilitate communication. Patients intubated for an exacerbation of MG can typically be liberated from mechanical ventilation in 1 to 2 weeks, so tracheostomy is deferred. Regardless of the underlying disease process and the weaning approach used, careful attention to the prevention of complications is essential.

ACCURACY

Data supporting specific strategies for the mechanical ventilation of neuroscience patients vary in quality. The scientific merit of these strategies is reflected in the level of support assigned to each recommendation. In addition, studies of patients with neuromuscular disease frequently describe the use of bedside pulmonary function parameters (FVC, MIP, and MEP; Table 1-1) to predict the need for the initiation or continuation of mechanical ventilation. Because of the prevalence of bulbar function and the impact of examiner technique, pulmonary function parameters can be both difficult to obtain and inconsistent in this patient population.

COMPETENCY

Patients with neurological injury or illness require nurses skilled in both neuroscience and critical care nursing to achieve optimal outcomes. Effective use of ventilation strategies in critically ill neuroscience patients requires an understanding of pulmonary and neuro anatomy and physiology, dynamics of brain injury and delivery of oxygen to prevent secondary ischemic injury, modes of mechanical ventilation, and the process of weaning patients from mechanical ventilation. Additionally, the nurse requires knowledge on the procedures and purposes of end-tidal carbon dioxide monitoring, and analysis of arterial blood gases. Finally, if brain tissue oxygenation monitoring is being utilized to assist in clinical management, the nurse requires knowledge of the procedures and purposes of this type of monitoring.

ETHICAL CONSIDERATIONS

As previously noted, patients with neurological illness sometimes maintain adequate oxygenation and ventilation, but remain intubated because they are unable to protect their airway. Many clinicians advocate early tracheostomy

placement in these patients. Because the presence of a tracheostomy may prolong the dying process in neurological patients, delaying tracheostomy may be appropriate in patients with a very poor prognosis while discussions about the patient's wishes are ongoing.

Patients with progressive neuromuscular disease such as amyotrophic lateral sclerosis or Duchenne muscular dystrophy pose a special challenge to the healthcare team. Mechanical ventilation represents end-stage disease in these patients. They are rarely admitted to the ICU because decisions regarding mechanical ventilation are usually made prior to the onset of respiratory failure. Although discussion of mechanical ventilation in progressive neuromuscular disease is outside of the scope of this protocol, critical care nurses should be aware that these patients have unique needs. When these patients are admitted to the ICU, the role of the critical care nurse focuses on communication, psychological support, and symptom management within the range of interventions desired by the patient.

OCCUPATIONAL HAZARDS

The primary occupational hazard associated with the use of mechanical ventilation is exposure to body fluids during airway management and suctioning. Use of universal precautions, including face mask and eye protection, is recommended. In-line suction devices also may decrease the risk of exposure to body fluids.

FUTURE RESEARCH

Most studies of mechanical ventilation and weaning exclude patients with neurological illness or injury. Because neurological patients are underrepresented in the literature on mechanical ventilation and weaning, many opportunities exist for research. Potential areas of investigation include the development of objective, validated bedside assessments of cough strength and the effects of high frequency ventilation on brain tissue oxygenation.

In addition, most research on extubation of neurological patients is based on retrospective data, with the decision for extubation left up to the individual physician. Prospective trials using specific protocols and criteria for extubation are needed. A related area of research is the use of sedation and analgesia in neurological patients undergoing ventilator weaning. Questions include the validity and reliability of sedation scales in patients with altered level of consciousness and the optimal agent to use for sedation during weaning.

Sedation scales such as the Richmond Agitation-Sedation Scale (RASS) have demonstrated excellent interrater reliability and validity in a broad range of medical and surgical ICU patients (Other References: 37), but very few have been adequately tested in neurological patients with decreased mental status. A unique feature of the RASS is that it uses the duration of eye contact following verbal stimulation (arousal) as the principal means of titrating sedation. This criterion can be assessed on neuroscience patients who may be candidates for ventilator weaning, even though they may not be able to consistently follow commands. A sedative agent that shows promise in this patient population is dexmedetomidine (Precedex), an alpha-2 agonist that does not significantly depress respirations and decreases agitation while leaving the patient able to respond to stimulation (Other References: 48, 113). Additional research is required to evaluate the potential advantages of this agent over more commonly used sedative medications.

The literature pertaining to mechanical ventilation and weaning of patients with acute neuromuscular disease is also limited. A small number of retrospective studies indicate that optimal ventilatory management of these patients may differ significantly from the management found to be effective for the general ICU population. Specifically, the use of high tidal volumes in patients with spinal cord injury (Other References: 88) and the use of pulmonary recruitment strategies such as periodic positive pressure breathing (Annotated Bibliography: 9) may have utility in this population, but this must be confirmed in prospective trials. The use of progressive ventilator-free periods (T-piece, tracheostomy collar, or spontaneous speaking valve trials) versus gradual reduction of pressure support in weaning patients with spinal cord injury promotes communication and patient comfort, and is supported by 1 retrospective analysis (Other References: 87). Further investigation of this strategy is warranted. Finally, while predictors of the need for mechanical ventilation have been identified in patients with acute neuromuscular disease, the optimal timing of intubation has not been established. Elective intubation of these patients before they exhibit overt respiratory failure may minimize complications associated with emergent intubation, and the impact of elective intubation on overall morbidity and mortality should be evaluated (Table 1-4).

Table 1-4   Agents Used in Rapid Sequence Intubation of Neuroscience Patients

Indication and Nursing Considerations

Pretreatment Agents	
Lidocaine	To attenuate the cardiovascular response to laryngoscopy, decrease airway reactivity, and prevent elevations in ICP. Given approximately 3 minutes prior to laryngoscopy.
Opioids (eg, fentanyl)	To attenuate the cardiovascular response to laryngoscopy and provide analgesia. May cause hypotension.
Defasciculating dose of a nondepolarizing neuromuscular blocking agent	Succinylcholine, a depolarizing neuromuscular blocking agent, causes fasciculations that may transiently increase ICP. A small dose of a nondepolarizing neuromuscular blocker (rocuronium and vecuronium) can be used to eliminate these fasciculations.
Beta blocker (eg, esmolol)	To block the sympathetic stimulation associated with laryngoscopy, thus attenuating tachycardia and hypertension. Only short-acting agents (ie, esmolol) should be used to avoid a prolonged effect on blood pressure. Avoid use in patients dependent on tachycardia to maintain cardiac output (eg, trauma patients).
Induction Agents	
Etomidate	Nonbarbiturate hypnotic. Less effect on blood pressure than other induction agents. Some practitioners avoid use due to inhibition of cortisol production.
Propofol	Benefit is rapid onset and short duration of action. Does not provide analgesia. May cause hypotension. Suppresses pharyngeal and laryngeal muscle tone/reflexes more than other induction agents, so may be used when paralysis is undesirable or contraindicated.
Thiopental	Barbiturate with rapid onset and short half-life. Used in patients with status epilepticus or elevated ICP. May cause significant hypotension.
*Neuromuscular Blocking Agents**	
Succinylcholine	Depolarizing neuromuscular blocking agent with rapid onset (30–60 seconds) and short duration (5–15 minutes). Causes transient fasciculations prior to paralysis (see Pretreatment Agents above). May cause an increase in potassium, which is more pronounced in patients with massive trauma, traumatic brain injury, neuromuscular disease, or sepsis. Avoid in patients with muscle weakness for longer than 24–48 hours, and in patients with neuromuscular disease.
Rocuronium	Nondepolarizing neuromuscular blocking agent with a short onset of action (1–2 minutes) and duration of 30–50 minutes. Decrease dose in patients with MG.
Vecuronium	Nondepolarizing neuromuscular blocking agent with a short onset of action (1.5–2 minutes) and duration of 20–30 minutes. Decrease dose in patients with MG.

*The duration of action of neuromuscular blocking agents generally exceeds the duration of action of the sedative agents used for induction. Patients require additional sedation and analgesia following intubation.

Source: Other References: 95, 99. *Martindale Complete Drug Reference*, electronic version, retrieved 9/24/2006 from Micromedex, University of Virginia Health System Intranet. Available at Thomson Micromedex, Greenwood, CO at http://www.micromedex.com/products/martindale/. Accessed August 2, 2007.

CLINICAL RECOMMENDATIONS

The rating scale for the Level of Recommendation ranges from I to VI, with levels indicated as follows: I, manufacturer's recommendations only; II, theory based, no research data to support recommendations; recommendations from expert consensus group may exist; III, laboratory data only, no clinical data to support recommendations; IV, limited clinical studies to support recommendations; V, clinical studies in more than 1 or 2 different populations and situations to support recommendations; VI, clinical studies in a variety of patient populations and situations to support recommendations.

Period of Use	Recommendation	Rationale for Recommendation	Level of Recommendation	Supporting References	Comments
Selection of Patients	Critically ill neuroscience patients may require intubation and mechanical ventilation because of loss of airway protection due to decreased mental status or bulbar weakness.	A decreased level of consciousness can cause relaxation of the oropharyngeal muscles, changing the contour of the upper airway and potentially causing obstruction. An adequate cough reflex, more so than gag reflex, is the final protective mechanism to clear the airway of any aspirated material. Patients with bulbar weakness due to neuromuscular disease or cranial nerve deficits may be unable to manage their oral secretions, compromising airway protection and placing them at risk for aspiration.	V	See Annotated Bibliography: 4 See Other References: 56, 61, 63, 67, 73, 93, 115	Airway protection during swallowing is accomplished through closure of the laryngeal sphincter, epiglottal covering of the laryngeal opening, and elevation of the larynx to effectively remove it from the path of the food bolus. Aspiration is generally defined as food entering the larynx below the true vocal cords. Signs of bulbar weakness include difficulty swallowing, accumulation of saliva, "wet" voice, nasal voice, and weak cough. Assessing bulbar weakness requires monitoring for these signs/symptoms and evaluation of bilateral facial movement, jaw strength, and tongue strength/movement. Decreased cough reflex, inability to clear secretions, and amount of endotracheal secretions can contribute to prolonged intubation. (Annotated Bibliography: 2, 3; Other References: 109)
	Critically ill neuroscience patients may require intubation and mechanical ventilation for management of concomitant pulmonary processes. a. Acute lung injury (ALI), acute respiratory distress syndrome (ARDS)	Hypoxia secondary to an underlying pulmonary process can affect oxygenation of brain tissue. The brain depends on an uninterrupted delivery of oxygen and glucose to prevent secondary ischemic injury. The proposed reason for the increase in brain tissue oxygenation associated with an increase in F_{IO_2} is the enhancement of the dissolved oxygen in plasma. Pa_{O_2} appears to be the driving force of oxygen movement from plasma to tissues.	V	See Other References: 7, 70, 83, 84, 103	The American-European Consensus Conference defines ALI as a partial pressure of oxygen/fraction of inspired oxygen (Pa_{O_2}/F_{IO_2}) ratio of <300 mm Hg, bilateral infiltrates on chest radiograph, and no clinical evidence of increased left atrial pressure (pulmonary capillary wedge pressure of <18 mm Hg).

Period of Use	Recommendation	Rationale for Recommendation	Level of Recommendation	Supporting References	Comments
Selection of Patients *(cont.)*		Correcting hypoxia is a crucial step in preventing secondary brain injury and worse neurological outcome. Adequate ventilation strategies to correct hypoxia while preventing further lung injury are essential.			ARDS is defined by the criteria above with a Pao_2/Fio_2 ratio of <200 mm Hg.
		Development of ALI correlates with mortality and with worse neurological outcome in patients with traumatic brain injury (TBI).		See Other References: 13, 55	
		In patients with TBI, there is an association between the use of induced elevations in mean arterial pressure to manage CPP and the development of ARDS.		See Other References: 12, 28, 97	
		In a recent study, patients with SAH who also met criteria for ALI had a statistically significant increase in hospital mortality and increased ICU length of stay. Risk factors for the development of ALI in SAH patients included severity of illness, clinical grade of SAH, packed red blood cell transfusion, and severe sepsis.		See Other References: 62	
	b. Neurogenic pulmonary edema (NPE)	NPE meets the criteria above for ALI. Unlike other mechanisms for ALI, NPE typically resolves in 48–72 hours and the treatment is supportive with oxygen, mechanical ventilation, and positive end-expiratory pressure (PEEP).	IV	See Other References: 41, 89, 114	NPE is thought to be a consequence of massive sympathetic discharge and catecholamine release following various types of brain injury. An increase in ICP or sympathetic tone gives rise to an increase in neurogenically-mediated pulmonary venoconstriction and increased capillary permeability. An increase in hydrostatic pulmonary pressure also occurs.
					In a retrospective review of patients with SAH, the incidence of vasospasm in SAH patients with NPE was higher than in those without NPE. This was thought to be the result of more conservative fluid management and the use of diuretics in the patients with NPE (Other References: 43).

Period of Use	Recommendation	Rationale for Recommendation	Level of Recommendation	Supporting References	Comments
Selection of Patients *(cont.)*	Critically ill neuroscience patients may require intubation and mechanical ventilation for management of underlying chronic pulmonary disease (ie, chronic obstructive pulmonary disease, asthma, pulmonary hypertension).	Any chronic underlying pulmonary conditions also should be addressed when mechanical ventilation is initiated in critically ill neuroscience patients. These conditions may impact ventilation strategies and extubation readiness.	II	See Other References: 19, 74	Pre-existing cardiac disease also impacts intubation, mechanical ventilation, and weaning.
	Critically ill neuroscience patients may require intubation and mechanical ventilation for weakness of inspiratory or expiratory respiratory muscles.	The diaphragm is the primary muscle of inspiration. The intercostal and scalene muscles also contribute to full inhalation. The abdominal muscles contribute to active exhalation. Weakness of the inspiratory muscles causes decreased tidal volume and loss of the ability to sigh. Atelectasis develops and the patient cannot generate an adequate inspiration to effectively cough. Weakness of the expiratory muscles results directly in decreased cough strength.	V	See Annotated Bibliography: 4, 7, 8 See Other References: 24, 25, 26, 56, 64, 86, 93, 107, 117	Common causes of acute neuromuscular respiratory failure include MG, GBS, and cervical or thoracic spinal cord injury (SCI).
	Patients with neuromuscular dysfunction who exhibit any of the following clinical signs of neuromuscular respiratory failure may require intubation and mechanical ventilation: 1. Tachypnea 2. Tachycardia 3. Paradoxical movement of the chest and abdomen 4. Staccato speech 5. Use of accessory muscles	Traditional indicators of the need for mechanical ventilation, such as hypoxia and hypercarbia, occur late in the course of acute neuromuscular respiratory failure.	IV	See Annotated Bibliography: 8 See Other References: 93, 98, 107	
	Obtain bedside pulmonary function parameters every 4–8 hours in patients at risk for neuromuscular respiratory failure. Parameters include: 1. FVC 2. MIP 3. MEP	These pulmonary function parameters can be measured at the bedside by the respiratory therapist or a specially trained nurse. Changes in FVC, MIP, and MEP, when used in combination with clinical assessment, assist the practitioner in identifying patients at risk for	II	See Annotated Bibliography: 4 See Other References: 24, 27, 47, 56, 67, 86, 93, 98	Table 1-1 describes these bedside pulmonary function parameters. Patients with significant bulbar weakness may have difficulty forming a seal around a mouthpiece when performing pulmonary function tests, thus decreasing the accuracy and utility of the tests.

Period of Use	Recommendation	Rationale for Recommendation	Level of Recommendation	Supporting References	Comments
Selection of Patients (*cont.*)		mechanical ventilation. Early identification (prior to overt respiratory failure) allows earlier intervention which may decrease complications. Serial monitoring every 4–8 hours allows for the identification of trends without causing undue fatigue.			Bedside pulmonary function parameters may be less useful in predicting the need for mechanical ventilation in patients with MG than in patients with GBS (Other References: 67, 93, 96, 107). This may be due to the highly variable course of MG, or the prevalence of bulbar symptoms.
					Literature describing the predictive value of bedside pulmonary function parameters in patients with SCI is sparse. The Consortium for Spinal Cord Medicine recommends periodic monitoring of volume capacity (VC), MIP, forced expiratory volume in 1 second (FeV_1), and peak cough flow (Other References: 27).
	Patients with GBS who exhibit the following findings on bedside pulmonary function testing are likely to progress to mechanical ventilation: 1. FVC <20 mL/kg 2. MIP >−30 cm H_2O 3. MEP <+40 cm H_2O 4. >30% reduction in FVC, MIP, or MEP	These parameters reflect inspiratory and expiratory weakness that may lead to inadequate ventilation or airway clearance. Early identification of patients at risk for mechanical ventilation allows increased monitoring, so that intubation can be performed prior to complete respiratory failure.	IV	See Annotated Bibliography: 4	In an older study of patients with GBS (Other References: 24), the need for mechanical ventilation was predicted by: 1. FVC <15 mL/kg 2. MIP >−20 cm H_2O 3. MEP <+40 cm H_2O
	For patients with GBS, the following are disease-specific predictors of the need for mechanical ventilation: 1. Rapid disease progression 2. Inability to lift elbows 3. Inability to stand 4. Inability to lift head 5. Cranial nerve dysfunction (bulbar weakness, bilateral facial weakness) 6. Dysautonomia 7. Areflexia	Research indicates that these criteria are associated with the need for mechanical ventilation. In general, the likelihood of neuromuscular respiratory failure requiring mechanical ventilation increases with the number of predictors present. Early identification of patients at risk for mechanical ventilation allows increased monitoring, so that intubation can be performed prior to complete respiratory failure.	IV	See Annotated Bibliography: 4, 7 See Other References: 23, 63	Mechanical ventilation is required in approximately 20%–30% of patients with GBS (Other References: 23, 42, 94). Elevated liver enzymes predicted the need for mechanical ventilation in 1 study (Annotated Bibliography: 7).

Period of Use	Recommendation	Rationale for Recommendation	Level of Recommendation	Supporting References	Comments
Selection of Patients (*cont.*)	Patients with MG who are infected, undergo a change in their medications (addition or withdrawal of steroid therapy, or withdrawal of pyridostigmine) or who undergo thymectomy are at increased risk for neuromuscular failure requiring mechanical ventilation.	One of the most common precipitating factors of myasthenic crisis is infection. Both steroids and thymectomy are used in the treatment of MG, but may cause a transient increase in the risk of myasthenic crisis. In addition, the withdrawal of steroids or pyridostigmine (an anticholinesterase inhibitor used in the management of MG) can precipitate myasthenic crisis.	IV	See Annotated Bibliography: 8, 9 See Other References: 10, 61, 91	Myasthenic crisis is defined by the need for mechanical ventilation in a patient not previously ventilated, or the requirement for greater than 24 hours of mechanical ventilation following surgery. In patients with MG, limb weakness may not correlate with respiratory muscle strength (Annotated Bibliography: 8).
	Patients with SCI at or above T6 are at risk for respiratory failure requiring mechanical ventilation, especially during the first 5 days after injury. Level of injury is highly correlated with the need for mechanical ventilation.	Unless the patient suffers a very high cervical SCI, he or she may be able to maintain oxygenation and ventilation initially. Deterioration often takes place over several days because of atelectasis and retained secretions. In a large study of patients with cervical or thoracic SCI (ASIA A, B, or C), ventilatory failure occurred an average of 4.5 days after injury. Although the risk of ventilatory failure decreases with lower levels of injury, patients with thoracic injury above the level of T6 have significantly decreased respiratory muscle strength (especially expiratory muscles) and warrant close monitoring.	IV	See Annotated Bibliography: 10 See Other References: 25, 26, 29, 60, 117 See Other References: 60	Copious sputum and the development of pneumonia are independent predictors of the need for mechanical ventilation in patients with cervical SCI (Other References: 25). In one study of patients with cervical SCI admitted to a large trauma center, all patients with complete SCI at or above C5 and 79% with complete cervical SCI at or below C6 required mechanical ventilation. The need for intubation and mechanical ventilation was lower among patients with incomplete SCI (Other References: 26).
	Consider elective intubation of patients with complete SCI above C5.	Patients with complete SCI at or above C5 almost always require mechanical ventilation. Emergency intubation may place the patient at risk for complications.	IV	See Annotated Bibliography: 10; See Other References: 25, 26, 102	Ninety-five percent of patients with complete SCI above C5 required intubation in 1 study (Annotated Bibliography: 10). In another study, all patients with complete injury at or above C5 required intubation (Other References: 26).
	Facilitate the transfer of patients with neuromuscular weakness and predictors of the need for intubation and mechanical ventilation to a unit that can provide ongoing monitoring, airway management and	Transfer facilitates monitoring and thus early intervention. Early intervention may decrease complications. A delay in transfer to a tertiary care center of more than 2 days has been	IV	See Annotated Bibliography: 8 See Other References: 40, 67, 86, 93 See Other References: 40	In most cases, patients with acute neuromuscular respiratory weakness and positive predictors of the need for mechanical ventilation will require transfer to an ICU or neurological special care

Period of Use	Recommendation	Rationale for Recommendation	Level of Recommendation	Supporting References	Comments
	ventilation, and definitive care for the underlying disease or injury.	associated with poor outcomes in patients with GBS.			unit at a tertiary care center.
Application of Device and Initial Use	When airway management is required, anticipate the use of rapid sequence intubation in patients with neurological injury or other intracranial process.	Intubation is recommended for patients with traumatic brain injury and a Glasgow Coma Scale (GCS) score ≤8. Use of rapid sequence intubation facilitates endotracheal tube placement.	II	See Other References: 11, 35, 95, 99	Rapid sequence intubation refers to the administration of an induction agent followed almost immediately by a neuromuscular blocking agent for the purpose of facilitating placement of an endotracheal tube. Medications commonly used in the intubation of neuroscience patients are described in Table 1-4.
	In patients with potential or actual elevations in ICP, anticipate the use of medications to attenuate elevations in ICP that occur with intubation.	Intubation transiently increases heart rate, blood pressure, and ICP. Medications such as lidocaine may lessen this response. Use of a depolarizing agent (ie, succinylcholine) for neuromuscular blockade may cause a transient rise in ICP due to the muscle fasciculations that precede paralysis. Some clinicians administer a small dose (defasciculating dose) of a nondepolarizing neuromuscular blocking agent (eg, rocuronium or vecuronium) to mediate this elevation in ICP.	IV	See Other References: 9, 49, 53, 69, 99	Esmolol or fentanyl also may be used to mitigate the hemodynamic response associated with intubation.
	Monitor the patient's hemodynamic response during and after intubation.	The increase in blood pressure associated with intubation may place patients with vascular anomalies (eg, aneurysm, arteriovenous malformation) at increased risk for hemorrhage. Some of the medications used can cause hypotension following intubation, placing patients at risk for cerebral hypoperfusion. The duration of action of some neuromuscular blocking agents exceeds the duration of the medications used for induction. Tachycardia and hypertension during the postintubation period may be indicators of inadequate sedation; additional sedation is necessary.	II	See Other References: 99	

Period of Use	Recommendation	Rationale for Recommendation	Level of Recommendation	Supporting References	Comments
Application of Device and Initial Use (*cont.*)	Anticipate the use of sedative agents without neuromuscular blockade in the intubation of patients with neuromuscular disease.	Patients with neuromuscular disease respond differently and somewhat unpredictably to neuromuscular blocking agents.	II	See Other References: 85, 99	Patients with diseases of the neuromuscular junction (eg, MG) require a much lower dose of nondepolarizing agents (ie, rocuronium or vecuronium).
	Avoid the administration of depolarizing neuromuscular blocking agents (succinylcholine) to patients with muscle weakness of >24 hours duration.	Patients with muscular weakness of >24–48 hours duration are at risk for hyperkalemia following succinylcholine administration.	IV	See Other References: 78, 85	Onset and duration of risk for hyperkalemia varies based on diagnosis and degree of immobility.
	Oral intubation of patients with cervical spine injury appears safe with manual in-line stabilization.	Manual in-line stabilization of the cervical spine helps prevent movement of the spinal column and potential further injury to the spinal cord. Discussion of the optimal method of intubation in spine patients is ongoing as there are no definitive studies.	IV	See Other References: 35, 101	Other factors to consider when intubating the patient with cervical spine injury include operator skill and comfort level.
	Ensure that equipment for the management of difficult airways is available when a patient with suspected spinal instability is intubated.	The need to avoid neck movement increases the difficulty of intubating the airway. Patients in a halo vest for management of spinal instability may be particularly difficult to intubate. Equipment for the management of difficult airways must be readily available.	II	See Other References: 102, 115	Examples of equipment used in the management of difficult airways include a variety of sizes of laryngoscopes and endotracheal tubes, fiberoptic bronchoscopes, lighted stylets, retrograde intubation equipment, alternative airway devices (eg, Combitube, laryngeal mask airway), and surgical airway devices (Other References: 2).
	Most patients with ALI or ARDS should be managed within the confines of a lung-protective strategy (respiration volume [V_T] <6 mL/kg predicted body weight, maintain plateau pressure <30 cm H_2O).	Lung protective ventilation strategy minimizes ventilator-induced lung injury by avoiding lung overdistension and providing adequate end-expiratory lung volume to avoid cyclical lung collapse. The plateau (alveolar) pressure is measured on the ventilator with a half-second inspiratory pause. High distending pressures (>30 cm H_2O) are associated with barotrauma and alveolar fractures. Studies evaluating computed tomography scans of patients with ARDS have demonstrated that alveolar filling in ARDS is	IV	See Other References: 16, 17, 18, 44, 72	The lower lung volumes during ventilation in patients with ALI/ARDS may reduce over-distension of the lung (volutrauma) and the release of inflammatory mediators.

Period of Use	Recommendation	Rationale for Recommendation	Level of Recommendation	Supporting References	Comments
Application of Device and Initial Use *(cont.)*		heterogeneous (ie, some areas of the lung are open and some are closed). The majority of the tidal volume breath from the ventilator is delivered to the compliant or open area of lung tissue. This puts the compliant lung at risk of over-distention that may be the mechanism associated with volutrauma.			
		Mechanical ventilation with a lower tidal volume (6 mL/kg of predicted body weight) in patients with ALI results in decreased mortality and an increase in the number of days without ventilator use.		See Other References: 16	
	Consider the use of lung protective strategies of mechanical ventilation in patients with acute brain injury and concomitant ALI/ARDS.	Ventilating patients with low tidal volumes can lead to respiratory acidosis (permissive hypercapnia). However, according to the ARDS network data, patients receiving small tidal volumes had a normal partial pressure of carbon dioxide in arterial blood ($Paco_2$; 40–41 mm Hg) on day 1, indicating that volutrauma can be avoided without causing hypercapnia in many cases.	IV	See Other References: 16, 62, 72	Refer to the ongoing monitoring section of this protocol for clinical parameters to continuously monitor when a neuroscience patient with ALI/ARDS is receiving ventilation with low tidal volumes.
		A recent retrospective study examined SAH patients with ALI who were ventilated with a lung protective strategy and found no significant differences in pH or $Paco_2$ in patients ventilated with low tidal volumes versus those that received conventional ventilation.		See Other References: 62	
	Use of moderate levels of PEEP (5–12 cm H_2O) in brain-injured patients with ALI/ARDS appears safe. The use of PEEP aids in lung recruitment and prevents repetitive opening injury.	PEEP improves oxygenation by increasing functional residual capacity, reduces the proportion of nonaerated lung, and minimizes the use of high levels of inspired oxygen.	IV	See Other References: 15	In addition to being caused by excessive stretch, lung injury also may result from repeated opening and closing of small airways or from excessive stress at margins between aerated and atelectatic regions of the lung. These types of lung injury may be prevented by the use of higher levels of PEEP.

Period of Use	Recommendation	Rationale for Recommendation	Level of Recommendation	Supporting References	Comments
Application of Device and Initial Use (*cont.*)		When noncompliant lungs are collapsed in patients with ARDS, high levels of PEEP may be required to reopen closed alveoli. Once reopened, the lung tissue remains at risk of closing again (derecruitment) unless adequate levels of PEEP are applied.		See Other References: 17, 18	Refer to the ongoing monitoring section of this protocol for clinical parameters to continuously monitor in critically ill neuroscience patients receiving high levels of PEEP.
		In patients who received mechanical ventilation with a tidal volume goal of 6 mL/kg predicted body weight and an end inspiratory plateau pressure limit of <30 cm H_2O, clinical outcomes were similar whether lower (8.3 ± 3.2 cm H_2O) or higher (13.2 ± 3.5 cm H_2O) levels of PEEP were used.		See Other References: 15	
		The increased respiratory rate used in the ARDSNet lower tidal volume strategy (to minimize respiratory acidosis) may lead to intrinsic (auto) PEEP, raising the total PEEP level. The reduced mortality observed with the ARDSNet strategy may have been due to the protective effect of a higher total PEEP.		See Other References: 31	Higher PEEP levels prevent repetitive alveolar recruitment-derecruitment.
		In a study examining patients with TBI and concomitant pulmonary dysfunction, the strategy of increasing PEEP (up to 15 cm H_2O) to optimize oxygenation did not increase ICP or reduce CPP.		See Other References: 59	
		One theory is that the intracranial effects of PEEP can be related to changes in respiratory system compliance. Hemodynamic effects of PEEP, including a reduced mean arterial pressure, were observed in patients with SAH with normal respiratory compliance. Those with reduced respiratory compliance (as commonly seen in patients with ALI/ARDS) were protected.		See Annotated Bibliography: 1	The degree to which cardiac output is affected during positive pressure ventilation depends on mean airway pressure, the extent to which the pressure is transmitted to the pleural space, and the patient's volume status. When lung compliance is reduced, the percentage of airway pressure transmitted to the pleural space is reduced.
		Another small study suggested that PEEP can be		See Other References: 80	

Period of Use	Recommendation	Rationale for Recommendation	Level of Recommendation	Supporting References	Comments
Application of Device and Initial Use (*cont.*)		used without affecting ICP if it is lower than the ICP. An increase in ICP associated with increased PEEP levels did not correspond to a change in CPP, questioning the clinical relevance of an increase in ICP.			
	Novel modes of ventilation such as high frequency oscillatory ventilation (HFOV) and high frequency percussive ventilation (HFPV) have been studied in general adult ICU patient populations with ARDS. These modes are not widely used as the initial ventilation strategy for ARDS patients, but are still being investigated for use in brain-injured patients.	HFOV appears to be a generally safe and effective mode of ventilation for the treatment of ARDS in adults, but studies are limited. The use of HFOV appears to improve oxygenation and has not been associated with adverse hemodynamic effects. As noted previously, systemic oxygenation has a profound effect on cerebral oxygenation. To date, HFOV has not been proven to have a beneficial effect on patient outcomes over conventional ventilation using a lung protective strategy, but research continues.	IV	See Other References: 32, 39, 81	HFOV delivers pressure oscillations to the lung around a constant mean airway pressure that is higher than typically applied with conventional ventilation. Gas is dispersed throughout the lung in very small volumes at very high frequencies. Maintenance of constant mean airway pressure during HFOV is believed to promote alveolar recruitment without high peak pressures (Other References: 32).
		One factor limiting the clinical use of high frequency ventilation in critically ill neuroscience patients with ARDS is that patients typically require prolonged chemical paralysis and sedation to tolerate this mode of ventilation. This makes it difficult to assess neurological status and may predispose patients to the development of a critical illness myopathy and potentially longer ventilation duration.			
		An early finding with HFOV was a reduction in ICP when utilized in patients with multisystem injuries. It is hypothesized that the lower intrathoracic pressures generated with HFOV leads to decreased ICP.		See Other References: 8, 58	
		The latest approach to high frequency ventilation is HFPV. Studies have demonstrated the same oxygenation and ventilation with HFPV at lower peak, mean, and end expiratory pressures than with		See Other References: 30, 112	HFPV delivers small tidal volumes at rapid rates (up to 500 bpm) superimposed on conventional ventilation. The cuff of the endotracheal tube is partially deflated,

Period of Use	Recommendation	Rationale for Recommendation	Level of Recommendation	Supporting References	Comments
Application of Device and Initial Use (*cont.*)		conventional ventilation. The impact of HFPV on long-term outcomes has not been evaluated.			preventing the build-up of potentially harmful levels of intra-alveolar pressure and promoting secretion clearance (Other References: 112).
		A small study using HFPV in head injured patients with ARDS showed a significant improvement in oxygenation and a reduction in ICP during the first 16 hours.		See Annotated Bibliography: 6	
	Carefully selected patients with neuromuscular respiratory failure and normal mental status may be successfully managed with noninvasive positive pressure ventilation (NPPV).	There are a limited number of reports of successful use of NPPV in patients with MG who are normocapnic ($Paco_2 \leq 50$ mm Hg) and in patients with SCI.	IV	See Other References: 6, 92, 108	NPPV should not be attempted in patients with decreased mental status due to the risk of aspiration. Many patients with progressive neurological diseases (eg, amyotrophic lateral sclerosis or Duchenne muscular dystrophy) opt for the use of noninvasive ventilation instead of ventilation through an artificial airway.
	NPPV should not be used in patients with GBS.	Patients with GBS who require mechanical ventilation typically have profound bulbar weakness. In addition, the course of GBS is characterized by continued decline until a nadir is reached, followed by slow improvement.	II	See Other References: 47, 116	
	While the use of lung protective strategies is suggested for most patients, the use of high tidal volumes may be helpful in weaning patients with high cervical SCI.	Peterson and colleagues evaluated the use of high (>20 mL/kg ideal body weight) versus low (<20 mL/kg ideal body weight) tidal volumes in weaning patients with C3 or C4 SCI. The mean V_T in the high V_T group was 25.3 mL/kg versus 15.5 mL/kg in the low V_T group. All patients were ventilated on assist control, and patients were weaned using increasing periods of ventilator-free breathing (starting with 2 minutes of ventilator-free breathing twice daily). The high V_T group weaned an average of 21 days faster than the low V_T group (37.6 days versus 58.7 days).	IV	See Other References: 27, 88	Differences may exist between patients with neuromuscular respiratory failure and patients with other types of acute respiratory failure requiring mechanical ventilation. Specifically, patients without concomitant lung disease or injury may have more compliant lungs, lessening the risk of volutrauma. To decrease the risk of lung injury, always monitor peak inspiratory pressures.

Period of Use	Recommendation	Rationale for Recommendation	Level of Recommendation	Supporting References	Comments
Application of Device and Initial Use *(cont.)*	Use of an abdominal binder or flat positioning may improve the pulmonary function of patients with cervical or high thoracic SCI.	Patients with cervical and high thoracic SCI lose function of the intercostal muscles and rely primarily on the diaphragm to provide muscle force for inspiration. Upright positioning places the diaphragm at a mechanical disadvantage because loss of abdominal muscle tone causes the abdomen to protrude and the diaphragm is in a lower position in the abdomen. Flat positioning and the use of abdominal binders improve the mechanics of respiration.	IV	See Other References: 51, 56, 71, 117	
	Use of progressive ventilator-free breathing (versus gradual reduction of pressure support) may be beneficial in weaning patients with cervical SCI.	Studies of weaning strategies indicate that there is no clear advantage to either of these methods. Use of gradually increasing periods of ventilator-free breathing (with complete rest between) provides a more obvious measure of success for patients and facilitates the use of a speaking valve for communication. Both of these factors may be psychologically beneficial for patients with cervical SCI.	IV	See Other References: 27, 87	One study of patients with high cervical spinal cord injury concluded that progressive ventilator-free breathing resulted in more rapid weaning than gradual reduction of pressure support. These findings are limited by numerous flaws in methodology; specifically, data are retrospective and based on observation of clinical practice following failed weaning attempts at other institutions. In addition, the study lacks information about weaning readiness indicators. Despite these limitations, Peterson et al. raise valid points regarding the theoretical benefits of progressive ventilator-free breathing (Other References: 87).
	In patients with GBS, monitor bedside pulmonary function parameters to guide weaning.	Bedside measurement of respiratory muscle strength allows monitoring of disease progression and similarly reflects recovery of function.	IV	See Other References: 24, 57	
		One small study suggests that brief T-piece trials can be initiated once the FVC reaches 7 mL/kg.		See Other References: 24	
	Avoid or limit the use of medications known to cause increased weakness in patients with MG.	Medications that cause increased weakness contribute to prolonged duration of mechanical ventilation.	II	See Other References: 67	Medications that may worsen weakness due to MG include magnesium preparations, quinidine, quinine sulfate, procainamide, beta blockers, calcium channel

Period of Use	Recommendation	Rationale for Recommendation	Level of Recommendation	Supporting References	Comments
					blockers, neuromuscular blockers, iodinated contrast agents, and certain antibiotics (aminoglycosides and quinolones; Other References: 67).
Ongoing Monitoring	Any neuroscience patient with an acute intracranial process who is receiving lung protective ventilation should receive continuous monitoring of ICP, CPP, end-tidal carbon dioxide, plateau pressure, oxygen saturation, and if available brain tissue oxygen monitoring, to correlate ventilatory changes with clinical impact.	Mechanical ventilation strategies that may alter F_{IO_2}, $Paco_2$, ICP, and CPP can affect cerebral oxygen delivery and/or consumption. Use of smaller tidal volumes can result in permissive hypercapnia, which potentially raises ICP through vasodilatation. Use of PEEP can increase intrathoracic pressure, which decreases venous return and potentially increases ICP.	V	See Other References: 7, 16, 72, 83, 110	
		Plateau pressures must be monitored when using PEEP. A PEEP level that results in lung recruitment will not change plateau pressure. However, an increase in PEEP that results in an increase in plateau pressure indicates that PEEP is contributing to alveolar over-distension.		See Other References: 17, 18, 76	
		Use of brain tissue oxygen ($Pbto_2$) monitoring adds another dimension in the management of patients with severe brain injury. This monitoring has the potential to detect early ischemic injury before alterations in other variables occur. The driving force that moves oxygen into tissues is the gradient between the dissolved oxygen in blood and $Pbto_2$ levels. Even if the oxygen saturation is 100%, the patient may still have inadequate brain tissue oxygenation and often requires F_{IO_2} of 100% for the first few hours during stabilization in the ICU.		See Other References: 7, 82, 83, 84, 111	

Period of Use	Recommendation	Rationale for Recommendation	Level of Recommendation	Supporting References	Comments
Ongoing Monitoring *(cont.)*	Transport patients on their established ventilator settings (versus manual ventilation or use of a transport ventilator) to prevent the deleterious effects of inadvertent hyperventilation.	Hyperventilation lowers $Paco_2$, producing vasoconstriction of the cerebral blood vessels, thus reducing blood flow and ultimately, oxygen delivery. Hyperventilation decreases ICP but may induce cerebral ischemia.	II	See Other References: 70, 72	This recommendation is consistent with American Association of Critical-Care Nurses (AACN) standards for the transport of critically ill patients (Other References: 1).
		The current recommendation is to avoid the use of chronic prophylactic hyperventilation. Establishing normocapnia is the routine target in brain injured patients; hyperventilation is used only transiently when ICP is elevated while other interventions are taking place.		See Other References: 11, 105	
	Prior to extubation of a neuroscience patient, consider the degree of mental status impairment.	The majority of critically ill neuroscience patients are intubated due to their primary neurological problem, and not because of a respiratory disorder. Many neuroscience patients can successfully pass a daily 2-hour spontaneous breathing trial, but remain intubated due to concerns about mental status and airway protection.	IV	See Annotated Bibliography: 5	A spontaneous breathing trial can be done with either a T-piece or CPAP. Successful completion of spontaneous breathing in the Namen trial consisted of respiratory rate <35, pulse oximetry >90 %, frequency/tidal volume (f/V_T) ratio of <100, and Pao_2/Fio_2 ratio (P/F) ratio of >200 (Annotated Bibliography: 5).
		A GCS score of ≥8 in neurosurgical patients may be associated with extubation success.		See Annotated Bibliography: 5	Conversely, another study found that 80% of the neurosurgical patients examined were successfully extubated despite a GCS score of <8 (Annotated Bibliography: 2).
		A chart review of SICU patients with blunt head trauma demonstrated that patients with a GCS score >7 and a Simplified Acute Physiology Score of <13 on the fourth day of ICU care were successfully extubated, while those with a GCS score of <7 and a Simplified Acute Physiology Score of >15 went on to have tracheostomy.		See Other References: 75	The Simplified Acute Physiology Score is impacted by the GCS score, but also factors in other indicators of severity of illness, including age, blood pressure, and laboratory values.
	Prior to extubation, consider the cough reflex, cough strength, amount of secretions, and suctioning frequency.	In patients who have successfully passed a spontaneous breathing trial, poor cough strength and increased endotracheal secretions (requiring	IV	See Annotated Bibliography: 3	Patients with a negative white card test were 3 times more likely to fail extubation then those with a positive white card test. A positive white card test

Period of Use	Recommendation	Rationale for Recommendation	Level of Recommendation	Supporting References	Comments
Ongoing Monitoring *(cont.)*		suctioning more frequently than every 2 hours) were synergistic in predicting a failed extubation.			means that the patient can spontaneously cough out secretions onto a card held 1–2 cm from the end of the endotracheal tube (Annotated Bibliography: 3).
		In another study, neurological patients had the highest rate of reintubation among patients who passed a 2-hour spontaneous breathing trial. Vallverdú et al. note that the ability to cough and clear secretions (measured objectively as MEP) may be useful when making decisions about extubating neurological patients.		See Other References: 109	
		Coplin and colleagues demonstrated that the presence of a spontaneous cough and low suctioning frequency were associated with successful extubation in brain injured patients. Of interest, 89% of successfully extubated study patients had a weak or absent gag.		See Annotated Bibliography: 2	This study did not support delaying extubation in patients when impaired neurological status and weak or absent gag were identified as the reasons for prolonging intubation. Delaying extubation was associated with higher incidence of pneumonias, longer ICU and hospital stays, and higher costs.
	The decision to perform an elective tracheostomy or tracheostomy after failed extubation is based on patient characteristics and predicted duration of mechanical ventilation. There are both benefits and risks associated with tracheostomy placement.	Tracheostomy placement improves patient comfort, improves communication, enhances patient mobility, decreases airway resistance, may improve pulmonary toilet, and contributes to decreased length of stay in the ICU. However, tracheostomy placement is not without risks, which include bleeding, infection, and scarring. The ideal timing of tracheostomy placement has not been determined for neuroscience patients.	II	See Other References: 52	In a study of early tracheostomy, critically ill patients (who had been assessed by their physicians as potentially requiring mechanical ventilation for >14 days) were randomly assigned to early percutaneous tracheostomy (48 hours) or routine tracheostomy (later tracheostomy). Those who received early tracheostomy demonstrated decreased mortality, rates of pneumonia, duration of mechanical ventilation, and ICU length of stay. It is difficult to determine the applicability of this study to the neurological patient because no neurological ICU patients were included in the study sample and mental status was not reported (Other References: 100).

Period of Use	Recommendation	Rationale for Recommendation	Level of Recommendation	Supporting References	Comments
Ongoing Monitoring *(cont.)*	An elective tracheostomy or tracheostomy after a failed extubation may be necessary in patients with lesions in the cerebellum or brainstem.	These patients showed a high frequency of unsuccessful extubations ultimately requiring tracheostomy. Lesions in these areas can cause damage to the primary respiratory center, damage to the cranial nerves involved in generation of protective cough reflexes, and damage to the reticular activating system impairing level of consciousness.	IV	See Other References: 90	
	Patients with MG do not routinely require tracheostomy placement.	Many patients with MG can be extubated within 2 weeks of intubation.	IV	See Annotated Bibliography: 8, 9 See Other References: 10, 61, 91	Studies of patients with myasthenic crisis report a median duration of mechanical ventilation of 5 to 13 days (Annotated Bibliography: 8, 9; Other References: 10, 91).
	Consider tracheostomy in patients with MG who have risk factors for prolonged intubation.	In a study independent risk factors for prolonged intubation (>14 days) included preintubation serum bicarbonate ≥30 mg/dL, peak VC on days 1 to 6 following intubation <25 mL/kg, and age >50 years.		See Annotated Bibliography: 8	
		Age, atelectasis, and pneumonia are associated with extubation failure in patients with MG.		See Other References: 91	
	Consider elective tracheostomy in patients with severe GBS.	Patients with GBS often require ventilation for more than 2 weeks, the time at which the decision to perform tracheostomy is often made.	IV	See Annotated Bibliography: 7 See Other References: 24, 42, 54, 57, 68, 94	The median duration of mechanical ventilation in a large study of patients with GBS was 21 days (Annotated Bibliography: 7).
	Consider early elective tracheostomy in patients with acute cervical SCI, especially those with higher levels of injury, increased age, or complicating pulmonary factors.	In patients with SCI, the average duration of mechanical ventilation (if required) is dependent on the level of injury.	IV	See Other References: 26, 50, 60	Jackson and Groomes (Other References: 60) found that patients with injuries at C4 remained on mechanical ventilation for an average of 66 days, while patients with injuries at C5 through C8 were weaned in approximately 23 days. Patients with thoracic injury who required mechanical ventilation weaned in an average of 13 days.
		In a study of cervical SCI patients admitted to a Level I trauma center, all patients with a complete injury above C5 received a tracheostomy.		See Other References: 26	
		In addition to level of injury, factors such as age, preexisting medical conditions, premorbid lung disease, and the presence of pneumonia impact the decision to place a tracheostomy in patients with SCI.		See Other References: 50	

Period of Use	Recommendation	Rationale for Recommendation	Level of Recommendation	Supporting References	Comments
Prevention of Complications	Use quality initiatives to prevent ventilator associated pneumonia.	Ventilator associated pneumonia (VAP) or health-care–associated pneumonia can be caused by adherence of microorganisms to epithelial cells in the upper and lower airways, aspiration of contaminated secretions, and/or bacterial colonization. VAP is associated with increased length of stay, increased mortality, and increased cost.	V	See Other References: 3, 22	
	Elevate the head of bed (HOB) 30° to 45° in all patients without contraindications.	HOB elevation is one of the most important nursing interventions to decrease aspiration risk and the risk of VAP.	V	See Other References: 3, 33, 34, 106	Audits of HOB elevation may be useful in identifying patients at risk for VAP.
		The Centers for Disease Control and Prevention recommend that healthcare institutions implement HOB elevation in all ventilated patients unless specific contraindications exist.		See Other References: 106	Education of staff on VAP prevention is also important (Other References: 5). In addition to HOB elevation, other VAP prevention strategies noted in the literature include scrupulous hand washing, use of noninvasive ventilation, prevention of accidental self-extubations, use of endotracheal tubes that offer continuous aspiration of subglottic secretions, stress ulcer prophylaxis, use of oral versus nasal feeding tubes (sinusitis prevention), ventilator circuit changes only with each new patient or if soiled, postpyloric feeding, use of kinetic therapy, oral care program for ventilated patients, and intensive insulin therapy.
	In patients with neuromuscular respiratory failure and no underlying lung disease or injury, consider strategies such as intermittent positive pressure breathing, sigh breaths, and chest physiotherapy.	Development of pneumonia contributes significantly to morbidity and mortality among patients with neuromuscular respiratory failure. In patients receiving mechanical ventilation for neuromuscular weakness versus lung pathology, these strategies may decrease the risk of atelectasis and pneumonia by minimizing alveolar collapse and	IV	See Annotated Bibliography: 9 See Other References: 27	Many of these measures have not been found to benefit most patients on mechanical ventilation. However, patients with neuromuscular disease typically require mechanical ventilation due to respiratory muscle weakness or bulbar weakness and do not have underlying lung injury. Because of the differences

Period of Use	Recommendation	Rationale for Recommendation	Level of Recommendation	Supporting References	Comments
Prevention of Complications *(cont.)*		promoting mobilization of secretions.			in pathophysiology, these patients may tolerate these interventions without volutrauma. These strategies provide increased lung volumes and mobilize secretions, which may help the neuromuscular patient who does not have the muscle strength to breathe deeply or cough effectively.
		Varelas and colleagues describe a program of intensive respiratory care based on patient condition and reports fewer pulmonary complications (atelectasis and pneumonia) compared to a previous study. This program included suctioning, intermittent positive pressure breathing or bronchodilator treatments, sigh breaths, and chest physiotherapy.		See Annotated Bibliography: 8, 9	
	Use manual and mechanical airway clearance strategies in patients who are unable to cough effectively due to neuromuscular respiratory weakness.	An effective cough is dependent on both inspiratory and expiratory muscle strength. Manual and mechanical airway clearance strategies promote secretion clearance.	II	See Other References: 79	
		Patients with neuromuscular weakness often experience paradoxical outward movement of the abdominal muscles when a cough is attempted, decreasing cough strength. Manual cough assistance consists of compressing the upper abdomen to decrease this paradoxical movement and support the patient's own cough effort.			
		Mechanical in-exsufflation works by supporting both inspiration and forced exhalation. The in-exsufflation machine applies positive pressure during the inspiratory phase, followed by an abrupt change to negative pressure for 1–3 seconds.			
	For prevention of deep vein thrombosis (DVT) and pulmonary embolism (PE) include the use of pneumatic sequential compression devices for all critically ill neuroscience patients without contraindications.	It is estimated that 60%–80% of SCI patients, 40%–80% of trauma patients, and 20%–50% of stroke patients will develop a DVT within the first to second week of admission WITHOUT prophylaxis.	IV	See Other References: 45	
		Sequential compression devices increase venous blood flow, stimulate endogenous fibrinolytic activity, and alter blood flow characteristics and perfusion pressure.		See Other References: 4	

Period of Use	Recommendation	Rationale for Recommendation	Level of Recommendation	Supporting References	Comments
Prevention of Complications *(cont.)*	Adhere to the most recent published guidelines for pharmacologic prophylaxis against venous thromboembolism.	Pharmacologic prophylaxis is an important adjunct to mechanical prophylaxis in neuroscience patients. The specific type of pharmacologic prophylaxis recommended is controversial and an area of ongoing research. New evidence is published frequently.	IV	See Other References: 45	In general, the use of subcutaneous unfractionated heparin or low-molecular weight heparin is recommended for neuroscience patients in the ICU. Inferior vena cava filter placement for PE prevention may be appropriate in patients with proximal DVT, absolute contraindications to prophylactic or therapeutic anticoagulation therapy, or in high-risk patients if surgery is planned in the near future.
	A program of progressive activity is recommended to help combat the effects of immobility and deconditioning.	Progressive activity and strengthening exercises may positively impact ventilator weaning.	IV	See Other References: 77, 104	Activity must be balanced with the need for rest, especially in patients with neuromuscular disease. Neuroscience patients often require inpatient rehabilitation following hospital discharge.
Quality Control Issues	Institutional outcomes measures and utilization of benchmarking data are helpful in monitoring the efficacy of evidence-based practice changes in the clinical setting.	Measuring care outcomes provides patients, payers, and institutions with quantifiable data on system interventions. Outcome measures depend on the system and the initiative. Some potential outcomes to measure for ventilated neuroscience ICU patients include: • VAP rates • Failed extubation rates • Emergency intubations • Unplanned extubations • Ventilator duration • Length of stay (LOS) • Discharge disposition • Quality of life	IV	See Other References: 20, 21	Reintubation rates among patients with MG were approximately 20% in 3 studies (Annotated Bibliography: 8, 9; Other References: 91).

ANNOTATED BIBLIOGRAPHY

1. **Caricato A, Conti G, Della Corte F, et al. Effects of PEEP on the intracranial system of patients with head injury and subarachnoid hemorrhage: the role of respiratory system compliance.** *J Trauma.* 2005;58:571–576.

Study Sample

Twenty-one comatose patients with severe head injury or SAH receiving ICP monitoring who required mechanical ventilation.

Comparison Studied

Patients were divided into those with normal respiratory system compliance (>45 mL/cm H_2O; n = 13) and those with low respiratory system compliance (<45 mL/cm H_2O; n = 8). Varying levels of PEEP were applied (0–12 cm H_2O) in random sequence. The authors investigated the effects of different PEEP levels on systemic and intracranial hemodynamics between the 2 groups.

Study Procedures

Jugular pressure, central venous pressure (CVP), CPP, ICP, cerebral compliance, mean velocity of the middle cerebral arteries (VmMCA), and jugular oxygen saturation (SjO_2)were evaluated in both study groups, while increasing PEEP levels from 0 to 12 cm H_2O.

Key Results

Increasing PEEP from 0 to 12 cm H_2O did not change ICP or cerebral compliance in either group.

When PEEP was increased from 0 to 12 cm H_2O in patients with normal respiratory system compliance, the mean arterial pressure (MAP), CPP, and VmMCA were reduced. When the same level of PEEP was applied to patients with low respiratory system compliance, no significant variation in MAP, CPP, or VmMCA occurred. After the PEEP application, SjO_2 monitoring never dropped below 50% in either study group.

Study Strengths and Weaknesses

The strengths of this prospective study include the specific population of patients studied with head injury and SAH, and good descriptions of the methods used. A major weakness was the very small number of study patients. Changes in cardiac output after PEEP application were not measured; therefore, the direct effect of PEEP on cardiac output and cerebral hemodynamics could not be quantified.

Clinical Implications

This study suggests that the transmission of PEEP into the thoracic cavity is variable, depending on the properties of the chest wall and lungs. Factors that reduce lung compliance (ie, pneumonia, ALI, atelectasis) have a protective effect with PEEP by minimizing airway pressure transmission. Among patients with low respiratory system compliance, PEEP up to 12 cm H_2O had no significant effect on cerebral and systemic hemodynamics in this study. When PEEP levels higher than 5 cm H_2O are applied to patients with brain injury, the authors recommend monitoring VmMCA and SjO_2, together with ICP and CPP.

2. **Coplin WM, Pierson DJ, Cooley KD, Newell DW, Rubenfeld GD. Implications of extubation delay in brain-injured patients meeting standard weaning criteria.** *Am J Respir Crit Care Med.* 2000;161:1530–1536.

Study Sample

One hundred thirty-six intubated patients with acute brain injury admitted to an ICU.

Comparison Studied

The purpose of the study was to identify reasons for and the implications of prolonging intubation in patients with acute brain injury who successfully met standard weaning criteria: MIP <−20 cm H_2O, rapid shallow breathing index (RSBI, frequency tidal volume) <105, spontaneous minute ventilation (VE) <12 L/min., PaO_2/FIO_2 >200 mm Hg, and PaO_2 >80 mm Hg on FIO_2 <0.5 (on 5 cm H_2O PEEP). Coplin et al. also examined the GCS score and the need for airway care (utilizing a semiquantitative assessment score of spontaneous cough, gag, sputum quantity, sputum viscosity, suctioning frequency, and sputum color) as potential reasons for delaying extubation.

Study Procedures

Spontaneous ventilatory parameters were measured daily on all study patients. These parameters included respiratory rate (number of breaths after disconnection of the ventilator), VT, RSBI, MIP, and VE. Patients did not have respiratory parameters done if 1 or more of the following were present: FIO_2 >0.7, PEEP >10 cm H_2O, VE >12 L/min while receiving ventilation, ICP >20 mm Hg, or use of neuromuscular blocking agents. The physician managing the patient was notified by the respiratory therapist when the patient successfully met all the extubation readiness criteria. Extubation delay was defined as the number of days that elapsed between the day that the patient met criteria for extubation and the day the patient was extubated minus 48 hours. The investigators subtracted 48 hours to provide a "grace period" to allow for communication among the team members managing the patient.

Key Results

Of 136 patients, 99 (73%) were extubated within 48 hours of meeting extubation readiness criteria. The other 37 patients (27%) remained intubated for a median of 3 days. Patients with delayed extubation developed more pneumonia and had longer ICU and hospital length of stays. Overall, reintubation occurred in 17% of patients without extubation delay and 19% of patients with extubation delay. The authors found that 51% of patients with a GCS score of <8 on extubation readiness day were extubated without delay. Higher airway care scores, indicating worse airway function, were associated with extubation delay. However, 89% of patients with absent or weak gag were successfully extubated. Eighty-two percent of patients with a weak or absent cough were successfully extubated.

Strengths and Weaknesses

The strengths of this prospective study include the specific neuro-ICU population examined, the good descriptions of methods used, and the relatively large number of patients studied. One weakness of the study was that the investigators permitted a 48-hour period between when the patient met extubation readiness criteria and the actual extubation day to allow for communication among the team members. Patients could have improved neurologically during that 48-hour period.

Clinical Implications

This study does not support delaying extubation in brain injured patients when impaired neurological status is the only concern prolonging intubation.

3. **Khaminees M, Raju P, DeGirolamo A, Amoateng-Adjepong Y, Manthous CA. Predictors of extubation outcome in patients who have successfully completed a spontaneous breathing trial.** *Chest.* **2001;120:1262–1269.**

Study Sample

Ninety-one adult patients treated in Medical-Cardiac ICUs who were recovering from respiratory failure.

Comparison Studied

All study patients who successfully completed a spontaneous breathing trial were evaluated for extubation. The authors evaluated factors of "airway competence" defined as cough strength, quantity of endotracheal secretions, and frequency of suctioning. These factors were then examined to measure the impact on extubation outcome.

Study Procedures

Study patients underwent a spontaneous breathing trial via unit protocol (T-piece, CPAP, or pressure support of <7 cm H_2O for 30 minutes to 2 hours). Patients who successfully completed the spontaneous breathing trial were then evaluated by investigators for voluntary cough strength (scale of 0–5), magnitude of endotracheal secretions (none–large), and an objective measure of cough strength termed the *white card test (WCT)*. A white file card was placed 1 to 2 cm from the end of the endotracheal tube. Patients were asked to

cough 3 to 4 times. Any wetness appearing on the card was classified as a positive WCT. Lastly, the frequency of suctioning was included in the assessment prior to the decision to extubate.

Key Results

The WCT results correlated with cough strength. Patients with a negative WCT were 3 times more likely to have unsuccessful extubations as those with a positive WCT. Patients with weak (grades 0–2) cough strengths were 4 times as likely to have unsuccessful extubations, compared to those with moderate to strong (grades 3–5) coughs. Patients with moderate-to-abundant secretions were more then 8 times as likely to have unsuccessful extubations as those with mild or no secretions.

Study Strengths and Weaknesses

The strengths of this study include the prospective design, the relatively large sample size, and the use of an objective marker to evaluate cough strength (the WCT). Weaknesses include the subjective measures of secretions and cough, and the fact that the decision to extubate was not based on explicit enforced protocols but by the individual physician caring for the patient.

Clinical Implications

Poor cough strength and increased endotracheal secretions were synergistic in predicting extubation failure.

4. **Lawn ND, Fletcher DD, Henderson RD, Wolter TD, Wijdicks EFM. Anticipating mechanical ventilation in Guillain-Barré syndrome.** *Arch Neurol.* **2001;58:893–898.**

Study Sample

One hundred fourteen patients with GBS admitted to the ICU of a tertiary care hospital between January 1976 and December 1996.

Comparison Studied

Patients who received mechanical ventilation (n = 60) were compared to patients who did not receive mechanical ventilation (n = 54).

Study Procedures

Data were collected through retrospective case review. Clinical assessments and pulmonary function parameters were recorded as well as the results of electrophysiological testing (when available).

Key Results

Clinical assessments associated with progression to mechanical ventilation included rapid onset of symptoms, bulbar dysfunction, bilateral facial weakness, and dysautonomia. Pulmonary parameters associated with progression to mechanical ventilation were VC <20 mL/kg, MIP >−30 cm H_2O, MEP <40 cm H_2O, and a decline of >30% in VC, MIP, or MEP. On multivariate analysis, bulbar dysfunction and VC <20 mL/kg at any point during admission were independent predictors of the need for intubation.

Study Strengths and Weaknesses

One weakness of this study is that some variables were excluded from multivariate analysis because of missing data (PaO_2, percent reduction in VC, MIP, and MEP).

Clinical Implications

Patients at risk for respiratory failure due to GBS can be identified using clinical assessment and serial measurement of pulmonary parameters. Lawn et al. recommend ICU admission for patients with VC <20 mL/kg, MIP >−30, MEP <40, more than a 30% reduction in VC from baseline, or significant bulbar weakness.

5. Namen AM, Ely EW, Tatter SB, et al. Predictors of successful extubation in neurosurgical patients. *Am J Respir Crit Care Med*. 2001; 163:658–664.

Study Sample

One hundred intubated patients with neurological injuries admitted to the ICU of a university medical center.

Comparison Studied

The purpose of this study was to determine if a respiratory care practitioner-driven ventilator weaning protocol previously validated in medical patients was useful in neurosurgery patients.

Study Procedures

Patients were randomized to intervention (n = 49) and control (n = 51) groups. All patients had daily screens of weaning parameters. If these were passed, a 2-hour spontaneous breathing trial was performed in the intervention group. Study physicians communicated if patients successfully passed the spontaneous breathing trial, and the decision to extubate was made by the primary neurosurgery team.

Key Results

Eighty-two percent of intervention patients successfully passed a 2-hour spontaneous breathing trial, but a median of 2 days passed before attempted extubation due to concerns about the patient's mental status. The median duration of mechanical ventilation was 6 days in both study groups and there was no difference in outcomes. Multivariate analysis showed that the GCS score (P <0.0001) and PaO_2/FiO_2 (PF) ratio (P <0.0001) were associated with extubation success. A GCS score of >8 at extubation was associated with success in 75% of cases. The odds of having a successful extubation increased by 39% for every increment in the GCS score.

Study Strengths and Weaknesses

One strength of this trial is that it was a prospective, randomized, controlled investigation. Patients in the intervention and control groups had similar demographic characteristics, illness severity, and neurological injuries. A weakness was that the protocol did not encompass neurological assessment parameters or assessments of cough and gag reflexes, which are specific needs in neurosurgical patients.

Clinical Implications

Implementation of a weaning protocol based on traditional respiratory parameters has practical limitations in neurosurgery patients that are related to concerns of neurological impairment.

6. Salim A, Miller K, Dangleben D, Cipolle M, Pasquale M. High-frequency percussive ventilation: an alternative mode of ventilation for head-injured patients with adult respiratory distress syndrome. *J Trauma*. 2004;57:542–546.

Study Sample

Ten patients with severe traumatic brain injury with a GCS score of 8 or lower, a ventriculostomy drain in place for ICP measurement and cerebrospinal fluid drainage, and ARDS.

Comparison Studied

Clinical data were collected retrospectively over a 1-year period on patients who met the above criteria. These patients were switched from conventional ventilation to HFPV at the discretion of the attending trauma surgeon.

Study Procedures

PF ratio, peak inspiratory pressure (PIP), ICP, $PaCO_2$, PEEP, and mean airway pressure were collected while patients were on conventional ventilation, and then 4 and 16 hours after institution of HFPV therapy.

Key Results

Therapy with HFPV produced a significant improvement in oxygenation. There was an increase in PF ratio (91.8 ± 13.2 versus 269.7 ± 34.6). Patients receiving HFPV had a reduction in ICP during the first 16 hours (30 ± 3.4 versus 17.4 ± 1.7). There was also a significant decrease in PIP and arterial CO_2 levels after institution of HFPV and a trend toward increased PEEP and mean airway pressures.

Strengths and Weaknesses

A strength of the study is that it incorporates a specific population of brain-injured patients with ARDS. Weaknesses include the retrospective design, no control group, and a very small number of patients. Because of these weaknesses, no conclusions can be made in regard to differences in outcome. There was no formal protocol for the timing of

HFPV initiation and, therefore, initiation was impacted by physician preference. Salim et al. note that the reduction in ICP may have been related to either a decrease in peak inspiratory pressure (intrathoracic pressure) or a drop in $Paco_2$. Lastly, data were only collected for 16 hours on HFPV. Measurements over a longer period of time are needed to demonstrate sustained impact on outcome measures.

Clinical Implications

HFPV may become an effective alternative mode of ventilation for traumatic brain injury patients with ARDS. Prospective randomized trials are needed to address the potential impact on clinical outcome.

7. **Sharshar T, Chevret S, Bourdain F, Raphaël JC, for the French Cooperative Group on Plasma Exchange in Guillain-Barré Syndrome. Early predictors of mechanical ventilation in Guillain-Barré syndrome. *Crit Care Med.* 2003;31:278–283.**

Study Sample

The study sample consisted of 722 patients with GBS enrolled in other clinical trials. Patients who were mechanically ventilated on admission were excluded.

Comparison Studied

Patients who received mechanical ventilation were compared to patients who did not progress to mechanical ventilation. The purpose of this study was to identify early predictors of the need for mechanical ventilation in patients with GBS.

Study Procedures

Sharshar et al. analyzed data obtained through retrospective chart review of patients who were enrolled in clinical trials of treatment with plasma exchange. Factors analyzed included demographic information, disease progression, clinical findings, laboratory values, and pulmonary function assessments. Univariate analysis was used to identify factors associated with mechanical ventilation; these factors were then investigated using a multivariate logistical regression model.

Key Results

Three hundred thirteen patients (43%) required mechanical ventilation within 30 days of hospital admission. The median duration of mechanical ventilation was 21 days. Six predictors of mechanical ventilation were identified: time of onset of symptoms to admission of <7 days, inability to cough effectively, inability to stand, inability to lift elbows, inability to lift head, and elevated liver enzymes. Using this model, mechanical ventilation was required in 63% of patients with 3 of 6 predictors, 85% with 4 of 6 predictors, and 98% with 5 of 6 predictors. Among the subset of patients in whom vital capacity was measured (n = 196), predictors of mechanical ventilation were time from the onset of symptoms to admission of <7 days, inability to lift head, and vital capacity <60% of the predicted value. Eighty-five percent of patients with all three of these predictors required mechanical ventilation.

Study Strengths and Weaknesses

Strengths of this study are the large sample size and the inclusion of patients from more than 1 institution. Weaknesses include the lack of an objective measurement of cough effectiveness, and the lack of objective criteria for intubation (the decision to intubate was made by the physician in charge of the patient).

Clinical Implications

This study allows clinicians to identify patients with GBS who are likely to require mechanical ventilation. Patients with at least 1 predictor should be closely monitored, and the authors recommend that these patients be transferred to an ICU. In addition, these early predictors can be used to identify patients for enrollment in future studies of the impact of early, elective intubation on pulmonary complications.

8. **Thomas CE, Mayer SA, Gungor Y, et al. Myasthenic crisis: clinical features, mortality, complications, and risk factors for prolonged intubation. *Neurology.* 1997;48:1253–1260.**

Study Sample

Data were collected on a total of 73 episodes of mechanical ventilation occurring in 53 patients admitted to a tertiary care center from 1983 to 1994.

Comparison Studied

Thomas et al. analyzed retrospective data to identify baseline characteristics of patients requiring mechanical ventilation for myasthenic crisis, mortality, morbidity, and risk factors for mechanical ventilation for longer than 2 weeks.

Study Procedure

Records of patients admitted to the neuro ICU with myasthenic crisis were retrospectively reviewed. One patient who was intubated in the emergency department following cardiac arrest and 2 patients intubated for sepsis and ARDS were excluded from data collection and analysis. Data included patient characteristics, events precipitating myasthenic crisis, duration of mechanical ventilation, and complications. Throughout the time period reviewed, the decision to intubate was made by the physician, but the authors noted that intubation was generally performed when

VC was less than 15 mL/kg, peak inspiratory force (ie, MIP) >–20 cm H_2O, and peak expiratory force (ie, MEP) <40 cm H_2O. The decision for weaning and extubation was based also on these parameters as well as the absence of medical complications. Independent predictors of the need for prolonged ventilation (longer than 2 weeks) were identified using statistical analysis. Complications associated with prolonged ventilation were recorded and analyzed.

Key Results

Infection was identified as a precipitating factor in 38% of all episodes. The median duration of mechanical ventilation was 13 days. Risk factors for prolonged mechanical ventilation (>14 days) included serum bicarbonate level ≥30 prior to intubation, peak vital capacity of less than 25 mL/kg on days 1 through 6 of intubation, and age greater than 50 years. Eighty-eight percent of patients with all 3 risk factors remained ventilated for at least 14 days. The need for prolonged mechanical ventilation correlated with an increased risk of atelectasis, anemia/transfusion, clostridium difficile infection, and congestive heart failure. Seven patients died, 3 while intubated; mortality was related to medical comorbidities in all cases.

Strengths and Weaknesses

Data for this study were collected using a retrospective chart review, which increases the potential for error. Another weakness is that the decision to intubate was made by the physician in charge of the patient versus objective criteria, although Thomas et al. included information about the criteria used by the physicians to guide decision-making. In addition, these episodes of myasthenic crisis occurred over a period of 11 years, during which time management strategies may have differed.

Clinical Implications

Tracheostomy may be warranted in patients with all 3 risk factors for prolonged mechanical ventilation. Patients with MG who develop an infection should be monitored for signs of respiratory compromise. Clinicians involved in the management of patients with myasthenic crisis must pay close attention to the prevention and management of medical complications and comorbidities.

9. **Varelas PN, Chua HC, Natterman J, et al. Ventilatory care in myasthenia gravis crisis: assessing the baseline adverse event rate.** *Crit Care Med.* 2002;30:2663–2668.

Study Sample

The study sample included 18 patients who received a total of 24 episodes of mechanical ventilation in the neuro-critical care unit of a tertiary medical center between January 1990 and July 1998. Patients requiring mechanical ventilation after thymectomy were excluded.

Comparison Studied

Rates of pneumonia and atelectasis in the study sample were collected and compared to the rates of pneumonia and atelectasis previously reported in a study at another institution (Annotated Bibliography: 8).

Study Procedure

Data were collected retrospectively. The investigators calculated a daily Lung Injury Score for each patient based on alveolar consolidation on chest x-ray, hypoxemia, level of PEEP required, and respiratory compliance. In addition, intensity of respiratory care was quantified using a respiratory intervention index reflecting the use of suctioning, intermittent positive pressure breathing or bronchodilator treatments, sigh breaths, and chest physiotherapy. A standard protocol for respiratory management was used, and interventions were increased based on the presence of atelectasis or pneumonia. Other data collected included demographic information, precipitating factors, ICU and hospital length of stay, duration of mechanical ventilation, tracheostomy placement, complications, and treatment strategies. Bedside measurements of FVC and negative inspiratory pressure were also recorded. Finally, the results (rates of atelectasis and pneumonia, duration of mechanical ventilation, and duration of ICU stay) were compared to the results of an earlier study at another institution (Annotated Bibliography: 8).

Key Results

Twenty-nine percent of patients developed atelectasis and 17% were diagnosed with pneumonia. Varelas et al. compared these rates to those detailed in Thomas et al.'s study (Annotated Bibliography: 8), in which 40% of patients developed atelectasis and 51% developed pneumonia. Infection and medication changes were common precipitating factors of myasthenic crisis. Patients received mechanical ventilation for a median duration of 6 days, and 14% received a tracheostomy. The intensity of respiratory interventions correlated with the severity of lung injury and was inversely related to FVC.

Strengths and Weaknesses

This study used a standardized approach to quantify lung injury and intensity of respiratory care. Weaknesses include the retrospective design, small sample size, and use of historical data for comparison. In addition, many of the respiratory interventions used have not proven beneficial in other populations.

Clinical Implications

This study supports the use of aggressive respiratory care to minimize complications such as atelectasis and pneumonia in patients experiencing myasthenic crisis. Routine tracheostomy is not indicated in this patient population because the median duration of mechanical ventilation was 6 days.

10. Velmahos GC, Toutouzas K, Chan L, et al. Intubation after cervical spinal cord injury: to be done selectively or routinely? *Am Surg.* 2003;69:891–894.

Study Sample

Sixty-eight patients with cervical SCI admitted to a Level I trauma center between July 1995 and July 2000.

Comparison Studied

The purpose of this study was to identify characteristics of patients who develop respiratory failure and require intubation following cervical SCI. Intubated patients were compared to patients who did not receive intubation and mechanical ventilation. In addition, the correlation between timing of intubation and morbidity was evaluated.

Study Procedures

A retrospective chart review was used for data collection. Information obtained for analysis included demographics, level of SCI, associated injuries, injury severity, details regarding intubation and duration of mechanical ventilation, hospital course, morbidity, and mortality.

Key Results

Fifty patients (74%) required intubation. Of patients with injuries above C5, 87.5% required intubation versus 61% of patients with injuries at the C5 to C8 levels. Ninety percent of patients with complete quadriplegia required intubation versus 48.5% of patients with incomplete injury or paraplegia. Three independent risk factors for intubation were identified: Injury Severity Score >16, SCI above C5, and complete quadriplegia. Twenty-one of 22 patients with complete quadriplegia above C5 required intubation. Thirteen of the 31 patients who did not present with overt respiratory failure later required intubation (up to 53 hours after admission). There was a trend toward fewer complications in patients who were intubated within 1 hour of admission compared to those who were intubated later in the hospital course, despite the fact that the first group had higher injury severity. This difference was not statistically significant.

Study Strengths and Weaknesses

One strength is that it was conducted in the clinical setting under conditions in which these patients are likely to be encountered. Weaknesses include the retrospective study design, small sample size, and lack of specific criteria upon which intubation decisions were based.

Clinical Implications

The results of this study suggest that patients with complete SCI above C5 will almost certainly require intubation and mechanical ventilation. Velmahos et al. recommend that these patients be offered elective intubation early in their hospital course. Avoiding emergent intubation may reduce morbidity.

OTHER REFERENCES

1. American Association of Critical Care Nurses. Guidelines for the transfer of critically ill patients. Aliso Viejo, CA: AACN, 1998.
2. American Society of Anesthesiologists Task Force on Management of the Difficult Airway. Practice guidelines for management of the difficult airway. *Anesthesiology.* 2003;98:1269–1277.
3. American Thoracic Society. Guidelines for the management of adults with hospital-acquired, ventilator-associated, and health care-associated pneumonia. *Am J Respir Crit Care Med.* 2005;171:388–416.
4. Attia J, Ray JG, Cook DJ, Douketis J, Ginsberg JS, Geerts WH. Deep vein thrombosis and its prevention in critically ill adults. *Arch Intern Med.* 2001;161:1268–1279.
5. Babcock HM, Zack JE, Garrison T, et al. An educational intervention to reduce ventilator-associated pneumonia in an integrated health system. *Chest.* 2004;125:2224–2231.
6. Bach JS, Hunt D, Horton JA. Traumatic tetraplegia: non-invasive respiratory management in the acute setting. *Am J Phys Med Rehabil.* 2002;81:792–797.
7. Bader, MK, Littlejohns L, March K. Brain tissue oxygen monitoring in severe brain injury, II. Implications for critical care teams and case study. *Crit Care Nurse.* 2003;23:29–38, 40–2, 44.
8. Barrette RR, Hurst JM, Branson RD, Davis K Jr. A comparison of conventional mechanical hyperventilation with two forms of high-frequency ventilation for the control of intracranial pressure in closed head injury. *Respir Care.* 1987;32:733–740.
9. Bedford RF, Persing JA, Pobereskin L, Butler A. Lidocaine or thiopental for rapid control of intracranial hypertension? *Anesth Analg.* 1980;59:435–437.
10. Berrouschot J, Baumann I, Kalischewski P, Sterker M, Schneider D. Therapy of myasthenic crisis. *Crit Care Med.* 1997;25:1228–1235.
11. Brain Trauma Foundation. Management and prognosis of severe traumatic brain injury. 2000. Available at: http://www2.braintrauma.org/guidelines /downloads/btf_guidelines_management.pdf. Accessed August 2, 2007.
12. Brain Trauma Foundation. Guidelines for the management of severe traumatic brain injury: cerebral perfusion pressure. 2003. Available at: http://www2 .braintrauma.org/guidelines/downloads/btf_guidelines _cpp_u1.pdf. Accessed August 2, 2007.
13. Bratton SL, Davis RL. Acute lung injury in isolated traumatic brain injury. *Neurosurgery.* 1997;40:707–712.
14. Brook AD, Ahrens TS, Schaiff R, et al. Effect of a nursing-implemented sedation protocol on the duration of mechanical ventilation. *Crit Care Med.* 1999;27:2609–2615.

15. Brower RG, Lanken PN, MacIntyre N, et al. (National Heart, Lung, and Blood Institute ARDS Clinical Trials Network). Higher versus lower positive end-expiratory pressures in patients with the acute respiratory distress syndrome. *N Engl J Med.* 2004;351:327–336.

16. Brower RG, Matthay MA, Morris A, Schoenfeld D, Thompson BT, Wheeler A (The Acute Respiratory Distress Syndrome Network). Ventilation with lower tidal volumes as compared with traditional tidal volumes for acute lung injury and the acute respiratory distress syndrome. *N Engl J Med.* 2000;342:1301–1308.

17. Brower RG, Morris A, MacIntyre N, et al. (National Heart, Lung, and Blood Institute ARDS Clinical Trials Network). Effects of recruitment maneuvers in patients with acute lung injury and acute respiratory distress syndrome ventilated with high positive end-expiratory pressure. *Crit Care Med.* 2003;31:2592–2597.

18. Burns SM. Mechanical ventilation of patients with acute respiratory distress syndrome and patients requiring weaning. *Crit Care Nurse.* 2005;25:14–23.

19. Burns SM. Weaning from mechanical ventilation. In Burns SM (ed). *AACN Protocols for Practice: Care of Mechanically Ventilated Patients*, 2nd ed. Sudbury, MA: Jones and Bartlett; 2007;97–154.

20. Burns SM, Earven S, Fisher C, et al. Implementation of an institutional program to improve clinical and financial outcomes of mechanically ventilated patients: one-year outcomes and lessons learned. *Crit Care Med.* 2003;31:2752–2763.

21. Burns SM, Marshall M, Burns JE, et al. Design, testing, and results of an outcomes-managed approach to patients requiring prolonged mechanical ventilation. *Am J Crit Care.* 1998;7:45–57.

22. Byers JF, Sole ML. Analysis of factors related to the development of ventilator-associated pneumonia: use of existing databases. *Am J Crit Care.* 2000;9:344–351.

23. Cheng BC, Chang WN, Chang CS, et al. Predictive factors and long-term outcome of respiratory failure after Guillain-Barré syndrome. *Am J Med Sci.* 2004;327:336–340.

24. Chevrolet J, Deléamont P. Repeated vital capacity measurements as predictive parameters for mechanical ventilation need and weaning success in the Guillain-Barré syndrome. *Am Rev Respir Dis.* 1991;144:814–818.

25. Claxton AR, Wong DT, Chung F, Fehlings MG. Predictors of hospital mortality and mechanical ventilation in patients with cervical spinal cord injury. *Can J Anaesth.* 1998;45:144–149.

26. Como JJ, Sutton ERH, McCunn M, et al. Characterizing the need for mechanical ventilation following cervical spine injury with neurologic deficit. *J Trauma.* 2005;59:912–916.

27. Consortium for Spinal Cord Medicine. Respiratory management following spinal cord injury: a clinical practice guideline for health-care professionals. Washington (DC): Paralyzed Veterans of America. 2005 Jan. Available at: http://www.guideline.gov /summary/summary.aspx?ss=15&doc_id=7198&nbr =4301. Accessed September 14, 2007.

28. Contant CF, Valadka AB, Gopinath SP, Hannay HJ, Robertson CS. Adult respiratory distress syndrome: a complication of induced hypertension after severe head injury. *J Neurosurg.* 2001;95:560–568.

29. Cotton BA, Pryor JP, Chinwalla I, Wiebe DJ, Reilly PM, Schwab CW. Respiratory complications and mortality risk associated with thoracic spine injury. *J Trauma.* 2005;59:1400–1409.

30. Davis K, Hurst JM, Branson RD. High-frequency percussive ventilation. *Respir Care.* 1989;2:39–47.

31. de Durante G, del Turco M, Rustichini L, et al. ARDS Net lower tidal volume ventilatory strategy may generate intrinsic positive end-expiratory pressure in patients with acute respiratory distress syndrome. *Am J Respir Crit Care Med.* 2002;165:1271–1274.

32. Derdak S, Mehta S, Stewart TE, et al. High-frequency oscillatory ventilation for acute respiratory distress syndrome in adults. *Am J Respir Crit Care Med.* 2002;166:801–808.

33. Dodek P, Keenan S, Cook D, et al. Evidence-based clinical practice guideline for the prevention of ventilator-associated pneumonia. *Ann Intern Med.* 2004;141:305–313.

34. Drakulovic MB, Torres A, Bauer TT, Nicolas JM, Noque S, Ferrer M. Supine body position as a risk factor for nosocomial pneumonia in mechanically ventilated patients: a randomised trial. *Lancet.* 1999;354:1851–1858.

35. Eastern Association for the Surgery of Trauma (EAST). Guidelines for emergency tracheal intubation immediately following traumatic injury. Allentown (PA): Eastern Association for the Surgery of Trauma (EAST). 2002. Available at: http://www.guideline .gov. Accessed August 2, 2007.

36. Ely EW, Baker AM, Dunagan DP, et al. Effect on the duration of mechanical ventilation of identifying patients capable of breathing spontaneously. *N Engl J Med.* 1996;335:1864–1869.

37. Ely EW, Truman B, Shintani A, et al. Monitoring sedation status over time in ICU patients; Reliability and validity of the Richmond Agitation-Sedation Scale (RASS). *JAMA.* 2003;289:2983–2991.

38. Esteban A, Alia I, Gordo F, et al. Extubation outcomes after spontaneous breathing trials with T-tube or pressure support ventilation. *Am J Respir Crit Care Med.* 1997;156:459–465.

39. Ferguson ND, Chiche JD, Kacmarek RM, et al. Combining high-frequency oscillatory ventilation and recruitment maneuvers in adults with early acute respiratory distress syndrome: the Treatment with

Oscillation and an Open Lung Strategy (TOOLS) Trial pilot study. *Crit Care Med.* 2005;33:479–486.

40. Fletcher DD, Lawn ND, Wolter TD, Wijdicks EF. Long-term outcome in patients with Guillain-Barré syndrome requiring mechanical ventilation. *Neurology.* 2000;54:2311–2315.

41. Fontes RB, Aquiar PH, Zanetti MV, Andrade F, Mandel M, Teixeira MJ. Acute neurogenic pulmonary edema: case reports and literature review. *J Neurosurg Anesthesiol.* 2003;15:144–50.

42. Forsberg A, Press R, Einarsson U, de Pedro-Cuesta J, Widén Holmqvist L. Impairment in Guillain-Barré syndrome during the first 2 years after onset: a prospective study. *J Neurol Sci.* 2004;227:131–138.

43. Friedman JA, Pichelmann MA, Piepgras DG, et al. Pulmonary complications of aneurysmal subarachnoid hemorrhage. *Neurosurgery.* 2003;52:1025–1032.

44. Gattinoni L, Presenti A, Torresin A, et al. Adult respiratory distress syndrome profiles by computed tomography. *J Thoracic Imaging.* 1986;1:25–30.

45. Geerts WH, Pineo GF, Heit JA, et al. Prevention of venous thromboembolism: the seventh ACCP conference on antithrombotic and thrombolytic therapy. *Chest.* 2004;126(3 Suppl):338s–400s.

46. Govoni V, Granieri E. Epidemiology of the Guillain-Barré syndrome. *Curr Opin Neurol.* 2001;14:605–613.

47. Green DM. Weakness in the ICU: Guillain-Barré syndrome, myasthenia gravis, and critical illness polyneuropathy/myopathy. *Neurologist.* 2005;11:338–347.

48. Hall JE, Uhrich TD, Barney JA, Arain SR, Ebert TJ. Sedative, amnestic, and analgesic properties of small-dose dexmedetomidine infusions. *Anesth Analg.* 2000;90:699–705.

49. Hamill JF, Bedford RF, Weaver DC, Colohan AR. Lidocaine before endotracheal intubation: intravenous or larygotracheal? *Anesthesiology.* 1981;55:578–581.

50. Harrop JS, Sharan AD, Scheid EH Jr, Vaccaro AR, Przybylski GJ. Tracheostomy placement in patients with complete spinal cord injuries: American Spinal Injury Association grade A. *J Neurosurg.* 2004;100 *(1 Suppl Spine)*:20–23.

51. Hart N, Laffont I, Perez de la Sota A, et al. Respiratory effects of combined truncal and abdominal support in patients with spinal cord injury. *Arch Phys Med Rehabil.* 2005;86:1447–1451.

52. Heffner JE. The role of tracheotomy in weaning. *Chest.* 2001;120(Suppl 6):477S–481S.

53. Helfman SM, Gold MI, DeLisser EA, Herrington CA. Which drug prevents tachycardia and hypertension associated with tracheal intubation: lidocaine, fentanyl, or esmolol? *Anesth Analg.* 1991;72:502–504.

54. Henderson RD, Lawn ND, Fletcher DD, McClelland RL, Wijdicks EFM. The morbidity of Guillain-Barré syndrome admitted to the intensive care unit. *Neurology.* 2003;60:17–21.

55. Holland MC, Mackersie RC, Morabito D, et al. The development of acute lung injury is associated with worse neurologic outcome in patients with severe traumatic brain injury. *J Trauma.* 2003;55:106–111.

56. Hughes RAC, Bihari D. Acute neuromuscular respiratory paralysis. *J Neurol Neurosurg Psychiatry.* 1993;56:334–343.

57. Hughes RAC, Wijdicks EFM, Benson E, et al. Supportive care for patients with Guillain-Barré syndrome. *Arch Neurol.* 2005;62:1194–1198.

58. Hurst JM, Saul TG, DeHaven CB Jr, Branson R. Use of high-frequency jet ventilation during mechanical hyperventilation to reduce intracranial pressure in patients with multiple organ system injury. *Neurosurgery.* 1984;15:530–534.

59. Huynh T, Messer M, Sing RF, Miles W, Jacobs DG, Thomason MH. Positive end-expiratory pressure alters intracranial and cerebral perfusion pressure in severe traumatic brain injury. *J Trauma.* 2002;53:488–493.

60. Jackson AB, Groomes TE. Incidence of respiratory complications following spinal cord injury. *Arch Phys Med Rehabil.* 1994;75:270–275.

61. Juel VC. Myasthenia gravis: management of myasthenic crisis and perioperative care. *Semin Neurol.* 2004;24:75–81.

62. Kahn JM, Caldwell EC, Deem S, Newell DW, Heckbert SR, Rubenfeld GD. Acute lung injury in patients with subarachnoid hemorrhage: incidence, risk factors, and outcome. *Crit Care Med.* 2006;34:196–202.

63. Kaida K, Kusunoki S, Kanzaki M, Kamakura K, Motoyoshi K, Kanazawa I. Anti-GQ1b antibody as a factor predictive of mechanical ventilation in Guillain-Barré syndrome. *Neurology.* 2004;62:821–824.

64. Kelly BJ, Luce JM. The diagnosis and management of neuromuscular diseases causing respiratory failure. *Chest.* 1991;99:1485–1494.

65. Kollef MH, Shapiro SD, Siler P, et al. A randomized, controlled trial of protocol-directed versus physician-directed weaning from mechanical ventilation. *Crit Care Med.* 1997;25:567–574.

66. Kress JP, Pohlman AS, O'Connor MF, Hall JB. Daily interruption of sedative infusions in critically ill patients undergoing mechanical ventilation. *N Engl J Med.* 2000;342:1471–1477.

67. Lacomis D. Myasthenic crisis. *Neurocrit Care.* 2005;3:189–194.

68. Lawn ND, Wijdicks EFM. Tracheostomy in Guillain-Barré syndrome. *Muscle Nerve.* 1999;22:1058–1062.

69. Levitt MA, Dresden GM. The efficacy of esmolol versus lidocaine to attenuate the hemodynamic response to intubation in isolated head trauma patients. *Acad Emerg Med.* 2001;8:19–24.

70. Littlejohns LR, Bader MK, March, K. Brain tissue oxygen monitoring in severe brain injury, I. Research and usefulness in critical care. *Crit Care Nurse.* 2003;23:17–25.

71. Loveridge B, Sanii R, Dubo HI. Breathing pattern adjustments during the first year following cervical spinal cord injury. *Paraplegia.* 1992;30:479–488.

72. Lowe GJ, Ferguson ND. Lung protective ventilation in neurosurgical patients. *Curr Opin Crit Care.* 2006;12:3–7.

73. Lundy DS, Smith C, Colangelo L, et al. Aspiration: cause and implications. *Otolaryngol Head Neck Surg.* 1999;120:474–478.

74. MacIntyre NR, Cook DJ, Ely EW Jr. et al. Evidenced-based guidelines for weaning and discontinuing ventilatory support: a collective task force facilitated by the American College of Chest Physicians, the American Association for Respiratory Care, and the American College of Critical Care Medicine. *Chest.* 2001;120(6 Suppl):375S–395S.

75. Major KM, Hui T, Wilson MT, Gaon MD, Shabot MM, Margulies DR. Objective indications for early tracheostomy after blunt head trauma. *Am J Surg.* 2003;186:615–619.

76. Marini JJ. Recruitment maneuvers to achieve an "open lung": whether and how? *Crit Care Med.* 2001;29:1647–1648.

77. Martin UJ, Hincapie L, Nimchuk M, Gaughan J, Criner GJ. Impact of whole-body rehabilitation in patients receiving mechanical ventilation. *Crit Care Med.* 2005;33:2259–2265.

78. Martyn JA, White DA, Gronert GA, Jaffe RS, Ward JM. Up-and-down regulation of skeletal muscle acetylcholine receptors. *Anesthesiology.* 1992; 76:822–843.

79. McCool FD, Rosen MJ. Nonpharmacologic airway clearance therapies: ACCP evidence-based clinical practice guidelines. *Chest.* 2006;129:250S–259S.

80. McGuire G, Crossley D, Richards J, Wong D. Effects of varying levels of positive end-expiratory pressure on intracranial pressure and cerebral perfusion pressure. *Crit Care Med.* 1997;25:1059–1062.

81. Mehta S, Lapinsky SE, Hallett DC, et al. A prospective trial of high frequency oscillatory ventilation in adults with acute respiratory distress syndrome. *Crit Care Med.* 2001;29:1360–1369.

82. Meixensberger J, Jaeger M, Vath A, Dings J, Kunze E, Roosen K. Brain tissue oxygen guided treatment supplementing ICP/CPP therapy after traumatic brain injury. *J Neurol Neurosurg Psychiatry.* 2003;74:760–764.

83. Menzel M, Doppenberg EM, Zauner A, Soukup J, Reinert MM, Bullock R. Increased inspired oxygen concentration as a factor in improved brain tissue oxygenation and tissue lactate levels after severe human head trauma. *J Neurosurg.* 1999;91:1–10.

84. Mulvey JM, Dorsch NW, Mudaliar Y, Lang EW. Multimodality monitoring in severe traumatic brain injury: the role of brain tissue oxygenation monitoring. *Neurocrit Care.* 2004;1:391–402.

85. Naguib M, Flood P, McArdle JJ, Brenner HR. Advances in neurobiology of the neuromuscular junction. *Anesthesiology.* 2002;96:202–231.

86. Orlikowski D, Prigent H, Sharshar T, Lofaso F, Raphael JC. Respiratory dysfunction in Guillain-Barré syndrome. *Neurocrit Care.* 2004;1:415–422.

87. Peterson W, Charlifue W, Gerhart A, Whiteneck G. Two methods of weaning persons with quadriplegia from mechanical ventilation. *Paraplegia.* 1994; 32:98–103.

88. Peterson WP, Barbalata L, Brooks CA, Gerhart KA, Mellick DC, Whiteneck GG. The effect of tidal volumes on the time to wean persons with high tetraplegia from ventilators. *Spinal Cord.* 1999;37:284–288.

89. Pyeron AM. Respiratory failure in the neurological patient: the diagnosis of neurogenic pulmonary edema. *J Neurosci Nurs.* 2001;33:203–207.

90. Qureshi AI, Suarez JI, Parekh PD, Bhardwaj A. Prediction and timing of tracheostomy in patients with infratentorial lesions requiring mechanical ventilatory support. *Crit Care Med.* 2000;28:1383–1387.

91. Rabinstein AA, Mueller-Kronast N. Risk of extubation failure in patients with myasthenic crisis. *Neurocrit Care.* 2005;3:213–215.

92. Rabinstein A, Wijdicks EFM. BiPAP in acute respiratory failure due to myasthenic crisis may prevent intubation. *Neurology.* 2002;59:1647–1649.

93. Rabinstein AA, Wijdicks EFM. Warning signs of imminent respiratory failure in neurological patients. *Sem Neurol.* 2003;23:97–104.

94. Rees JH, Thompson RD, Smeeton NC, Hughes RAC. Epidemiological study of Guillain-Barré syndrome in south east England. *J Neurol Neurosurg Psychiatry.* 1998;64:74–77.

95. Reynolds SF, Heffner J. Airway management of the critically ill patient: rapid-sequence intubation. *Chest.* 2005;127:1397–1412.

96. Rieder P, Louis M, Jolliet P, Chevrolet JC. The repeated measure of vital capacity is a poor predictor of the need for mechanical ventilation in myasthenia gravis. *Intensive Care Med.* 1995;21:663–668.

97. Robertson CS, Valadka AB, Hannay HJ, et al. Prevention of secondary ischemic insults after severe head injury. *Crit Care Med.* 1999;27:2086–2095.

98. Ropper AH, Kehne SM. Guillain-Barré syndrome: management of respiratory failure. *Neurology.* 1985;35:1662–1665.

99. Roppolo LP, Walters K. Airway management in neurological emergencies. *Neurocrit Care.* 2004;1:405–414.

100. Rumbak MJ, Newton M, Truncale T, Schwartz SW, Adams JW, Hazard PB. A prospective, randomized, study comparing early percutaneous dilational tracheotomy to prolonged translaryngeal intubation (delayed tracheotomy) in critically ill medical patients. *Crit Care Med.* 2004;32:1689–1694.

101. Shatney CH, Brunner RD, NguyenTQ. The safety of orotracheal intubation in patients with highly unstable cervical spine fracture or high spinal cord injury. *Am J Surg.* 1995;170:676–680.

102. Sims CA, Berger DL. Airway risk in hospitalized trauma patients with cervical injuries requiring halo fixation. *Ann Surg.* 2002;235:280–284.

103. Stevens WJ. Multimodal monitoring: head injury management using $SjvO_2$ and Licox. *J Neurosci Nurs.* 2004;36:332–337.

104. Stiller K. Physiotherapy in intensive care: towards an evidence-based practice. *Chest.* 2000;118:1801–1813.

105. Stocchetti N, Maas AIR, Chieregato A, van der Plas AA. Hyperventilation in head injury: a review. *Chest.* 2005;127:1812–1827.

106. Tablan OC, Anderson LJ, Besser R, Bridges C, Hajjeh R. Guidelines for the prevention of health-care-associated pneumonia, 2003: recommendations of the CDC and the Healthcare Infection Control Practices Advisory Committee [electronic version]. *MMMR Recomm Rep.* 2004;53(RR-3):1–36. Available at: http://www.guideline.gov (search under first author's name). Accessed August 2, 2007.

107. Thieben MJ, Blacker DJ, Liu PY, Harper CM Jr, Wijdicks EF. Pulmonary function tests and blood gases in worsening myasthenia gravis. *Muscle Nerve.* 2005;32:664–667.

108. Tromans AM, Mecci M, Barrett FH, Ward TA, Grundy DJ. The use of BiPAP® biphasic positive airway pressure system in acute spinal cord injury. *Spinal Cord.* 1998;36:481–484.

109. Vallverdú I, Calaf N, Subirana M, Net A, Benito S, Mancebo J. Clinical characteristics, respiratory functional parameters, and outcome of a 2-hour T-piece trial in patients weaning from mechanical ventilation. *Am J Respir Crit Care Med.* 1998;158:1855–1862.

110. van den Brink WA, van Santbrink H, Steyerberg EW, et al. Brain oxygen tension in severe head injury. *Neurosurgery.* 2000;36:868–878.

111. van Santbrink H, Maas AL, Avezaat CJ. Continuous monitoring of partial pressure of brain tissue oxygen in patients with severe head injury. *Neurosurgery.* 1996;38:21–31.

112. Velmahos GC, Chan LS, Tatevossian R, et al. High-frequency percussive ventilation improves oxygenation in patients with ARDS. *Chest.* 1999;116:440–446.

113. Venn RM, Grounds RM. Comparison between dexmedetomidine and propofol for sedation in the intensive care unit: patient and clinician preferences. *Br J Anaesth.* 2001; 87:684–690.

114. Vespa PM, Bleck TP. Neurogenic pulmonary edema and other mechanisms of impaired oxygenation after aneurysmal subarachnoid hemorrhage. *Neurocrit Care.* 2004;1:157–170.

115. Wijdicks EF, Borel CO. Respiratory management in acute neurologic illness. *Neurology.* 1998;50:11–20.

116. Wijdicks EFM, Roy TK. BiPAP in early Guillain-Barré syndrome may fail. *Can J Neurol Sci.* 2006;33:105–106.

117. Winslow C, Rozovsky J. Effect of spinal cord injury on the respiratory system. *Am J Phys Med Rehabil.* 2003;82:803–814.

CHAPTER TWO 2

Intracranial Pressure Management

Karen March, RN, MN, CCRN, CNRN
and Lori Madden, RN, MS, CCRN, CNRN, ACNP-C

CASE STUDY

H.H. is a 23-year-old man who sustained a 3-story fall. He was verbal at the scene but subsequently had a rapid decrease in his level of consciousness. H.H. was transported by emergency medical services after his airway was secured. Once evaluated in the emergency department, he underwent emergent head computed tomographic (CT) scan that revealed a large, 3-cm left frontotemporoparietal epidural hematoma, right rim subdural hematoma, and intraparenchymal contusions. He was emergently taken to the operating room for evacuation of the epidural hematoma. Intraoperatively, a left linear skull fracture was identified in the temporal area overlying the lacerated left middle meningeal artery.

H.H. did well postoperatively with a Glasgow coma scale (GCS) score of 10 (E3V1M6) and pupils at 3-mm reacting briskly to light, bilaterally. He was extubated given his improved level of consciousness. His exam progressively deteriorated by the next morning (GCS 4 = E1V1M2, pupils 6-mm nonreactive bilaterally), and he was reintubated. A right frontal ventriculostomy with a fiberoptic intracranial pressure (ICP) monitor was placed that afternoon with an initial ICP of 24 mm Hg. Figure 2-1 shows examples of ICP monitors. Mildly elevated ICPs initially responded to sedation, chemical paralysis, mannitol infusion, and cerebrospinal fluid (CSF) drainage. Brain tissue oxygen monitoring also was performed during this time in order to maximize medical management and minimize

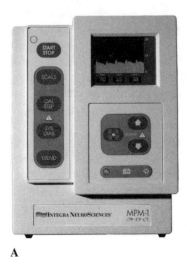
A

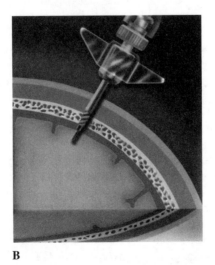
B

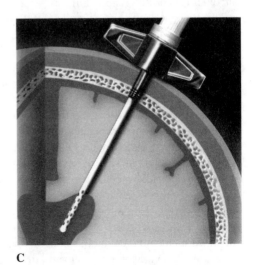
C

Figure 2-1 **(A) Camino MPM intracranial pressure monitor and catheters, (B) parenchymal and (C) bolted ventricular catheter.**

Source: © Integra LifeSciences Corporation 2006. Compliments of Integra LifeSciences

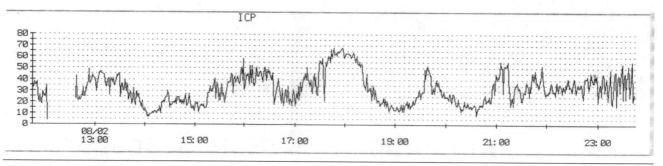

Figure 2-2   Printout of a monitor showing an intracranial pressure trend.

cerebral ischemia. Despite these measures, ICP continued to rise further and he became nonresponsive to medical management. ICP ranged from 29 to 51 mm Hg during that period. Figure 2-2 is an example of an ICP trend. Head CT scan was repeated and revealed worsening right to left shift and obliteration of the basal cisterns. He was brought back to the operating room for craniectomy. ICP improved subsequently to a goal of <20 mm Hg. Therapies were weaned gradually, and H.H.'s neurological exam results improved progressively. Ten days after injury, H.H. once again followed commands and 2 weeks after injury, his GCS was 15. The bone flap was replaced 3 weeks after injury. H.H. is now in acute inpatient rehabilitation.

GENERAL DESCRIPTION

ICP monitoring devices measure the sum of the pressures exerted by the intracranial contents (blood, brain, CSF) within the skull. When expansion of intracranial volume exceeds the brain's the ability to compensate (ie, shunting of venous blood and CSF into the spinal canal) for this increase, the ICP will increase. Increases in ICP contribute to secondary brain injury and a worsening of neurologic outcomes (Other References: 50).

The type of monitoring device used and location in which the device is placed will influence the usability, accuracy, and incidence of complications. Types of ICP monitors can be divided into fluid-filled systems or advanced technology. Fluid-filled systems require the monitoring device to be connected to preservative-free saline-filled pressurized tubing connected to an external strain-gauge pressure transducer. Advanced technology consists of 3 types of technology all with implantable transducers: fiberoptics, miniaturized strain-gauge transducers (or micro-electrical mechanical systems), and air pouch devices. All of these devices create an electrical signal that is transmitted to a monitor that converts the signal into a pressure reading. The locations where each device can be implanted include the epidural, subdural, and subarachnoid spaces, and the intraparenchymal and intraventricular compartments. Intraventricular monitors have a distinct advantage to the other systems in that CSF can be drained to treat

elevations in ICP as well as monitor pressure (Other References: 61).

Monitoring ICP consists of measuring the mean pressure exerted within the cranium. Under normal circumstances, ICP in the supine position is 0 to 15 mm Hg and may be less than 0 in the upright position. As volume increases and normal compensatory mechanisms fail (shunting of venous blood and CSF out of the cranium), pressure increases, which results in greater neuronal injury (Other References: 60). Thresholds for treatment still vary but the Guidelines for the Management of Adult Severe Traumatic Brain Injury Patient and the Guidelines for the Acute Medical Management of Severe Traumatic Brain Injury in Infants, Children, and Adolescents recommend 20 to 25 mm Hg as the treatment threshold (Other References: 1, 14).

Along with the digital ICP measurement, these devices also transmit a waveform. The waveform represents the pressure pulse wave being transmitted into the intracranial compartment by systemic hemodynamics. Alteration in the normal waveform pattern is thought to represent changes in the patient's compliance or ability to adjust to changes in intracranial volume without always impacting pressure. Without a reliable ICP waveform, the reliability of the digital data may be questionable because of improper placement, debris, or other impediment to proper transmission of the ICP signal, or pathophysiology (ie, pneumocephalus, craniectomy; Other References: 55, 60).

Without monitoring ICP, the clinician must wait for external signs of increased ICP such as deterioration in the neurologic examination (ie, decreased level of consciousness or change in pupils) or changes in the neurodiagnostic imaging studies (evidence of herniation or swelling on CT or magnetic resonance imaging [MRI]). By this time, neuronal damage may already have occurred. ICP monitoring allows the clinician to react early before significant secondary neurologic injury has occurred.

ACCURACY

Accuracy of ICP monitors is influenced by the location of the placement of the device, heterogeneity of the brain, focal factors, and the technology of the device. Pressure

Table 2-1   Product Specifications

Technology Reference	Zero Drift	Temperature Drift
Camino (Integra LifeSciences, Plainsboro, NJ) (Other References: 15)	±2 mm Hg/1st 24 hours and <1 mm Hg/day for next 4 days = total 5 days	Maximum of 3 mm Hg over temperature range of 22°C–38°C (70°F–100°F)
Codman (Johnson & Johnson, Raynham, MA) (Other References: 19)	3 mm Hg/day	<0.15 mm Hg/°C (Other References: 8)
Neurovent (Raumedic Systems, Münchberg, Germany) (Other References: 61)	1–2 mm Hg over 5 days	<0.15 mm Hg/°C (Other References: 8)
Ventrix (Integra LifeSciences, Plainsboro, NJ) (Other References: 108)	±2 mm Hg/1st 24 hours and <1 mm Hg/day for next 48 hours	5 mm Hg maximum change over operating range of Ventrix ICP monitor
Fluid-filled transducers (Other References: 24, 65)	±2 mm Hg/8 hours	<±0.3 mm Hg/°C

within the intracranial compartment is not homogeneous and is compartmentalized. Pressures on the surface may not represent pressures deep in the cerebral hemisphere or within the posterior fossa. Pressure gradients may develop within the tissues as a result of hematomas or edema. Other factors that influence accuracy include debris, blood, or blockage within the system or device altering the transmission of the pressure frequency by the transducer. A dampened ICP waveform is a factor that the clinician may assess where the information being transmitted may be inaccurate.

The Association for the Advancement of Medical Instrumentation has established standards for ICP technology. These standards include specifications for the measure ranges, accuracy, and maximum error. Pressure range measures should be between 0 and 100 mm Hg, accuracy ±2 mm Hg over a range of 0 to 20 mm Hg, and maximum error of 10% over a range of 20 to 100 mm Hg (Other References: 1, 14, 55).

Accuracy of a device is most often described as drift. *Drift* is defined in 2 ways: the offset of zero (positive or negative readings from zero) and error in the reading in response to changes in temperature. Temperature drift occurs when an implantable device is zeroed to atmosphere in a cold room and then implanted into a warm head. The temperature difference may exceed 15°C (Annotated Bibliography: 9, 10). Manufacturers establish and report their products' expected drift in use and specifications literature packaged with the device. Table 2-1 lists a few examples of product specifications. Many studies have examined commonly used product devices for in vivo and in vitro applications. Caution should be taken when evaluating in vitro studies to determine drift in relation to dwelling time of catheter.

COMPETENCY

Effective use of ICP monitoring requires knowledge of intracranial anatomy and physiology as well as the Monro-Kellie doctrine; understanding of the pathophysiology of the disease process that prompts ICP monitoring; and nursing, medical, and surgical interventions and their implications on ICP and cerebral perfusion pressure (CPP). Additional aspects needed for competency verification include the following:

- Identify the clinical indications for ICP monitor placement.
- Identify the correct anatomical location of ICP monitor insertion.
- Demonstrate proper assembly of all supplies necessary for ICP monitor placement.
- Demonstrate proper assembly and placement of all monitor and drainage devices used within the patient care area/institution.
- Identify the tasks involved in assisting with the insertion of an ICP monitor.
- Correctly level and calibrate device.
- Perform maintenance tasks (eg, zero the transducer of a fluid-filled ventriculostomy) related to each device.
- Demonstrate proper drainage of CSF (per institutional policy).
- Demonstrate collection of CSF specimen for low/normal CSF output, infected CSF. State how often and the time when the specimen is generally collected.
- Document the ICP and CPP every hour, or as ordered, and with changes in the patient's neurological status.
- Identify a normal and an abnormal ICP waveform.
- Identify therapeutic interventions that can alter ICP compliance.
- Troubleshoot dampened or absent ICP waveform and irrigate (per institutional policy).
- Maintain a closed ventricular monitoring system and intact dressing or performance of site care per institutional policy.
- Demonstrate/discuss troubleshooting of each type of ICP monitoring device.
- Discuss indications for removal of a device.

ETHICAL CONSIDERATIONS

The ethical principles of beneficence and nonmalfeasance are often referred to in difficult medical situations. The medical team seeks to "do no harm" to patients when providing treatment and withdrawing or withholding treatment. *Benefi-cence* is defined as (1) prevention of evil or harm, (2) removal of evil or harm, and (3) do or promote good. The term *non-malfeasance* means that one ought not to inflict evil or harm (Other References: 9).

Providing ICP Monitoring

ICP monitoring is provided to patients in whom elevated ICP is suspected or anticipated. ICP levels are monitored to identify if ICP is elevated; if it is elevated, then the response to treatment can be evaluated. This is done with the understanding that elevated ICP is harmful to patients and that lowering of elevated ICP will result in avoiding or minimizing harm to the patients, who then experience a better outcome. Some patient populations have been found to have no benefit with ICP monitoring while others do seem to benefit (Table 2-1).

Despite the lack of randomized controlled trials, treatment of the same sets of patients (see Clinical Recommendations, pp. 40–60) with ICP monitoring and treatment of elevated ICP has resulted in these strategies becoming the standard of care for those populations. To avoid any professional or legal criticism about the provision of substandard care, many patients for whom an ICP monitor may not be indicated may have a monitor inserted.

Clinicians must consider whether potential injury or complications might occur in patients with an elevated ICP, as the use of ICP monitoring and treatment of elevated ICP should change the outcome for the patient positively. Further research on this issue is needed. ICP monitoring has not been proven to clearly improve outcomes in all patient populations in which it is utilized. Lack of funding, grouping of participating medical centers, and a sufficiently large number of patients for data analysis are all factors impeding a definitive conclusion. One preliminary study on this issue found no difference in outcome for patients treated according to common ICP management principles compared to a group in whom clinical findings alone prompted treatment (Other References: 20). The only difference between groups was the increase in length of stay for patients receiving ICP monitoring and ICP-based treatment.

Withdrawal or Withholding of ICP Monitoring

Several concerns exist regarding futility of care that prompts the withdrawal (stopping) of ICP monitoring or withholding (not starting) ICP monitor placement. Consider whether harm will be inflicted onto patients who would not survive regardless of treatment. For example, a patient may come in to the hospital after a motor vehicle crash with a severe traumatic brain injury (TBI) and 90% body surface area burns, including most of the scalp. In this scenario, considering the high mortality rate for such injuries and the significant risk of infection after placement of an ICP device, if a neurosurgeon opts to not place an ICP monitoring device, would it be considered care withheld? Would placement of the device change the outcome for this unfortunate individual?

ICP monitoring has not been proven to significantly improve morbidity and/or mortality in any patient population because it has not been subjected to a large randomized control study. As ICP monitoring is an integral part of the management of many disease processes, for example, TBI, ethically it is difficult to design a study in which a group of patients would not receive ICP monitoring or would be treated irrespective of ICP values. ICP monitoring has helped to detect intracranial mass lesions more rapidly, limited indiscriminate use of therapies that by themselves can be harmful, reduced ICP levels by CSF drainage thereby improving cerebral perfusion, and helped to determine prognosis.

The World Medical Association adopted the Declaration of Helsinki to guide ethical principles for medical research involving human subjects. This Declaration, which is regularly updated, sets forth clear principles that are used by institutional review boards and ethical committees when evaluating research. Trials that involve ICP diagnostic and/or therapeutic efficacy would need to adhere to such guidelines (available at http://www.wma.net/e/policy/b3.htm; accessed August 4, 2007).

Ultimately, each case should be considered individually. Ethical issues should be discussed by the team of providers involved together with the patient, family, social services, and possibly with the hospital ethics committee if concerns remain.

OCCUPATIONAL HAZARDS

In 1991, the Occupational Safety and Health Administration issued standards to reduce the risk of exposure of healthcare workers to bloodborne pathogens (hepatitis, human immunodeficiency virus). These standards have focused on reducing needlesticks and accidental sharps injuries from objects contaminated by blood or other body fluids, and to limit exposure to blood and body fluids. ICP monitors are implanted into or onto the surface of the brain and thus require special handling to prevent exposure or transmission of bloodborne pathogens. Strict sterile technique and use of personal protective devices are crucial prophylactic measures when inserting an ICP monitoring device, both to prevent contamination and exposure to infections for the patient, and to protect the clinician from potential exposure to bloodborne pathogens from the patient. Proper handling and disposal of these implantable devices when removed will limit healthcare worker exposure.

Upon removal of the monitor, all 1-time use items (as recommended by the manufacturer) should be disposed of as hazardous material. All reusable items, such as the monitor and cables, should be decontaminated as recommended by the manufacturer before being used for another patient (Other References: 104).

ICP monitoring using advanced techniques has other safety concerns. These devices are linked to electronic monitors that require routine safety checks to ensure they are working correctly and safely. Routine maintenance should be carried out according to manufacturer's recommendations. Not only do these checks ensure electrical safety, but they assure the proper calibration of the device and accurate interpretation of the displayed values.

FUTURE RESEARCH

Despite multiple studies investigating ICP monitoring, a lack of evidence persists on multiple issues. The impact of each treatment for elevated ICP should be evaluated. ICP values and the timing of such values could be evaluated relative to outcome. Further testing of ICP versus CPP as treatment goals is another area for research. ICP treatment versus nontreatment or nonmonitoring should be considered on a larger, randomized scale.

How the type of ICP monitor is selected for a particular patient population is another consideration. In particular, device selection and pathology could be better coupled. Perhaps some monitor types are better suited to certain disease or injury processes.

Rigorous analysis of scientific data is the most powerful way to change or affirm practice. Multicenter trials are needed to evaluate the issues surrounding the various types of ICP monitors as well as clinically important infection and complication rates. Surveillance practices related to these 2 issues also remain to be elucidated. The use of antibiotic impregnated catheters as well as different insertion techniques of monitors (eg, tunneled versus bolted catheters) should be evaluated to identify if there is truly a difference in infection rates. CSF drainage techniques vary among centers and should be evaluated to discover the best method(s) to treat patients with this intervention.

Waveform analysis may provide more information than is currently considered in clinical practice. Clinical studies identifying correlations among waveform findings, interventions/treatment, nursing care, and outcome should be pursued. Further, the predictive value of waveform changes might be evaluated relative to clinical events or outcome.

CLINICAL RECOMMENDATIONS

The rating scale for the Level of Recommendation ranges from I to VI, with levels indicated as follows: I, manufacturer's recommendations only; II, theory based, no research data to support recommendations; recommendations from expert consensus group may exist; III, laboratory data only, no clinical data to support recommendations; IV, limited clinical studies to support recommendations; V, clinical studies in more than 1 or 2 different populations and situations to support recommendations; VI, clinical studies in a variety of patient populations and situations to support recommendations.

Period of Use	Recommendations	Rationale for Recommendation	Level of Recommendation	Supporting References	Comments
Selection of Patients ICP monitoring is an appropriate strategy for several patient populations.	**Traumatic brain injury patients** GCS ≤8 with an abnormal head CT scan, even with open fontanels and sutures. GCS ≤8 with a normal CT with 2 or more of the following: • Hypotension • >40 years of age • Exhibit decorticate or decerebrate motor posturing GCS >9 with a mass lesion may benefit from ICP monitoring, or a pediatric patient who cannot participate in serial assessments. MD may choose to monitor conscious patient with mass lesion or patient who cannot perform serial exam.	Strong evidence supports the association of intracranial hypertension and poor neurological outcome. ICP monitoring and aggressive treatment of intracranial hypertension are associated with the best reported clinical outcomes.	VI	See Other References: 1, 36	Brain Trauma Foundation Guidelines provide review of literature with no studies providing standard-level evidence. Guidelines are provided based upon multiple publications. Severe head injury is defined as a GCS score of 3 to 8 after cardiopulmonary resuscitation. An abnormal CT scan of the head is one that reveals hematomas, contusions, edema, or compressed basal cisterns.
	CT scan may not identify opening ICP.	Admission of head CT scan does not predict opening ICP.	IV	See Other References: 35, 64	Do not use admission head CT scan findings alone to identify patients for monitoring. Retrospective chart review at an institution.
	Intracranial hemorrhage patients Limited evidence suggests that ICP monitoring in this patient population may improve outcome.	Patients with intracerebral hemorrhage, subarachnoid hemorrhage, subdural hemorrhage, hemorrhagic intracerebral contusions, epidural hemorrhage, and isolated intraventricular hemorrhage were retrospectively reviewed in the context of ICP monitor use and standardized mortality ratios were evaluated. A beneficial effect of ICP monitoring in patients	IV	See Other References: 106	Retrospective single-center comparison of standardized mortality ratios between ICP monitored group and group without ICP monitoring (selection bias in outcome).

Period of Use	Recommendations	Rationale for Recommendation	Level of Recommendation	Supporting References	Comments
Selection of Patients (*cont.*)		with intracranial hemorrhage may be reflected in an improved standardized mortality ratio.			
	Ventricular drain placement with intraventricular instillation of tissue plasminogen activator (tPA) may accelerate clot lysis and potentially improve outcome for patients with intraventricular hemorrhage.	Intraventricular instillation of urokinase within 12 to 48 hours in intraventricular hemorrhage patients looked at 30-day survival rates. Urokinase is no longer available and tPA is used in its place. Subsequent research involves tPA for treatment.	IV	See Other References: 119	
	Subarachnoid hemorrhage patients				
	ICP monitoring may allow for treatment of intracranial hypertension present in some patients.	Some patients may have an elevated ICP, even those with good clinical grade. Those with ICP <20 mm Hg have a better outcome than those with ICP >20 mm Hg, especially if ICP does not respond to treatment. This association may be more dependent upon the overall subarachnoid hemorrhage severity rather than ICP alone.	IV	See Other References: 40	Retrospective database review.
		Most commonly, ICP is monitored in higher Hunt & Hess grade patients. These patients have longer length of stay and higher morbidity and mortality. However, they may have improved quality of survival if intracranial hypertension is avoided and cerebral perfusion is optimized.			
	ICP monitoring in subararchnoid hemorrhage patients may prove to be beneficial.		IV	See Other References: 58	Retrospective chart review at an institution.
	Hydrocephalus patients				
	ICP monitoring can be used to identify some of the problems in the management of children with hydrocephalus, both before and after the insertion of shunt systems.	In a study, intraparenchymal fiberoptic ICP monitoring led to the more accurate selection of patients for surgical intervention and the avoidance of making some children shunt-dependent who did not require CSF diversion. It also enabled more confident diagnosis	IV	See Other References: 29, 77	

Period of Use	Recommendations	Rationale for Recommendation	Level of Recommendation	Supporting References	Comments
Selection of Patients *(cont.)*		of intracranial hypotension (ie, overdrainage of CSF in patients who present with a multitude of previously unexplained symptoms and signs).			
	Sylvian arachnoid cysts	Prolonged ICP monitoring proved an important pre-operative tool to rule out unnecessary surgery on children with type I cysts. ICP elevation is almost always present in children with type III Sylvian fissure arachnoid cysts.	IV	See Other References: 25	
	Cerebral fat embolism				
	Patients with cerebral fat embolism syndromes with a neurological deterioration (decrease in GCS of $\geq$5 points) and limited neurological exam (during anesthesia or sedation) may benefit from ICP monitoring.	One report noted that ICP monitoring will allow earlier detection and treatment of intracranial hypertension.	II	See Other References: 95	
	Fulminant hepatic failure (FHF)				
	ICP monitoring should be performed in patients with FHF with clinical signs of stage III or early stage IV encephalopathy once coagulopathies have been corrected with fresh frozen plasma (FFP) and platelets (goal international normalized ratio [INR] <1.7, prothrombin time <3 seconds, and platelets $\geq$50,000 at time of insertion).		IV	See Other References: 7, 44, 54, 84, 107	Elevated ICP is reported to occur in 75% to 80% of FHF cases that progress to stage IV encephalopathy. Intracranial hypertension is thought to be related to cerebral edema (vasogenic and cellular).
	ICP and CPP should be interpreted within the context of other variables in this patient population.	Case report of 2 FHF patients with false-positive elevated ICP suggests that ICP/CPP is less accurate in isolation; consider within context of patient condition, examination, and other parameters.	II		
	Ischemic stroke				
	ICP monitoring may be considered in some centers for major territorial infarctions.	Most major territorial infarctions will produce cytotoxic edema and consecutive rise in ICP	II	See Other References: 38	Literature review, 1 center's methods.

Period of Use	Recommendations	Rationale for Recommendation	Level of Recommendation	Supporting References	Comments
Selection of Patients *(cont.)*		leading to some space occupying effects. Early ICP monitoring in these patients is necessary.			
	ICP monitoring and treatment is unlikely to have a positive influence on clinical outcome in patients with large hemispheric or middle cerebral artery ischemic strokes.	In all patients clinical signs of herniation preceded the increase in ICP. Patients with ICP values >35 mm Hg did not survive. CT changes did not always correspond with the measured ICP values. ICP monitoring of large hemispheric infarction can predict clinical outcome. ICP monitoring was not helpful in guiding long-term treatment of increased ICP.	IV	See Other References: 92	The clinical course of 48 patients with the clinical signs of increased ICP due to large hemispheric or middle cerebral artery territory infarction defined by CT and subjected to ICP monitoring was prospectively evaluated.
	ICP monitoring may be beneficial in patients with malignant middle cerebral artery infarctions. It identifies patients who may benefit from craniectomy and/or additional anterior temporal lobectomy.	Patients with malignant middle cerebral artery infarctions were divided into 3 groups: ultra-early craniectomy, craniectomy beyond 6 hours, and no operation. Those treated with craniectomy were provided anterior temporal lobectomy if ICP was sustained at >30 mm Hg. Those patients had improved outcomes versus those without surgery. Patients with ultra-early craniectomy fared better than those with delayed or no surgery.	IV	See Other References: 17	Consecutive patients admitted to one facility. Patients were not randomly assigned. They were divided into 3 groups: A (dx within 6 hours and tx consented); B (presentation at study facility >6 hrs after dx or dx initially smaller territory); or C (no family consent for surgical treatment).
	Meningitis				
	ICP monitoring may be helpful in the management of patients with bacterial meningitis.	Head CT scan in patients with bacterial meningitis may not rule out the possibility of elevated ICP or herniation syndromes. ICP monitoring should be considered in comatose patients with bacterial meningitis.	IV	See Other References: 113	Limited case report.
		Patients presenting with bacterial meningitis may have intracranial hypertension and should be considered candidates for ICP monitoring. Patients responsive to treatment in a small group were noted to have a high survival rate.	IV	See Other References: 35	Report of retrospective review of 12 cases.
	ICP monitoring and management of elevated ICP may prevent	Theoretically, pathological changes (such as cerebral edema and alterations in	II	See Other References: 67	

Period of Use	Recommendations	Rationale for Recommendation	Level of Recommendation	Supporting References	Comments
Selection of Patients *(cont.)*	secondary insults and improve outcome in patients with tuberculous meningitis.	blood flow regulation) which occur during tuberculous meningitis may result in elevated ICP. ICP elevation should be treated in order to avoid poorer outcome resulting from secondary insults which would occur due to elevated ICP.			
	ICP monitoring does not influence outcome in children with meningitis.	Retrospective review found that there was no influence on mortality when ICP monitoring was used in children with meningitis.	IV	See Other References: 72, 73	Two retrospective reviews of mortality between 2 groups; not well controlled regarding treatment or looking at morbidity or quality of survival.
Application of Device and Initial Use					
Selecting the type of device:	**Ventriculostomy** A hollow ventricular catheter (connected to an external strain gauge or with a fiberoptic or microchip sensor tip). • Most accurate and reliable method of monitoring ICP • Allows for therapeutic CSF drainage	Not only allows for ICP monitoring, but provides for CSF drainage. This may be of therapeutic (eg, to decrease ICP) and diagnostic value (eg, specimen sampling for glucose, protein, and culture). It is also believed that by reducing CSF volume, there is an increase in cerebral blood flow (CBF) and therefore an improvement in cerebral perfusion.	II	See Annotated Bibliography: 8 See Other References: 10, 19, 45, 76	Cost of these devices varies.
	External strain-gauge transducers.	These devices are connected to the fluid-filled ventriculostomies to measure the pressure transmitted from the CSF in the ventricles. These transducers typically measure the electrical resistance caused by a change in the strain present in a length of thin metal foil. The strain-gauge pressure sensing element sits atop a mechanical diaphragm. The ventricular catheter and pressure tubing conduct fluid, and therefore ICP, to the rear side of the diaphragm. Changes in ICP cause changes in the pressure exerted on the diaphragm and hence the strain on the sensor element. Simple electrical circuits are used to measure the resistance of the sensor element, which is proportional to ICP.	III	See Other References: 23, 55, 61, 71, 105, 117	

Period of Use	Recommendations	Rationale for Recommendation	Level of Recommendation	Supporting References	Comments
Application of Device and Initial Use *(cont.)*		Considered the most accurate method of monitoring ICP.	IV	See Other References: 117	
	Fiberoptic ("transducer tipped") catheters	Catheters have a primary pressure transducer mounted on the distal tip of the implanted catheter. With fiberoptic technology, the primary sensor is a mechanical diaphragm that moves with changes in pressure. The position of the diaphragm changes the intensity of the light reflected from its rear surface. The amount of light that is refracted is translated by the electronics into pressure. These systems may be used to measure intraventricular, parenchymal, subdural, or epidural pressure.		See Other References: 42, 61, 117	
	Microchip (internal strain-gauge) catheters	Changes in the position of the diaphragm cause changes in the electrical resistance that are recorded, transformed, and displayed as ICP readings. These systems may be used to measure intraventricular, parenchymal, subdural or epidural pressure.		See Other References: 61, 117	
	Air pouch technology	Senses ICP by filling a balloon that surrounds the end of the catheter with a set volume of air (0.05–0.1 cc). The pressure exerted on the balloon pouch is the pressure of the surrounding tissue. The catheter re-zeros itself hourly by deflating and re-inflating the balloon to maintain a constant balloon volume. This system may be used to measure intraventricular, parenchymal, or epidural pressure.	IV	See Other References: 69, 117	
	• Set up: All devices should include povidone-iodine scrub solution, povidone-iodine swabs, sterile gloves, surgical caps, masks, sterile surgical gowns, sterile towels, drapes, local anesthetic (1%–2% lidocaine without			See Other References: 15, 19, 34, 63, 69	

Period of Use	Recommendations	Rationale for Recommendation	Level of Recommendation	Supporting References	Comments
Application of Device and Initial Use *(cont.)*	epinephrine), 5–10-cc syringe with an 18-gauge needle to draw up lidocaine, 23-gauge needle to administer lidocaine, drill and bits, sutures, scalpel with blade, scalp retractor, sterile scissors and needle holder, razor, intraventricular catheter, sterile occlusive dressing, stapler (optional).				
	1. External strain-gauge transducers: Transducer cable, external strain-gauge transducer, sterile preservative-free normal saline, sterile CSF drainage system, system holder, device to secure transducer to the bed or IV pole.				
	2. Fiberoptic ("transducer tipped") catheters: Stand-alone monitor, cable to connect stand-alone monitor to bedside monitor, fiberoptic intraventricular catheter or intra-parenchymal catheter with calibration device, sterile CSF drainage system (if drainage exists).				
	3. Microchip (internal strain-gauge) catheters: Stand-alone monitor, cable to connect stand-alone monitor to bedside monitor, fiberoptic intraventricular catheter or intra-parenchymal catheter with calibration device, sterile CSF drainage system (if drainage exists).				
	4. Air pouch technology: Stand-alone monitor, cable to connect stand-alone monitor to bedside monitor, fiberoptic intraventricular				

Period of Use	Recommendations	Rationale for Recommendation	Level of Recommendation	Supporting References	Comments
Application of Device and Initial Use *(cont.)*	catheter or intraparenchymal catheter with calibration device, sterile CSF drainage system (if drainage exists).				
Insertion of device by anatomic location	**Anatomical location**				
	Pressures within the various locations (hemispheres, supratentorial, and infratentorial) in the cranium vary.	Location of parenchymal and ventricular catheters to pathology gives different pressures—the closer the catheter to the pathology, the higher the ICP.	IV	See Annotated Bibliography: 3 See Other References: 87, 97, 114	
	Ventricular catheter, external strain-gauge transducer, or catheter tip pressure transducer device is an accurate and reliable method of ICP monitoring in pediatric patients.		V	See Other References: 1	
	Generally, surface monitors are less accurate as they do not represent pressures in the deeper tissues.		IV		
	In patients with FHF, subdural or parenchymal placement is more accurate. However, epidural placement may be safer.	While subdural or parenchymal monitor is more accurate, epidural placement is safer in FHF patients.	IV		
		One report of ICP monitoring in FHF patients recommends subdural or subarachnoid catheter placement under general anesthesia.	IV	See Other References: 84	
	Ventricular	The gold standard of ICP monitoring is ventriculostomy. A burr hole is made in the skull after an incision is made in the scalp, usually in the midpupillary line anterior to the coronal suture of the skull. An opening is made in the dura, and a small flexible tube over a stylet is passed through the parenchyma into the lateral ventricle. The trajectory of the catheter from the insertion site is perpendicular to the brain surface. Often these catheters are tunneled under the scalp a short distance away from the burr hole insertion site before	VI	See Other References: 71, 114	

Period of Use	Recommendations	Rationale for Recommendation	Level of Recommendation	Supporting References	Comments
Application of Device and Initial Use (*cont.*)		they exit the scalp. Others are secured using a bolt. The tunneling under the scalp is thought to decrease infection.			
		Complications related to the use of a ventriculostomy include an approximate 1% to 10% risk of infection (causing ventriculitis or meningitis) and a 1% to 2% risk of bleeding.	VI		
	Parenchymal	Fiberoptic intraparenchymal ICP monitoring devices are safe for use in children with severe TBI. However, some investigators have found that this does not always correlate with ventricular ICP.	V	See Other References: 1, 43	Prospective review of 98 children.
		Parenchymal ICP monitoring involves a fiberoptic or strain-gauge device placed within the brain tissue for pressure monitoring. It may be placed in patients in whom CSF sampling or drainage is unnecessary or in patients with significant coagulopathies. Complications still include infection and bleeding (2%), although the incidence is lower with these devices in comparison with the ventricular catheter. Dislodgement of the cable/fiberoptics has been reported at a rate of 4%.	VI		
	Subdural	Drains or monitors are placed between the dura and the subarachnoid space. Monitors placed are usually fluid-filled or fiberoptic. Unfortunately, the fluid-filled devices can collapse and impair the waveform. Monitors placed in the subdural space have a lower rate of infection compared with ventriculostomy, but because of problems associated with subdural catheters, monitoring at this site is less common.		See Other References: 13, 63, 117	
	Epidural	Monitors are placed between the skull and the dura and provide an indirect measurement of ICP. As a			

Period of Use	Recommendations	Rationale for Recommendation	Level of Recommendation	Supporting References	Comments
Application of Device and Initial Use *(cont.)*		result, they are less accurate and do not represent pressures in the deeper tissues. These devices are rarely used.			
Facility location of insertion	The operating room is the best location in which to place an ICP catheter in a patient. Alternate locations include the emergency department and the intensive care unit (ICU).	ICP catheters placed in the patient while in the operating room have the lowest incidence of infection.	II	See Other References: 43	
		Seven percent positive culture rate (*Staphylococcus epidermidis*) in review of 98 children with fiberoptic devices: no clinical signs of infection; believed to be colonization. All positive cultures were from devices placed outside of OR.	IV		Prospective review of 98 children.
		Ventriculostomy-associated infections increase in frequency when monitors are placed outside of the OR.	IV	See Other References: 3	
Ongoing Monitoring					
ICP treatment threshold	Goal ICP in adults should be less than 20–25 mm Hg.	It appears that keeping ICP <20–25 mm Hg improves outcomes.	VI	See Other References: 1, 109	
	Goal ICP in infants, children, and adolescents should be <20 mm Hg. Interpretation and treatment of ICP based upon any threshold should be corroborated by frequent clinical examination and CPP data.	No prospective study has addressed the treatment threshold of ICP in children. Retrospective studies conclude ICP ≥20 mm Hg is associated with worse outcome. It has been suggested that lower ICP values for younger children should be used for treatment thresholds, but there is no data to support such recommendations.	VI	See Other References: 7, 36, 84	
	Standard management of elevated ICP is done in a step-wise approach and may include the following measures: • Evacuation of mass lesions • CSF drainage • Sedation • Chemical paralysis • Osmotic diuretic bolus • Hypertonic saline	Reducing intracranial hypertension can be achieved by reducing the space occupied by any of the 4 components: • Reduce brain size using mannitol or other hypertonic substances. • Reduce CSF using drainage. • Reduce blood by inducing hyperventilation to induce vasoconstriction.		See Other References: 116	

Period of Use	Recommendations	Rationale for Recommendation	Level of Recommendation	Supporting References	Comments
Ongoing Monitoring *(cont.)*	• Moderate hyperventilation • Drug (barbiturate or Propofol) coma • Hemicraniectomy • Moderate hypothermia	• Surgical removal of a pathologic process (tumor, hematoma). Alternatively, one may open the skull to allow expansion of the structures (decompressive craniectomy).			
	Lund concept for management of elevated ICP: • Once normovolemia is established, antihypertensive treatment with both β-blocker (eg, metoprolol) and an β-2 agonist (eg, clonidine). • Decrease cerebral blood volume with dihyroergotamine and thiopental. • Reduce brain metabolism and stress with opiates and benzodiazepines. • Balanced or slightly negative fluid volume balance. • Volume substitution with plasma/albumin infusion and blood transfusion to maintain normovolemia and normal plasma osmotic pressure. • Volume-controlled mechanical ventilation		IV	See Other References: 98	Prospective observational study in 1 center.
	Specific management for patients with FHF: • Elective endotracheal (ET) intubation • Moderate head of bed (HOB) elevation • Normovolemia • Dialysis ultrafiltration • Mannitol 0.5 g/kg bolus dose; do not repeat more frequently than every hour • Mannitol is contraindicated in anuric patients unless followed by continuous ultrafiltration during	Elective ET tube intubation; avoid ICP spike with ET tube; avoid hypercapnia with decreased loss of consciousness (LOC) and secure airway. Continuous renal-replacement therapy improves hemodynamic stability. Cooling to "subnormal" temperatures in FHF patients reduced ICP but patients must have transplant prior to rewarming or mortality is 100%. Arterial and cerebral uptake of ammonia are both lowered with cooling.	IV		

Period of Use	Recommendations	Rationale for Recommendation	Level of Recommendation	Supporting References	Comments
Ongoing Monitoring *(cont.)*	renal-replacement therapy • Barbiturates with careful hemodynamic monitoring; some regard as unsafe practice • Continuous renal-replacement therapy • Cooling				

	Standard management of CPP is generally done in a step-wise approach and may include the following measures:
	• Achieve adequate ICP
	• Elevate mean arterial pressure (MAP)
	  1. Infusion of crystalloids or colloids to achieve euvolemia or slight hypervolemia
	  2. Inotrope infusion (eg, phenylephrine, norepinephrine, dopamine)
		CPP is a calculated value derived from ICP and MAP (MAP – ICP = CPP); it is an indirect method of evaluating cerebral perfusion and blood flow. Generally, CPP is considered adequate if 50–70 mm Hg.	VI	See Other References: 36	

	CPP-focused therapy despite elevated ICP can lead to good neurological outcomes.	CPP-focused therapy rather than ICP-focused therapy was used at a center for severe TBI patients.	IV		
Nursing interventions and ICP	**Bed position**				
	Although ICP may be higher than in other positions, horizontal position may provide optimal CPP.	On the whole, stroke patients may benefit from horizontal backrest positions rather than backrest/HOB positioning at 15° or 30° as is standard in many institutions. Patient positioning ultimately should be tailored to the individual patient.	V	See Other References: 93	Eighteen patients with complete or subtotal middle cerebral artery territory stroke were monitored in various positions on 43 total occasions.
	HOB at 30° in TBI patients reduces ICP and improves CPP without concomitant decrease in cerebral oxygenation.	ICP was significantly lower in HOB 30° group in comparison to group in supine position. CPP was slightly but not significantly higher in the 30° HOB group in comparison to those in the supine position. Oxygenation values were above critical thresholds in both groups.	V	See Other References: 70, 112	
	ICP is improved with HOB 30°. CPP is not	Literature review of 11 articles.	V	See Other References: 26	

Period of Use	Recommendations	Rationale for Recommendation	Level of Recommendation	Supporting References	Comments
Ongoing Monitoring *(cont.)*	significantly different in flat supine position versus HOB 30°.				
	ET suctioning				
	Deepen the level of sedation in patients with head injury to avoid cerebral ischemia associated with ICP elevation related to suctioning.	ICP commonly increases with endotracheal suctioning. One study monitored ICP, CPP, and jugular oxygen saturation (Sjo_2) during suctioning with and without an increase in sedation. Patients suctioned with adequate sedation had an increase in ICP, CPP, and Sjo_2 without evidence of ischemia. Patients who coughed or moved in response to suctioning had a significant decrease in CPP and Sjo_2 with the concomitant increase in ICP, resulting in ischemia.	IV	See Annotated Bibliography: 4	
	ET suctioning protocols consisting of pre-suctioning increased tidal volume breaths and 100% fraction of inspired oxygen (Fio_2) delivery before and after suctioning results in ICP return to baseline within minutes.	A set protocol as described in 1 ICU resulted in return of ICP to baseline within 2 minutes of endotracheal suction (ETS).	IV	See Annotated Bibliography: 7	Prospective, descriptive with repeat assessments for each patient.
Waveform interpretation	Increased amplitude of ICP waveform and peak waveform level 2 (P2) elevation is clinically relevant and has been found to provide a rough indicator of decreased adaptive capacity.	Analysis of various ICP waveforms has provoked much discussion, yet the importance of the waveform is clear, whether or not it is present. If a good waveform is present, the pressure reading displayed on the monitor is more reliable. If the waveform is dampened, it reflects a mean pressure that is reasonably, if not completely, accurate. An exception is the fluid-filled system (ie, for ventriculostomy) in which a blood clot or brain tissue has blocked the tubing. In this situation, the reading is inaccurate and may require troubleshooting to clear the obstruction.	VI	See Other References: 49	Multiple clinical studies.
		The real-time waveform appears slightly similar to a vascular pressure reading. It has 3 to 4 peaks. The first peak (P1), called the *percussion wave*, is attributed			

Period of Use	Recommendations	Rationale for Recommendation	Level of Recommendation	Supporting References	Comments
Ongoing Monitoring *(cont.)*		to transmitted arterial pressure. Two or 3 smaller peaks (P2, P3, and P4) have been attributed to choroid plexus or venous pressure artifact. Usually these peaks occur in a stairstep fashion. However, P2 may become prominent as compliance decreases and/or ICP increases. The separate peaks may be less distinct or unnoticeable if the waveform is dampened.			
		A waves (plateau waves) are visible on analysis of larger spans of time with elevation of ICP to ≥60 mm Hg for 5 to 20 minutes. B waves appear as sharp rhythmic oscillations of pressure values every 30 to 120 seconds and are seen in relation to respiratory patterns such as Cheyne-Stokes breathing. They are thought to progress to A waves. C waves occur every 4 to 8 minutes and relate to changes in blood pressure. Their effect is unknown.			
Prevention of Complications				See Other References: 13, 28, 63, 110, 117	
Infection	Use strict aseptic techniques during insertion (gown, glove, mask) and when manipulating the device is essential to prevent contamination.	Infection is defined as: a positive CSF culture obtained from ventricular or lumbar catheter; positive culture with CSF pleocytosis, low glucose level, or high protein level; CSF pleocytosis or low glucose level alone without a positive culture; presence of clinical symptoms as fever or mental status changes; and 2 positive cultures with the same organisms. Contamination has been identified as an isolated CSF culture with normal CSF cell counts and absent clinical symptoms or a Gram-negative stain with a positive culture. It is difficult to ascertain the incidence of CNS infections resulting from ICP monitoring devices because of the variability in what is defined as an infection. Some suggest that	VI	See Annotated Bibliography: 5 See Other References: 2, 5, 18, 21, 37, 41–43, 46–48, 53, 57, 61, 62, 66, 75, 80–82, 85, 86, 88–91, 93, 99–101, 109, 111, 115, 118	

Period of Use	Recommendations	Rationale for Recommendation	Level of Recommendation	Supporting References	Comments
Prevention of Complications (*cont.*)		device colonization should be followed as it increases significantly after 5 days of implantation. If detected, removal of the device is sufficient treatment.			
		Overall infection rates reported in the literature regardless of definition ranged from 0%–27%; many of these had poor or no definition of infection.	V		
		Zingale reported a 53% infection rate with externalized shunts. Of those who clearly defined a CNS infection, an overall incidence of ventricular catheter infection of 5.6% to 20.5% was reported. Infection rates for tunneled ventricular catheters appear to be between 0%–4%. Reported infection rates for intraparenchymal devices ranged from 0.3%–3.7%. Jensen reported a 7% incidence of positive tip culture from intraparenchymal devices but no evidence of clinical infection. The time the device was indwelling (greater than 5 days) and location in the hospital the catheter was inserted (outside of operating room) correlate with higher infection rates. The most commonly reported pathogens are *Staphylococcus aureus* and *S. epidermis*, *E. coli*, *Klebsiella*, and *Streptococcus*.		See Other References: 118 See Other References: 43	
		Seven percent positive culture rate (*Staphylococcus epider-midis*) in a review of 98 children with fiberoptic devices, no clinical signs of infection; believed to be colonization. All positive cultures were from devices placed outside of operating room.		See Other References: 43	Prospective review of 98 cases meeting criteria.
		Eight and one-half percent of cases with positive probe tip cultures (*S. epidermidis* was the pathogen in 47.8% of these cases; others had *E. coli* and *Corynebacterium*).		See Other References: 33	Chart review of 1000 cases.

Period of Use	Recommendations	Rationale for Recommendation	Level of Recommendation	Supporting References	Comments
Prevention of Complications *(cont.)*		0.3% infection		See Other References: 80	Prospective data collection for 303 children at 1 center
	Antibiotic prophylaxis to prevent infection is not supported by any literature and may result in development of resistant organisms.	Use of antibiotic prophylaxis during placement of intracerebral monitoring devices is controversial. There are no randomized, controlled trial data to support or refute their use, although a retrospective study suggested that antibiotic prophylaxis has no effect on rates of infection, and concerns remain regarding the risks of encouraging the development of antibiotic resistance.		See Other References: 82, 89	
	CSF cultures should be obtained only when clinically indicated, rather than as routine surveillance.	Routine surveillance cultures of CSF are no more likely to detect infection than cultures obtained when clinically indicated.		See Other References: 3	
Hemorrhage	Proper insertion minimizes risk of bleeding.	Hemorrhages are often not reported or may be clinically insignificant. Recent studies have attempted to classify the significance of hemorrhages.	V	See Annotated Bibliography: 1 See Other References: 2, 5, 11, 37, 46, 61, 66, 85, 91, 93, 96, 102, 103, 115	
		Overall hemorrhage rates have been reported as 6.4%–9.2% with intraparenchymal devices. One study reported a hemorrhage rate of 17.6% with intraventricular catheters, including 1 requiring surgical intervention.	V	See Other References: 80	Prospective data collection of 303 children.
		Three-tenths percent hemorrhage in 1 child with low platelet count.	IV	See Other References: 33	Chart review of 1000 cases.
		Eight and seven-tenths percent rate of coagulation abnormality, only 8% rate of postoperative bleeding. However, these data have no clinical relevance.	IV		
	Coagulopathies should be corrected prior to device insertion.	The role of coagulopathy as a contributing factor in hemorrhage is often a concern, particularly in patients with acute trauma and liver failure. It is recommended the coagulopathy be corrected	VI	See Annotated Bibliography: 3	

Period of Use	Recommendations	Rationale for Recommendation	Level of Recommendation	Supporting References	Comments
Prevention of Complications *(cont.)*		before placing an ICP monitor. Correcting coagulation factors is a difficult issue in patients with FHF who may have an elevated ICP.			
	In patients with INR ≤1.6, use of FFP to "normalize" INR below that level is not necessary.	Retrospective chart review at 1 institution looked at TBI patients with parenchymal ICP monitor placement. In patients with INR <1.6, hemorrhagic complications after ICP monitor were infrequent. Delays in monitor placement and treatment occurred in patients given component therapy.	IV	See Annotated Bibliography: 3	
	FHF patients have been reported to have complication rates of 3.8% with epidural monitors; 20% (mainly bleeding) with subdural bolts and 22% with parenchymal monitors. Fatal hemorrhages occurred in 1% of epidural monitor case, 5% of subdural devices, and 4% of intraparenchymal devices.	Monitoring of ICP in acute liver failure is controversial as a result of the reported complication risk (~20%) and limited therapeutic options for intracranial hypertension. A survey performed in a subset of these patients revealed intracranial hemorrhage in 10.3% of the cohort, half of the complications being incidental radiological findings. However, intracranial bleeding could have contributed to the demise of 2 patients. In subjects listed for liver transplant, ICP monitoring was associated with a higher proportion of subjects receiving vasopressors and ICP-related medications. The 30-day survival after liver transplant was similar in both monitored and nonmonitored groups (85% vs 85%).	IV	See Other References: 19, 107	
Quality Control Issues					
Accuracy	External strain-gauge-coupled devices are accurate and can be recalibrated, but obstruction of the fluid-filled line can cause inaccuracy. In addition, the external transducer must be consistently maintained at a fixed reference point relative to the patient's head (usually the external auditory	Standards for ICP technology have been established by the Advancement of Medical Instrumentation. These standards include the following specifications: pressure range measures between 0 to 100 mm Hg; accuracy of ±2 mm Hg over a range of 0 to 20 mm Hg; maximum error of 10% over a range of 20 to 100 mm Hg. Drift is defined as offset of	VI	See Annotated Bibliography: 9, 10 See Other References: 1, 6, 8, 13, 15, 16, 19, 21, 27, 31, 34, 42, 61, 66, 68, 69, 76, 77, 80, 89, 91, 93, 96, 108, 110, 117	

Period of Use	Recommendations	Rationale for Recommendation	Level of Recommendation	Supporting References	Comments
Quality Control Issues *(cont.)*	canal) to avoid measurement error.	zero and error in reading in response to changes in temperature. There is considerable variability of data among studies evaluating drift. When interpreting ICP recordings, the clinician must consider its proximity to pathology (ICP may be higher when closer to pathology), clinical condition, and proper insertion.			
	Ventricular catheters may become obstructed by blood clots. Intraventricular instillation of tPA may be used to lyse clots obstructing the tip of a ventricular catheter.	Blood clot at the tip of a ventricular catheter will dampen the ICP waveform and may diminish the accuracy of the measurement. The obstruction also inhibits CSF drainage. Urokinase has been studied in the treatment of intraventricular hemorrhage. While urokinase is no longer available, tPA is often used for clot lysis in patients with intraventricular blood which blocks the ventricular catheter.	IV	See Other References: 119	
	Catheter tip strain-gauge or fiberoptic devices are calibrated prior to intracranial insertion (without an associated ventricular catheter). If a device drifts and is not recalibrated, there is potential for inaccurate measurement.	Thirteen percent mechanical failure rate of intraparenchymal fiberoptic device in review of 98 severe TBI children.	IV	See Other References: 80	Prospective data collection of 303 children.
	Cumulative drift may be acceptable in those situations where patient monitoring exceeded manufacturer's recommendations (ie, >5 days). Proper placement and recording of the location of the catheter may impact reliability of the data.	Two and sixth-tenths percent monitor malfunction rate reported in the literature. Manufacturers generally recommend changing device after 5 days due to potential increase in infection and drift.	IV	See Other References: 33	Chart review of 1000 cases.
	Secure system so that the ICP monitor is not displaced.	One percent rate of monitor displacement. Dislocation or optical fiber breakage in 4.5% of cases with fiberoptic technology; most occurred during nursing activities, patient transport	IV		

Period of Use	Recommendations	Rationale for Recommendation	Level of Recommendation	Supporting References	Comments
Quality Control Issues *(cont.)*		(eg, to CT scanner), or patient activity.			
	To be accurate, preservative-free saline-filled systems must use short, unobstructed, nonflexible tubing without air bubbles and connected to a nonflush strain-gauge transducer.	Traditional flush transducers used for cardiovascular hemodynamic monitoring deliver a continuous infusion of ~3 cc of solution from a pressurized intravenous bag (usually heparinized saline). The flush system is intended to prevent clotting of the line and backflow of blood into the transducer in cardiovascular applications. Continuous pressurized infusion of (heparinized) saline may raise ICP and cause bleeding. There are several key elements to obtaining an accurate measurement using a fluid-filled system. These include the in situ catheter; low-compliant, unobstructed tubing; and the appropriate transducer connection to the bedside monitor. Small, intraluminal size (<7F) of the in situ catheter increases the frictional resistance of the CSF fluid and impacts pressure. The length, diameter, and flexibility of the tubing used can alter the fidelity of the recording. Flexible, soft tubing (compliant), a large diameter tube, and excessive length in the tubing (>4 feet) dampen or blunt the pressure recording, resulting in an underestimation of ICP. Debris in the catheter or tubing (brain matter, blood clots) and increased viscosity of the fluid (blood, infection, increased protein content) also can affect the reading. Air bubbles in the transducer, tubing, or stopcocks will dampen the pressure waveform, potentially leading to ICP measurement errors.	IV	See Annotated Bibliography: 2 See Other References: 4, 16, 23, 67, 80, 117	
	Proper leveling of the CSF drainage chamber and the transducer are important aspects of ICP monitor use.	The transducer is leveled or zeroed at an external reference point that represents the level of the foramen of Monro. The transducer must be leveled and re-zeroed at		See Annotated Bibliography: 2 See Other References: 4, 23, 24, 61, 65, 83	

Period of Use	Recommendations	Rationale for Recommendation	Level of Recommendation	Supporting References	Comments
Quality Control Issues (*cont.*)	Protocols outlining both the proper procedure (including proper use of leveling devices) and a standard reference for the foramen of Monro, and regular educational sessions are key to accurate use of this technique.	regular intervals to maintain accuracy. Current transducers drift ±2 mm Hg per 8 hours. Some methods used to reference the foramen of Monro are: 1. Measuring halfway between the outer canthus of the eye and the tragus. 2. Measuring 1 centimeter posterior to the eye or 2 cm above the pterion. 3. Drawing a line between the 2 eternal auditory meatus and determining the midpoint. 4. Using the external auditory meatus as the reference. If the transducer and external ventricular drain (EVD) are not referenced to the foramen of Monro correctly using a carpenter levels, bubbleline level, or laser level, there can be a significant error. For every inch of deviation above or below the reference, there is a 1.86 mm Hg error (or 0.73 mm Hg for every centimeter). As the transducer falls below zero, the pressure increases and it decreases when it is raised above zero. Inaccurate leveling and positioning of the drainage chamber and transducer drift all can lead to a cumulative error of several millimeters of mercury.			
Duration of use	FHF ICP monitoring may be used up to 24 hours post-transplantation		IV	See Other References: 7	
	Evaluate necessity to change ICP monitor at day 5.	Bacterial colonization generally occurs by day 5 after insertion. Documentation of bacterial colonization and actual infection varies from 0 infection rate regardless of length of time implanted to elevated infection rate after 5 days. Manufacturers generally recommend changing devices after 5 days because of the potential increase in infection and drift.	IV	See Other References: 74	Longer duration of use increases risk of infectious complication and diminished accuracy.

Period of Use	Recommendations	Rationale for Recommendation	Level of Recommendation	Supporting References	Comments
Outcome of treatment	ICP-targeted therapy may not improve outcome in patients with TBI.	ICP/CPP-targeted intensive care results in prolonged mechanical ventilation and increased levels of therapy intensity, without evidence for improved outcome in patients who survive beyond 24 hours following severe head injury. Intracranial hypertension after severe head injury is associated with case fatality, but there is no prospective randomized controlled trial proving that monitoring of ICP and targeted management of CPP improve outcome, despite widespread recommendation by experts in the field. One study in adult severe TBI sought to determine the effect of ICP/CPP-targeted intensive care on functional outcome and therapy intensity levels in this population. Multiple factors were observed in 2 groups. In center A (supportive intensive care), mean arterial pressure was maintained at approximately 90 mm Hg, and therapeutic interventions were based on clinical observations and CT findings. In center B (ICP/CPP-targeted intensive care), management was aimed at maintaining ICP <20 mm Hg and CPP >70 mm Hg.	IV	See Other References: 20	Retrospective cohort study of 333 severely head-injured adults who survived for >24 hours with prospective assessment of outcome in 2 level I trauma centers.
	ICP monitor insertion is associated with a lower death rate in severe TBI patients.	Trauma registry files were reviewed in Ontario, Canada. Statistical analyses controlling for various other factors found that insertion of an ICP monitor is associated with a significant decrease in death rate among patients with severe TBI.	IV	See Other References: 52	Retrospective database review.
	ICP monitoring and treatment in FHF patients does not improve outcome in comparison to patients who are not monitored.	No difference in 85 FHF patients who underwent emergency LT (½ with ICP monitoring vs ½ without ICP monitoring).	IV	See Other References: 107	Multi-center U.S. Acute Liver Failure Study Group database review/survey.

ANNOTATED BIBLIOGRAPHY

1. **Blaha M, Lazar D, Winn R, Ghatan S. Hemorrhagic complications of intracranial pressure monitors in children.** *Ped Neurosurg.* **2003;39:27–31.**

Study Sample
The sample was 112 pediatric patients (ages 5 months to 16 years) who underwent intraparenchymal fiberoptic ICP monitoring.

Comparison Studied
The purpose was to determine the incidence of intracranial hemorrhage after insertion of an intraparenchymal ICP monitor and to grade the clinical significance of the hemorrhages.

Study Procedures
This was a retrospective review of the patients' charts and radiographic records. All patients with hemorrhage were graded by the investigator and coagulation profiles assessed.

Key Results
All of the children received ICP monitoring; 19 had more than 1 monitor placed, resulting in 134 procedures being performed. A total of 119 procedures demonstrated no hemorrhagic complications (grade 0), 10 had punctate hemorrhage or localized subarachnoid hemorrhage (grade 1), and 3 had an intracerebral hemorrhage that did not require evacuation (grade 2). There were no intracerebral hemorrhages that required evacuation (grade 3). Stratification of complications did not show an increased risk related to age of patients.

Study Strengths and Weaknesses
The strength of this study is the systematic evaluation of hemorrhages and the correlation to clinical significance. Weaknesses include the limitation to the pediatric population and no correlation of complication rate to the skills of the practitioner.

Clinical Implications
Intraparenchymal ICP monitoring is a safe method of ICP monitoring in children with a low risk of significant hemorrhagic complications.

2. **Brisnaire, D, Robinson, L. Accuracy of leveling intraventricular collection drainage systems.** *J Neuroscience Nurs.* **1997;29:261–268.**

Study Sample
Nurses participated from an ICU, a neuroscience special care unit, and the acute care unit of an academic medical center in Ontario, Canada. Thirty-three nurses participated in part I, and 31 different nurses participated in part II of the study.

Comparison Studied
Accuracy of leveling practices (visual leveling, use of a carpenter level, and use of a laser level) were evaluated as well as identification of an appropriate anatomical landmark.

Study Procedures
Part I of the study tested 6 leveling practices. Each nurse leveled an external CSF drainage system to 3 mannequins without an anatomical mark to represent the Foramen of Monro and 3 with a mark. Participants' leveling practices were observed and noted (bend down to eye level; use of tubing extended between mannequin and drainage system). Accuracy was verified by the researchers using a carpenter level and a set square. For part II, a different group of nurses were asked to level the CSF drainage system 3 times with a carpenter level and 3 times with a laser level. Participants were observed for ease of use, dexterity, and safety. Accuracy of measurement was rechecked using the same procedure.

Key Results
Part I showed that the leveling practices using visualization were inaccurate. Practices were worse if there was no anatomic landmark identified. It was also noted that several nurses did not know the proper anatomic landmark for leveling, which added to the inaccuracy. Part II results demonstrated that leveling accuracy improved significantly.

Study Strengths and Weaknesses
A strength of this study is that it shows that use of a tool improves accuracy regardless of age and experience of the participant. Weaknesses include the poor generalizability of the data because the study was performed at a single site; only 1 drainage system was assessed, and the definition of acceptable accuracy may have been too loose (2 cm).

Clinical Implications
Brisnaire and Robinson showed that the addition of tools helped the accuracy of leveling practices for CSF drainage systems. The laser tool was easier to use than the carpenter level. Knowledge deficits regarding use of CSF drainage systems may influence the accuracy of leveling practices.

3. **Davis JW, Davis IC, Bennink LD, Hysell SE, Curtis BV, Kaups KL, Bilello JF. Placement of ICP monitors: are "normal" coagulation parameters necessary?** *J Trauma.* **2004;57: 1173–1177.**

Study Sample
A retrospective chart review was performed of severe head injury patients admitted to a Level I trauma center over a

3-year period who underwent fiberoptic intraparenchymal ICP monitoring. One hundred fifty-seven patients met inclusion criteria and were included in the study.

Comparison Studied

This study examined the hemorrhagic complication rates from ICP monitor placement and the need to give FFP to correct coagulation parameters to "normal."

Study Procedures

Patients included in the study were to have coagulation studies (prothrombin time, partial thromboplastin time, INR, and platelet count) before the insertion of the ICP monitor, and a head CT scan to assess for hemorrhage before and after the monitor was placed. Additional data collected were age, GCS, head region abbreviated injury score, time to ICP monitor placement, complications, and outcomes. Patients were grouped by INR: normal (0.8–1.2), borderline (1.2–1.6), and increased (1.7).

Key Results

One hundred three patients were categorized as having normal INRs, 42 were borderline, and 12 were increased. Twenty-two patients received component therapy (FFP and platelets) to improve or correct coagulation. All but 1 patient received the component therapy for INR >1.2.

Component therapy resulted in a delay in ICP monitoring. Three patients, 1 in each group (INRs 1.2, 1.3, and 2.5), had clinically insignificant hemorrhages (1.9%). No patient required an intervention.

Study Strengths and Weaknesses

A strength of this study was its significant sample size and the stratification of the patient groups by INR. Weaknesses are the retrospective nature of the study and the single population.

Clinical Implications

Complications associated with an INR greater than 1.6 are low, and the use of component therapy to normalize the INR is not supported by this study and only served to delay monitoring ICP.

4. Gemma M, Tommasino C, Cerri M, Giannotti A, Piazzi B, Borghi T. Intracranial effects of endotracheal suctioning in the acute phase of head injury. *J Neurosurg Anesthesia.* 2002; 14:50–54.

Study Sample

Seventeen consecutive severe head injury patients aged 44 ± 18 years (17–77) were included in this study.

Comparison Studied

This prospective nonrandomized study evaluated the effect of routine ET suctioning on intracranial dynamics in head injuries.

Study Procedures

The impact of routine ET suction on ICP, systemic blood pressure, heart rate, saturation of jugular oxygen, and arterial blood gases was continuously assessed before, during, and immediately after suctioning. Patients were placed on 100% oxygen for 60 seconds prior to single-pass ET suctioning using a 16F disposable multilumen catheter with a negative pressure of 100 mm Hg. The duration of the suctioning was less than 30 seconds. After suctioning, oxygen was maintained at 100% for 30 seconds. ICP and MAP were recorded, and a blood sample was drawn.

Key Results

ET suctioning resulted in an increase in ICP, the jugular oxygen saturation decreased, and CPP fell. These suctioning effects were greatest in patients whose sedation was inadequate.

Study Strengths and Weaknesses

This was an observation study and not well defined. The pre- and postsuction times for data collection were not clearly defined.

Clinical Implications

Increases in ICP with suctioning are small and insignificant if patients are adequately sedated.

5. Hader W, Steinbok P. The value of routine cultures of the cerebrospinal fluid in patients with external ventricular drains. *Neurosurgery.* 2000;46:1149–1155.

Study Sample

Charts from 157 patients with 160 extraventricular drains were reviewed from a tertiary care pediatric neurosurgical center between 1984 and 1997. Patients were between newborn and 17 years of age.

Comparison Studied

This study evaluated if infections can be identified early and therefore complications related to bacterial ventriculitis could be prevented by performing routine CSF cultures in patients with EVDs.

Study Procedures

A single-center database retrospective review of all patients in whom an EVD was placed during a 13-year period extracted the following information in 157 pediatric patients: diagnosis, reason for EVD placement (no infection), surgical procedures performed, and complications. Other information was gathered about the extraventricular drainage: location of catheter placement (operating room or intensive care), duration of catheter placement, number of catheters placed, reason for removal, prophylactic antibiotic coverage, whether routine culture of CSF was performed, and microbiology reports.

Key Results

Seven of 48 positive cultures were identified, defined as a gram-positive stain, positive culture, and a subsequent positive culture. The majority of the positive cultures were contaminants. None of the 7 infected patients were identified as having an infection before clinical changes occurred despite routine cultures. Each developed a fever (>38.5°C) and peripheral leukocytosis value (>$11^3 \times 10^3/mm^3$) on the day the infection was identified, and 1 had a change in CSF appearance. No infections occurred in catheters inserted for less than 2 days. Patients who developed a CSF infection within 3 days of the EVD insertion all had a CSF leak; all others developed after prolonged indwelling (5–17 days).

Study Strengths and Weaknesses

Data were retrospective and some clinical information was not available in all patients. Generalizability is limited because of its small sample size, single site, and age of patients (especially to the adult population).

Clinical Implications

This study suggests that routine CSF cultures may not be beneficial in pediatric patients with EVDs. A protocol identifying key clinical indicators (new fever [>38.5°C], peripheral leukocytosis, neurological deterioration, or development of turbid CSF) may be better markers of when CSF cultures should be performed.

6. Kaups K, Parks S, Morris C. Intracranial pressure monitor placement by midlevel practitioners. *J Trauma*. 1998;45:884–886.

Study Sample

Two hundred fifteen ICP monitors were inserted between December 1993 to June 1997 at a Level I trauma center by neurosurgeons, midlevel practitioners, and general surgery residents.

Comparison Studied

The risk-benefit of midlevel practitioners (physician assistants and nurse practitioners) was evaluated.

Study Procedures

Medical records and trauma registry data were reviewed on all patients who had an ICP monitor placed. The following data were collected: age, sex, mechanism of injury, injury type, reason for ICP monitor placement, duration of placement, GCS score at admission and discharge, who placed the ICP monitor, complications related to the ICP monitor, and patient outcome. Computed tomographic scans before placement and after removal were reviewed for hematoma development.

Key Results

Two hundred fifteen monitors were placed in 210 patients: 105 by neurosurgeons, 97 by midlevel practitioners, and 13 by general surgery residents. There were no major compli-

cations resulting from the placement of the ICP monitors; however, 19 minor complications (malfunction, dislodgment) were seen, of which 11 were placed by neurosurgeons (10%), 7 by midlevel practitioners (7%), and 1 by a resident (8%).

Study Strengths and Weaknesses

The strength of this study is that all practitioners underwent a similar training. The weakness of this study was that it lacked randomization and was a single-site study.

Clinical Implications

Placement of ICP monitors by midlevel practitioners is safe and may facilitate prompt placement.

7. Kerr ME, Weber BB, Sereika SM, Darby J, Marion DW, Orndoff PA. Effect of endotracheal suctioning on cerebral oxygenation in traumatic brain-injured patients. *Crit Care Med*. 1999;27:2776–2781.

Study Sample

Sixty-six severe adult head-injured patients were included, 29 subjects for the first part of the study and 37 for the second.

Comparison Studied

This study is a repeated measure, randomized within-group design that looked at the efficacy of 2 methods of controlled short-duration hyperventilation, blunting the rise in ICP that occurs with ET suctioning.

Study Procedures

Each experimental hyperventilation hyperoxygenation ET suctioning protocol was tested against the control hyperventilation ET suctioning protocol. The control protocol used a rate of 12 breaths per minute (4 breaths in 20 seconds) between and following ET suctioning, using a tidal volume (V_T) of 135% with 100% fraction of oxygen. The first study used 4 breaths/20 seconds before ET suctioning, 8 breaths/40 seconds between each catheter insertion, and 4 breaths/20 seconds following ET suctioning. The manual sigh control was used on the ventilator, which was set at 135% of the V_T and 100% oxygen. The suction procedure consisted of a catheter inserted twice per protocol for 10 seconds per insertion.

The second protocol increased both the number of breaths and the rate to 4 breaths/8 seconds before suctioning, and 30 breaths/60 seconds between each catheter insertion and following suctioning. Physiologic parameters (ICP, airway pressure, electrocardiogram, arterial oxygen saturation [Sao_2], and end-tidal carbon dioxide pressure [$PETco_2$]) were collected 5 minutes prior to, during, and 10 minutes after suctioning.

Key Results

Four basic patterns were seen: (1) an increase from baseline that began with ET suctioning and continuing throughout the sequences, (2) spikes in the ICP during suctioning, (3) a combination of a rise from baseline of the ICP and spiking, and (4) no response in ICP. There were no significant changes in the physiologic parameter during any of the procedures. No significant differences were found between the 4- and the 8-cycle breath protocols. ICP values were significantly lower with the 30-breath cycle protocol.

Study Strengths and Weaknesses

The strength of this study is that it is a well-controlled study. Weaknesses are the limitation of small sample size and that it cannot be generalized to populations other than patients with severe head injury.

Clinical Implications

Hyperoxygenation in combination with short-term hyperventilation with ET suctioning may control increases in ICP during the procedure.

8. Kerr ME, Weber BB, Sereika SM, Wilberger J, Marion, DW. Dose response to cerebrospinal fluid drainage on cerebral perfusion in traumatic brain-injured adults. *Neurosurg Focus*. 2001;11:1–12.

Study Sample

Fifty-eight TBI patients, aged 16 to 65 years, with a GCS score of ≤8, each with a ventriculostomy, participated in this study. Other parameters measured were systemic arterial pressure, CPP, cerebral blood flow velocity (CBFV), and near infrared spectroscopy determined regional cerebral oxygenation (rSo_2). Sjo_2 was measured in 20 patients. The sample is representative of TBI patients.

Comparison Studied

The purpose of the study was to determine if there is a dose response of the ICP when CSF is drained from a ventriculostomy in patients with increased ICP. Secondarily, the impact of CSF drainage on CBFV (surrogate for cerebral blood flow) and cerebral oxygenation was assessed.

Study Procedures

Patients who developed intracranial hypertension of greater than 20 mm Hg were randomly treated by draining 1 mL of CSF (16 drops), 2 mL of CSF (32 drops), and 3 mL (48 drops). A drip counter was placed on the drip chamber to count the number of drops. All data were continuously collected and analyzed by Gould software (Gould Instrument Systems, Inc., Valley View, OH) or with a BioPac (BioPAC Systems, Inc., Goleta, CA) and AcKnowledge software (BioPAC Systems, Inc., Goleta, CA). All monitored physiological variables (ICP, arterial pressure, CPP, CBFV, rSo_2, end-tidal carbon dioxide concentration in expired air [$etCO_2$], and heart rate) were time-averaged and calculated into 11 phases: a 1-minute baseline and minute-

by-minute segment for 10 minutes following CSF drainage (P1–P10). The relationship between the volume of CSF drainage and the time elapsed (1–10 minutes) was analyzed as to its impact on ICP, flow velocity, and oxygenation.

Key Results

There was a relationship between the amount of CSF drained (1, 2, or 3 mL) and the time (1 minute or 10 minutes). One milliliter drainage resulted in a 2.4 mm Hg drop in ICP at 1 minute and 1 mm Hg at 10 minutes after CSF drainage. Two milliliters drainage in CSF produced a drop of 3.4 mm Hg at 1 minute and a 1.7 mm Hg drop in the ICP at 10 minutes. Draining 3 mL of CSF resulted in a 4.5 and 2.4 mm Hg drop in ICP at 1 and 10 minutes, respectively. No significant change was seen in cerebral blood flow or oxygen parameters. No significant ordering effect of treatment was noted.

Study Strengths and Weaknesses

The strength of this study is that the design is easily reproducible. Weaknesses include the lack of generalizabilty to other populations and the limitation of very small volumes of CSF drainage. The amount of CSF drained prior to implementation of the study may have had an impact on the response of the patients.

Clinical Implications

CSF drainage as a method to treat patients with intracranial hypertension is widely used. It has been thought that draining the CSF will not only lower ICP but improve cerebral blood flow and oxygenation. This study demonstrated that even though ICP may decrease transiently, there is no benefit to blood flow and oxygenation.

9. Morgalla M, Mettenleiter H, Katzenberger T. ICP measurement accuracy: the effect of temperature drift. Design of a laboratory test for assessment of ICP transducers. *J Med Eng Technol*. 1999;23:10–14.

Study Sample

Seven Camino (Integra LifeSciences, Plainsboro, NJ), 7 Codman (Johnson & Johnson Raynham, MA), 5 Gaeltec (Novotronic GmbH, Bonn, Germany), 5 Epidyn (Braun Melsungen, Melsungen, Germany), and 7 Rehau (Rehau AG, Rehau, Germany) catheters were tested in a water chamber for drift between 20°C and 45°C.

Comparison Studied

A laboratory test evaluated the impact of temperature drift on 5 different ICP monitors.

Study Procedures

Each probe was tested in a pressure chamber filled with water that underwent 5 consecutive heating or cooling cycles. Four probes were evaluated simultaneously. Pressure was examined at 10 mm Hg increments between 0 and 50 mm Hg.

Key Results

The impact of temperature varied slightly between manufacturers, with Camino catheters being affected most by temperature drift: Camino 0.2 mm Hg/(C); Gaeltec [5] 0.18 mm Hg/(C); Codman, Epidyn, and Rehau <0.15 mm Hg/(C).

Study Strengths and Weaknesses

This is a well-controlled experimental study. The weakness is the small sample size of each probe.

Clinical implications

The accuracy of ICP probes that are zeroed to atmosphere in room air (~22°C) and then placed into a warm head (~36°C–40°C) may be impacted by temperature drift.

10. Morgalla M, Mettenleiter H, Britzer M, Fretschner R, Grote E. ICP measurement control: laboratory test of 7 intracranial transducers. *J Med Eng Technol.* 1999;23:144–151.

Study Sample

Twelve Camino (Integra LifeSciences, Plainsboro, NJ), 7 Codman (Johnson & Johnson Raynham, MA), 7 Gaeltec (Novotronic GmbH, Bonn, Germany), 5 Epidyn (Braun Melsungen, Melsungen, Germany), 10 HanniSet (pvb medizintechnik GmbH, Kirchseeson/Eglharting, Germany), 9 Medex (Medex Medical GmbH, Ratingen, Germany), and 7 Spiegelberg (Spiegelberg, Hamburg, Germany) catheters were evaluated.

Comparison Studied

Seven currently used ICP monitoring devices were evaluated for measurement accuracy, 24-hour drift, and 10-day drift.

Study Procedures

The catheters were placed in a pressure chamber in which the temperature was maintained at a constant 37°C. Hydrostatic pressure changes were made ranging between 0 and 100 mm Hg. Five catheters were tested simultaneously. Absolute measurement accuracy was tested at 5-minute increments between 0 and 80 mm Hg. Twenty-four–hour drift and 10-day drift were measured at 10 mm Hg increments from 0 to 50 mm Hg.

Key Results

Measurement accuracy ranged from 2 to 3 mm Hg for Camino and up to 5 mm Hg for Codman devices; Gaeltec were up to 8 mm Hg low, Epidyn were also too low, HanniSet catheters were 1 to 3 mm Hg off, Medex were 2 to 4 mm Hg off, and Spiegelberg was up to 6 mm Hg off.

Camino catheters had 0.8 mm Hg/24 hr and 0.8 mm Hg average daily drift; Codman catheters had 0.95 mm Hg/24 hr and 0.2 mm Hg average daily drift; Gaeltec catheters had 1.5 mm Hg/24 hr and 1.0 mm Hg average daily drift; Epidyn catheters had 1.2 mm Hg/24 hr and 1.5 mm Hg average daily drift; HanniSet catheters had 0.2 mm Hg/24 hr and 0.8 mm Hg average daily drift; Medex catheters had 1.8 mm Hg/24 hr and 0.35 mm Hg average daily drift; and Spiegelberg catheters had 2.1 mm Hg/24 hr and 0.7 mm Hg average daily drift. Drift also varied between catheters at various pressures.

Study Strengthes and Weaknesses

A strength was the systematic controlled approach to testing all parameters. The weakness is the limited number of individual catheters tested.

Clinical Implications

ICP management depends on obtaining accurate information. Many factors influence accuracy, and it is difficult to assess the accuracy when the catheter is in the patient. This study provides a systematic assessment of simulated information about the accuracy of these 7 catheters. HanniSet, Camino and Codman brands were found to be the most accurate.

OTHER REFERENCES

1. Adelson PD, Bratton SL, Carney NA, et al. Guidelines for the acute medical management of severe traumatic brain injury in infants, children, and adolescents. *Crit Care Med.* 2003;4(Suppl).
2. Anderson RC, Kan P, Kilmo P, Brockmeyer DL, Walker M, Kestle JR. Complications of intracranial pressure monitoring in children with head trauma. *J Neurosurg (Pediatr 1).* 2004;101:53–58.
3. Arabi Y, Memish ZA, Balkhy HH, Francis C, Ferayan A, Al Shimemeri A, Almuneef MA. Ventriculostomy-associated infections: incidence and risk factors. *Am J Infect Control.* 2005;33:137–143.
4. Attia J. Moving beyond sensitivity and specificity: using likelihood ratios to help interpret diagnostic tests. *Aust Prescr* 2003;23:111–113.
5. Bader M, Littlejohns L, Palmer, S. Ventriculostomy and intracranial pressure monitoring: in search of a 0% infection rate. *Heart Lung.* 1995;24:166–172.
6. Bannister K, Chambers I, Siddique M, Fernandes M, Mendelow A. Intracranial pressure and clinical status: assessment of two intracranial pressure transducers. *Physiol Meas.* 2000;21:473–479.
7. Bass NM. Monitoring and treatment of intracranial hypertension. *Liver Transplant.* 2000;6(Suppl 1): S21–S26.
8. Bavetta S, Norris J, Wyatt M, Sutcliffe J, Hamlyn P. Prospective study of zero drift in fiberoptic pressure monitors used in clinical practice. *J Neurosurg.* 1997;86:927–930.

9. Beauchamp TL, Childress JF. *Principles of Biomedical Ethics*, 4th ed. New York: Oxford University Press; 1994.

10. Bland JM, Altman D. Comparing methods of measurement: why plotting difference against standard method is misleading. *Lancet.* 1995;346:1085–1087.

11. Blei A, Olafsson S, Webster S, Levy R. Complications of intracranial pressure monitoring in fulminant hepatic failure. *Lancet.* 1993;8838:157–159.

12. Bochicchio M. Iatronico N, Zappa S, Beindorf A, Candiani A. Bedside burr hole for intracranial pressure monitoring performed by intensive care physicians. A 5-year experience. *Intensive Care Med.* 1996;22:1070–1074.

13. Bruder N, N'Zoghe P, Graziani N, Petissier D, Grisoli F, François G. A comparison of extradural and intraparenchyma intracranial pressures in head injured patients. *Intensive Care Med.* 1995;21:850–852.

14. Bullock R, Chesnut RM, Clifton G, Ghajar J, Marion DW, Narajan RK, et al. Guidelines for the management of severe traumatic brain injury. *J Neurotrauma.* 2000;17:451–553.

15. *Camino Directions for Use* (package insert). Integra NeuroScience, 311 Enterprise Drive, Plainsboro, New Jersey.

16. Chambers I, Kane P, Choksey M, Mendelow A. An evaluation of the Camino ventricular bolt system in clinical practice instrumentation and application. *Neurosurgery.* 1993;33:866–868.

17. Cho D-Y, Chen T-C, Lee H-C. Ultra-early decompressive craniectomy for malignant middle cerebral artery infarction. *Surg Neurol.* 2003;60:227–233.

18. Clark W, Muhlbauer M, Lowrey R, Hartman M, Ray M, Watridge C. Complications of intracranial pressure monitoring in trauma patients. *Neurosurgery.* 1989;25:20–24.

19. *Codman Directions for Use* (package insert). Johnson & Johnson, 325 Paramount Drive, Raynham, Massachusetts.

20. Cremer OL, van Dijk GW, van Wensen E, et al. Effect of intracranial pressure monitoring and targeted intensive care on functional outcome after severe head injury. *Crit Care Med.* 2005;33:2207–2213.

21. Crutchfield J, Narayan R, Robertson C, Michael L. Evaluation of a fiberoptic intracranial pressure monitor. *J Neurosurg.* 1990;72:482–487.

22. D'Ambrosio A, Hoh D, Mack W, Winfee CJ, Fair MN. Interhemisoheric intracranial pressure gradients in nonhuman primate strokes. *Surg Neurol.* 2002;58:295–301.

23. Darovic, G, Zbilut, J. Fluid-filled monitoring systems: types of monitoring systems. In Darovic G (ed). *Hemodynamic Monitoring: Invasive and Noninvasive Clinical Application.* Philadelphia: Saunders; 2002;111–131.

24. Dextran Transducers. Utah Medical Products, Ltd., 7043 South 300 West, Midvale, Utah.

25. Di Rocco C, Tamburrini G, Caldarelli M, Velardi F, Santini P. Prolonged ICP monitoring in Sylvian arachnoid cysts. *Surg Neurol.* 2003;60:211–218.

26. Fan JY. Effect of backrest position on intracranial pressure and cerebral perfusion pressure in individuals with brain injury: a systematic review. *J Neurosci Nurs.* 2004;36;278–288.

27. Fernandes H, Bingham K, Chambers I, Mendelow A. Clinical evaluation of the Codman Microsensor intracranial pressure monitoring system. *Acta Neurochir.* 1998;71:44–46.

28. Fortune J, Feustel P, Graca L, Hasselbarth J, Kuehler D. Effect of hyperventilation, Mannitol, and ventriculostomy drainage on cerebral blood flow after head injury. *J Trauma.* 1995;39:1091–1099.

29. Fouyas IP, Casey ATH, Thompson D, Harkness WF, Hayward RD. Use of intracranial pressure monitoring in the management of childhood hydrocephalus and shunt-related problems. *Neurosurgery.* 1996;726–732.

30. Friedman W, Vries J. Percutaneous tunnel ventriculostomy. *J Neurosurg.* 1980;53:662–665.

31. Gambardella G, d'Avella D, Tomasello F. Monitoring of brain tissue pressure with a fiberoptic device. *Neurosurgery.* 1992;31:918–922.

32. Gardner R. Accuracy and reliability of disposable pressure transducers coupled with modern pressure monitors. *Crit Care Med.* 1996;24:879–882

33. Gelabert-Gonzalez M, Ginesta-Galan V, Sernamito-Garcia R, Allut AG, Bandin-Diéguez J, Rumbo RM. The Camino intracranial pressure device in clinical practice. Assessment in 1000 cases. *Acta Neurochir (Wien).* 2006;148:435–441.

34. Gopinath S, Cherian L, Robertson C, Narayan RK, Grossman RG. Evaluation of a microsensor intracranial pressure transducer. *J Neurosci Methods.* 1993;49:11–15.

35. Grande P-O, Myhre EB, Nordstrom C-H, Schliamser. Treatment of intracranial hypertension and aspects on lumbar dural puncture in severe bacterial meningitis. *Acta Anaesthesiol Scand.* 2002;46:264–270.

36. Guidelines for the Management and Prognosis of Severe Traumatic Brain Injury. Brain Trauma Foundation. Available at: http://www2.braintrauma.org/guidelines. Accessed August 6, 2007.

37. Guyot L, Dowling C, Diaz F, Michael D. Cerebral monitoring devices: analysis of complications. *Acta Neurochir.* 1998;71(Suppl):47–49.

38. Hacke W, Stingele R, Steiner T, Schuchardt V, Schwab S. Critical care of acute ischemic stroke. *Intensive Care Med.* 1995;21:856–862.

39. Harris CH, Smith RS, Helmet SD, Gerick JP, Rody, RB. Placement of intracranial pressure monitors by non-neurosurgeons. *Am Surg.* 2002;68:787–790.

40. Heuer G, Smith M, Elliott J, Winn HR, Le Roux PD. Relationship between intracranial pressure and other clinical variables in patients with aneurysmal subarachnoid hemorrhage. *J Neurosurg.* 2004;101:408–416.

41. Holloway K, Barnes T, Choi S, Bullock R, Marshall LF, et al. Ventriculostomy infections: the effect of monitoring duration and catheter exchange in 584 patients. *J Neurosurg.* 1996;85:419–424.

42. Holzschuch M, Woertgen C, Metz C, Brawanshi A. Clinical evaluation of InnerSpace fiberoptic intracranial pressure monitoring device. *Brain Injury.* 2000;12:191–198.

43. Jenson R, Hahn Y, Ciro E. Risk factors of intracranial pressure monitoring in children with fiberoptic devices: a critical review. *Surg Neurol.* 1997;47:16–22.

44. Jones EA, Weissenborn K. Neurology and the liver. *J Neurol Neurosurg Psychiatry.* 1997;63:279–293.

45. Kerr ME, Marion D, Sereika S, Weber B, Orndoff P, Henker R, Wilberger J. The effects of cerebrospinal fluid drainage on cerebral perfusion in traumatic brain-injured adults. *J Neurosurg Anesth.* 2000;12:324–333.

46. Khan S, Kureshi IU, Mulgrew T, Ho SY, Onyiuke HC. Comparison of percutaneous ventriculostomies and intraparenchymal monitor: a retrospective evaluation of 156 patients. *Acta Neurochir.* 1998;71(Suppl):50–52.

47. Khanna R., Rosenblum M, Rock J, Malik G. Prolonged external ventricular drainage with percutaneous long-tunnel ventriculostomies. *J Neurosurg.* 1995;83:791–794.

48. Kim D, Uttley D, Bell B, Marsh HT, Moore AJ. Comparison of rates of infection of two methods of emergency ventricular drainage. *J Neurol Neurosurg Psychiatr.* 1995;58:444–446.

49. Kirkness CJ, Mitchell PH, Burr RL, March KS, Newell DW. Intracranial pressure waveform analysis: clinical and research implications. *J Neurosci Nurs.* 2000;32:271–277.

50. Kirkness C, March K. Intracranial pressure management (chapt 9; Mitchell P, section ed). In Bader MK, Littlejohns L (eds). *AANN Core Curriculum for Neuroscience Nursing.* St Louis, MO: Saunders; 2004.

51. Ko K, Conforti A. Training protocol for intracranial pressure monitor placement by non-neurosurgeons: 5-year experience. *J Trauma.* 2003;55:480–484.

52. Lane PL, Skoretz TG, Doig G, Girotti MJ. Intracranial pressure monitoring and outcomes after traumatic brain injury. *Can J Surg.* 2000;43:442–448.

53. Lang J, Beck J, Zimmerman M, Seifert V, Raabe A. Clinical evaluation of intraparenchymal Spiegelberg pressure sensor. *Neurosurgery.* 2003;52:1455–1459.

54. Larsen FS, Ranek L, Hansen BA. Pitfalls in intracranial pressure monitoring in fulminant hepatic failure. *J Hepatol.* 1997;26:451–452 (letter to editor).

55. Lieberman D, Matz P, Rosegay H. History of the strain gauge in measurement of the intracranial pressure: from engineers to physiologists and clinicians. *J Trauma.* 2002;52:172–178.

56. Lundberg N. Continuous recording and control of ventricular fluid pressure in neurosurgical practice. *Acta Psychiatr Neurol Scand.* 1960;36(Suppl 149):1–193.

57. Lyke K, Obasanjo O, Williams M, O'Brien M, Chotani R, Perl T. Ventriculitis complicating use of intraventricular catheters in adult neurosurgical patients. *Clin Infect Dis.* 2001;33:2028–2033.

58. Mack WJ, King RG, Ducruet AF, Kreiter K, Mocco J, Magjoub A, Mayer S, Connoly ES Jr. Intracranial pressure following aneurismal subarachnoid hemorrhage: monitoring practices and outcome data. *Neurosurg Focus.* 2003;14:1–5.

59. March K, Arbour R, Wellwood J. Technology (chapt 7; March K, section ed). In Bader MK, Littlejohns L (eds). *AANN Core Curriculum for Neuroscience Nursing.* St Louis, MO: Saunders; 2004.

60. March K, Wellwood J. Intracranial pressure concepts and cerebral blood flow (chapt 3; March K, section ed). In Bader MK, Littlejohns L (eds). *AANN Core Curriculum for Neuroscience Nursing.* St Louis, MO: Saunders; 2004.

61. Martínez-Mañas R, Santamarta D, de Campos J, Ferrer E. Camino intracranial pressure monitor: prospective study of accuracy and complications *J Neurol Neurosurg Psychiatr.* 2000;69:82–86.

62. Mayhall C, Archer N, Lamb A, Spadora AC, Baggett JW, Ward JD, Narayan RK. Ventriculostomy-related infections. *N Engl J Med.* 1984;310:553–559.

63. Miller MT, Pasquale M, Kurek S, White J, Martin, P, Bannon K, Wasser T, Li M. Initial head computed tomographic scan characteristics have a linear relationship with initial intracranial pressure after trauma. *J Trauma.* 2004;56:967–973.

64. Miller J, Hunt B, Kappa J. Inaccurate pressure readings for subarachnoid bolts. *Neurosurgery.* 1986;19:253–255.

65. MLT0670 Disposable BP Transducer (sterile) ADInstruments Transducers. Available at: http://www.ADInstruments.com. Accessed August 6, 2007.

66. Munch E, Weigel R, Schmiedek P, Schurer L. The Camino intracranial pressure device in clinical practice: reliability, handling characteristics and complications. *Acta Neurochir.* 1998;140:1113–1119.

67. Murthy JMK. Management of intracranial pressure in tuberculous meningitis. *Neurocrit Care.* 2005;2:306–312.

68. Narayan R, Bray R, Robertson C, et al. Experience with new fiberoptic devices for intracranial pressure monitoring. Abstract presented at American Association of Neurological Surgeons, May 3–7, 1987, Dallas, Texas.

69. *Neurovent (Rehau) Directions for Use.* Rehau Company, Ytterbium 4 91058, Erlangen-Eltersdorf, Germany.

70. Ng I, Lim J, Wong HB. Effects of head posture on cerebral hemodynamics: its influences on intracranial pressure, cerebral perfusion pressure, and cerebral oxygenation. *Neurosurgery*. 2004;54:593–597.

71. North B. Intracranial pressure monitoring (chapt 10). In Reilly P, Bullock R (eds). *Head Injury*, 2nd ed. London, UK: Hodder Arnold; 2005.

72. Odetola F, Bratton S. Characteristics and immediate outcome of childhood meningitis treated in the pediatrixc intensive care unit. *Intensive Care Med*. 2005;31:92–97.

73. Odetola O, Tilford J, Davis M. Variation in the use of intracranial monitoring and mortality in critically ill children with meningitis in the United States. *Pediatrics*. 2006;117:1893–1900.

74. Paramore CG, Turner DA. Relative risks of ventriculostomy infection and morbidity. *Acta Neurochir (Wien)*. 1994;127:79–84.

75. Park, P, Garton, H, Kocan, M, Thompson, B. Risk of infection with prolonged ventricular catheterization. *Neurosurgery*. 2004;55:594–601.

76. Piper I, Barnes A, Smith D, Dunn L. The Camino intracranial pressure sensor: is it optimal technology? An internal audit with a review of current intracranial pressure monitoring technologies. *Neurosurgery*. 2001;49:1158–1165.

77. Poca MA, Sahuquillo J, Barba MA, Anez JD, Arikan F. Prospective study of methodological issues in intracranial pressure monitoring in patients with hydrocephalus. *J Neurosurg*. 2004;100:260–265.

78. Poca M, Sahuquillo J, Arribas M, Báguena M, Amorós M, Rubio E. Fiberoptic intraparenchymal brain pressure monitoring with the Camino V420 Monitor: reflections on our experience in 163 severely head-injured patients. *J Neurotrauma*. 2002;19:439–448.

79. Poon W, Ng S, Wai S. CSF antibiotic prophylaxis for neurosurgical patients' ventriculostomy: a randomized study. *Acta Neurochir Suppl*. 1998;71:146–148.

80. Pople I, Muhlbauer M, Sanford R, Kirk E. Results and complications of intracranial pressure monitoring in 303 children. *Pediatr Neurosurg*. 1995;23:64–67.

81. Prabhu V, Kaufman H, Voelker J, Aronoff SC, Niewiadomska-Buqaj M, Hobbs GR. Prophylactic antibiotics with intracranial pressure monitors and external ventricular drains: a review of the evidence. *Surg Neurol*.1999;52:226–237.

82. Rebuck J, Murry K, Rhoney D, Michael D, Coplin W. Infection related to intracranial pressure monitors in adults: analysis of risk factors and antibiotic prophylaxis. *J Neurol Neurosurg Psychiatry*. 2000;69:381–384.

83. Rice W, Fernandez E, Jarog D, Jensen A. A comparison of hydrostatic leveling methods in invasive pressure monitoring. *Crit Care Nurse*. 2000;20:20–30.

84. Richardson D, Bellamy M. Intracranial hypertension in acute liver failure. *Nephrol Dial Transplant*. 2002;17:23–27.

85. Rossi S, Buzzi F, Paparella A, Mainini P, Stocchetti N. Complications and safety associated with ICP monitoring: a study of 542 patients. *Acta Neurochir*. 1998;71(Suppl 71):91–93.

86. Ruchholtz S, Waydhas C, Müller A, et al. Percutaneous computer tomographic-controlled ventriculostomy in severe traumatic brain injury. *J Trauma*. 1998;45:505–511.

87. Sahuquillo J, Poca M, Arribas M, Garnacho A, Rubio E. Interhemispheric supratentorial intracranial pressure gradients in head-injured patients: are they clinically important? *J Neurosurg*. 1999;90:16–26.

88. Saunders R, Lyons T. External ventricular drainage. *Crit Care Med*. 1979;7:556–558.

89. Schickner D, Young R. Intracranial pressure monitoring: fiberoptic monitor compared with the ventricular catheter. *Surg Neurol*. 1992;37:251–254.

90. Schultz M, Moore K, Foote A. Bacterial ventriculitis and duration of ventriculostomy catheter insertion. *J Neuroscience Nurs*. 1993;23:158–164.

91. Schurer L, Munch E, Piepgras A. Assessment of the Camino intracranial pressure device in clinical practice. *Acta Neurochir*. 1997;296–298.

92. Schwab S, Aschoff A, Spranger M, Albert F, Hacke W. The value of intracranial pressure monitoring in acute hemispheric stroke. *Neurology*. 1996;47:393–398.

93. Schwarz S, Georagiadis D, Aschoff A, Schwab A. Effects of body position on intracranial pressure and cerebral perfusion in patients with large hemispheric stroke. *Stroke*. 2002:33:497–501.

94. Shapiro S, Bowman R, Callahan J, Wolfa C. The fiberoptic intraparenchymal cerebral pressure monitor in 244 patients. *Surg Neurol*. 1996;45:278–282.

95. Sie MY, Toh KW, Rajeev K. Cerebral fat embolism: an indication for ICP monitor? *J Trauma*. 2003; 55:1185–1186 (letter to editor).

96. Signorini D, Shad A, Piper I, Statham P. A clinical evaluation of the Codman Microsensor for intracranial pressure monitoring. *Br J Neurosurg*. 1998;12:223–227.

97. Slavin K, Misra M. Infratentorial intracranial pressure monitoring in neurosurgical intensive care unit. *Neurol Res*. 2003;25:880–884.

98. Stahl N, Ungerstedt U, Nordstrom C-H. Brain energy metabolism during controlled reduction of cerebral perfusion pressure in severe head injuries. *Intensive Care Med*. 2001;27:1215–1223.

99. Stangl A, Meyer B, Zentner J, Schramm J. Continuous external CSF drainage—a perpetual problem in neurosurgery. *Surg Neurol*. 1998;50:77–82.

100. Stenager E, Gerner-Smidt P, Kock-Jensen C. Ventriculostomy-related infections—an epidemiological study. *Acta Neurochir*. 1986;83:20–23.

101. Taylor W, Todd N, Leighton S. CSF drainage in patients with posterior fossa tumours. *Acta Neurochir.* 1992;117:1–6.

102. Tofteng F, Jorgensen L, Hansen B, Ott P, Kondrup J, Larsen F. Cerebral microdialysis in patients with fulminant hepatic failure. *Hepatology.* 2002;36:1333–1340.

103. Tofteng F, Larsen F. The effect of indomethacin on intracranial pressure, cerebral perfusion and extracellular lactate and glutamate concentrations in patients with fulminant hepatic failure. *J Cereb Blood Flow Metab.* 2004;24:798–804.

104. Transducers for hemodynamic measurements. Hugo Sachs Electronik-Harvard Apparatus GmbH, Hugstetten, Germany. Available at: http://www.hugo-sachs.de/transd~1/bp_trans.htm. Accessed August 6, 2007.

105. U.S. Department of Occupational Safety and Health Administration, Regulations (Standards—29 CRF) Bloodborne Pathogens 1910.1030. Available at: http://www.osha.gov/pls/oshaweb/owadisp.show_document?p_table=STANDARDS&p_id=10051. Accessed September 17, 2007.

106. Valentin A, Lang T, Karnik R, Ammerer H, Ploder J, Slany J. Intracranial pressure monitoring and case mix-adjusted mortality in intracranial hemorrhage. *Crit Care Med.* 2003;31:1539–1542.

107. Vaquero J, Fontana RJ, Larson AM, et al. Complications and use of intracranial pressure monitoring in patients with acute liver failure and severe encephalopathy. *Liver Transplant.* 2005;11:1581–1589.

108. *Ventrix Directions for Use* (package insert). Integra NeuroScience, 311 Enterprise Drive, Plainsboro, New Jersey.

109. Walter, H, Steinbok, P. The value of routine cultures in the cerebrospinal fluid in patients with external ventricular drains. *Neurosurgery.*2000;46:1149–1155.

110. Weinstabl C, Richling B, Plainer B, Czech T, Spiss C. Comparative analysis between epidural (Gaeltec) and subdural (Camino) intracranial pressure probes. *J Clin Monitor.* 1992;8:116–120.

111. Winfield J, Rosenthal P, Kanter R, Casella G. Duration of intracranial pressure monitoring does not predict daily risk of infectious complications clinical study. *Neurosurgery.* 1993;33:424–431.

112. Winkelman C. Effect of backrest position on intracranial and cerebral perfusion pressures in traumatically brain-injured adults. *Am J Crit Care.* 2000;9:373–380.

113. Winkler F, Kastenbauer S, Yousry TA, Maerz U, Pfister H-W. Discrepancies between brain CT imaging and severely raised intracrnail pressure proven by ventriculostomy in adults with pneumococcal meningitis. *J Neurol.* 2002;249:1292–1297.

114. Wolfa C, Luerssen T, Bowman R, Putty T. Brain tissue pressure gradients created by expanding frontal epidural mass lesion. *J Neurosurg.* 1996;84:642–647.

115. Yablon J, Lantner H, McCormack T, Nair S, Barker E, Black P. Clinical experience with a fiberooptic intracranial pressure monitor. *J Clin Monitor.* 1993;9:171–175.

116. Young JS, Blow O, Turrentine F, Claridge JA, Schulman A. Is there an upper limit of intracranial pressure in patients with severe head injury if cerebral perfusion pressure is maintained? *Neurosurg Focus.* 2003;15:E2.

117. Zhong J, Dujovny M, Park HK, Perez E, Perlin AR, Diaz FG. Advances in ICP monitoring techniques. *Neurol Res.* 2003;25:339–350.

118. Zingale A, Ippolito S, Pappalardo P, Chibbaro S, Amoroso R. Infections and re-infections in long-term external ventricular drainage. *J Neurosurg Sci.* 1999;43:125–133.

119. Naff N, Carhuapoma J, Williams M, et al. Intraventricular hemorrhage with urokinase: effects on 30-day survival. *Stroke.* 2000;31:841–847.

Cerebrospinal Drainage Systems: External Ventricular and Lumbar Drains

Barbara Leeper, RN, MN, CCRN
and Darlene Lovasik, RN, MN, CCRN, CNRN

EXTERNAL VENTRICULAR DRAINS

CASE STUDY

Mrs J. is a 57-year-old woman transferred from an outlying hospital with a diagnosis of subarachnoid hemorrhage. She has a history of mild hypertension and had been in her usual state of health until she was lifting large rocks to use as a border for her garden. She complained to her daughter of a sudden, severe headache, "the worst headache I've ever had," followed by projectile vomiting and then a loss of consciousness. She was taken by ambulance to her local hospital where a computed tomography (CT) scan revealed a right-sided subarachnoid hemorrhage. Mrs J. was transferred to the university teaching hospital for further treatment. Upon arrival, she was drowsy, but awakened to peripheral stimuli (pressure applied to her trapezius muscle to elicit a response in an unresponsive patient). She was oriented to name only. She described a severe headache, nausea, and sensitivity to light. Her pupils were equal and reactive to light. She had a left facial weakness and 2/5 strength in her left arm and leg. Physician examination also revealed nuchal rigidity. She went for a magnetic resonance image (MRI) and magnetic resonance angiogram (MRA) that confirmed the presence of a subarachnoid hemorrhage with a probable rupture of a right middle cerebral artery (MCA) aneurysm. A ventriculostomy catheter was inserted without difficulty by the neurosurgeon in the emergency department, and it was connected to an external ventricular drainage (EVD) system and intracranial pressure (ICP) monitor via a fluid-coupled system. The initial ICP was 18 mm Hg (normal range is 0–10 mm Hg, although 15 is considered the upper limit of normal). The cerebrospinal fluid (CSF) was bright red and drained rapidly into the CSF collection bag. With a mean arterial pressure (MAP) of 104, her cerebral perfusion pressure (CPP) registered 86 mm Hg (normal range is 60–100 mm Hg). An angiogram was performed that confirmed the presence of a right MCA aneurysm and she was taken urgently to the operating room for surgical clipping of aneurysm.

Immediately following surgery, Mrs J. was admitted to the neuroscience intensive care unit (ICU). She was on a ventilator, had an EVD and ICP monitor, and was on a neosynephrine drip to maintain her systolic blood pressure above 160 mm Hg. She was arousable and obeyed commands slowly. Pupils were equal and reactive to light, and she had a left facial weakness with 3/5 strength in her left arm and leg. The EVD was open to drain with ICP measured hourly. The ICP ranged from 13 to 18 mm Hg, with CPP between 82 and 94 mm Hg. She was ordered hypervolemic, hypertensive, and hemodilution (triple H) therapy and magnesium intravenously (IV) to prevent vasospasm. She remained on the ventilator for the first 14 hours after surgery and was extubated without difficulty. On her third postoperative day, she became more difficult to arouse and did not follow commands, and her left-sided weakness progressed to 1/5. An angiogram confirmed mild vasospasm and the neosynephrine was increased to maintain her systolic blood pressure above 180 mm Hg. Serial transcutaneous cerebral Doppler sonographies (TCD) were performed daily and her neurologic function improved. On postoperative day 8, the EVD was clamped and then removed on day 9. She was transferred to the neuro intermediate unit for 3 days and then to the neuro floor for 4 days. On postoperative day 18, she was moved to a rehabilitation facility for physical and occupational therapy.

On her return to the clinic for her 8-week evaluation, she had little recall of her hospital stay, was oriented times 3, and had a mild left facial weakness. Muscle strength in her left arm and leg was 4/5, and she walked with the assistance of a walker. She was able to feed herself and performed her activities of daily living with some assistance.

GENERAL DESCRIPTION

Long before the advent of ICP monitoring, trephination was performed to relieve increasing pressure inside the skull. ICP monitoring is the cornerstone of neurosurgical critical care and is recognized as the most significant factor in determining the outcome for many neurologic events. Ventriculostomy remains the "gold standard" of ICP monitoring for accuracy of ICP monitoring and the ability to drain CSF.[1-4] In some situations, such as meningitis, medication also can be instilled through the ventriculostomy catheter. At this time, it is also the least expensive system.

The procedure can be performed in the emergency department, ICU, or operating room. Before inserting the catheter, laboratory results, including a coagulation profile, must be reviewed. The site, anterior to the coronal suture at the level of the mid-pupillary line, is shaved, prepped, and draped, and a local anesthetic is injected. Using sterile technique, the catheter is placed in the anterior horn of a lateral ventricle, usually in the nondominant hemisphere, but this option may be limited due to the location of the neurologic incident. The neurosurgeon (or other credentialed practitioner) makes an incision down to the skull and then uses a small twist drill to create a burr hole. The dura is opened and the catheter is inserted through a burr hole, using anatomic landmarks anterior to the coronal suture, 3 to 4 cm from midline. When the ventricle is reached, CSF will usually flow freely. The catheter may be tunneled through the scalp via a separate incision to help secure it. Some practitioners believe that this technique may decrease the risk of infection, although this has not been confirmed through research. The dressing is applied, which may be an occlusive clear dressing, gauze pads with tape, or a full craniotomy dressing per the unit or institutional policy. If a fluid-coupled system is used, the tubing must be primed with nonbacteriostatic (without preservative) saline. After priming the tubing, the flush bag or syringe must be removed to prevent inadvertent administration of saline through the catheter into the ventricle. Some newer, hybrid (fiberoptic or microchip) catheters have a pressure sensor at the tip of the catheter and must be zeroed to atmosphere prior to insertion. This type of catheter is never rezeroed after it is inserted. The catheter is then attached to an EVD system and generally also connected to an ICP monitoring system, either a fluid-coupled system with a flushless transducer or via a hybrid catheter with a microchip or fiberoptic transducer. The tranducer is leveled at the foramen of Monro following the reference points of the external auditory meatus, midpoint of a line joining the two external auditory meatuses or 2 cm above the pterion. After attaching the tubing to the ICP system, it is calibrated to zero. Zero balancing includes opening the transducer to air, recalibrating with the monitor, then closing the system (refer to unit or institution policy and manufacturer's instructions). The waveform is assessed, and ICP and CPP (MAP – ICP = CPP) are noted (refer to ICP section in this chapter). The color and volume of the CSF are also documented.[3,4]

The patient must be carefully monitored for complications of EVD. There is a risk of hemorrhage from the process of inserting the catheter. The drainage of CSF may become obstructed from brain tissue or a blood clot in the catheter. Excessive drainage from an EVD can occur when the drainage bag is inadvertently dropped below the prescribed level or onto the floor. If a large amount of CSF drains quickly, it can cause the ventricles to collapse, increasing negative pressure within the skull, and tearing the blood vessels in the dura. This will cause hemorrhage, increase ICP, and result in herniation and death in a very short time span. Ventriculostomy-related infections are reported to be between 5% and 10%, but there is not clear consensus on treatment practices to decrease or prevent infection.[5-21] The duration of catheter placement is correlated with an increased risk of CSF infection during the first 10 days post-procedure.[6,8,9,11,12] Prophylactic antibiotics and/or catheters that have been impregnated with antibiotics do not appear to change the infection rate.[5,6,10-13,16,19,21] CSF specimen collection remains controversial; although specimen collection provides useful information, it requires that the system be broached and may increase the risk of infection.[8,12,18]

ACCURACY

As previously mentioned, ventriculostomy continues to be the "gold standard" for accuracy in ICP monitoring. There are some mechanical situations that may affect the precision of the reading. First, the EVD must be leveled correctly at the foramen of Monro. When the collection system is set at the prescribed point and the ICP surpasses the established level, it will flow into the collection system. Look for kinks in the system, especially around the catheter connection. Air bubbles in the system will actually decrease the flow of CSF and trigger a dampened waveform. The air can be removed following unit or institutional practices and manufacturer's recommendations. The air vent on the drip chamber must remain dry; if it becomes wet, some systems require that the entire system must be changed while other systems have a hydrophilic system. The catheter may be blocked by brain tissue or a blood clot at the end of the catheter. Notify the physician if the system is not functioning properly as evidenced by either a lack of drainage or a lack of or dampened waveform.

COMPETENCY

Effective and safe use of a ventriculostomy catheter and EVD system requires:

- Knowledge of the ventricular system of the brain.
- Expertise in working with the ventriculostomy catheter and EVD system.
- Understanding of the unit or institutional policies and practices related to a ventriculostomy catheter and EVD.
- Familiarity with the equipment and supplies that are used to insert the catheter and maintain the system.
- Awareness of the complications of and potential hazards to the patient with an EVD.

FUTURE RESEARCH

There are multiple opportunities for research related to ventriculostomies and EVD systems. Many of the studies in the current literature are retrospective and may be confounded by other variables that impact the study.

A few suggested topics for future research include:

- Is there value in collecting routine cultures of the CSF in patients with external ventricular drains?
- Obtaining a specimen requires a break in the system that may place the patient at risk for an infection. Do the cultures identify the infection before clinical signs appear?
- Should specimens be drawn based on clinical signs only?
- Is it safe to give heparin to a patient with an intraventricular catheter? What is the safe dose/range for these critically ill patients?
- Should CSF drainage be continuous or intermittent? Are there preferred methods based on the diagnosis? Do other, subtle changes exist that may be a result of the method of drainage?
- The time limit for EVDs remains controversial, although several reports have shown that there is no advantage to changing the catheter at 5-day intervals. Further study of the EVD duration would be useful.
- Which type of dressing (over the catheter) is the safest for the patient?
- When is the best time to insert the EVD?

REFERENCES

1. Recommendations for intracranial pressure monitoring technology. In Bullock R, Chesnut RM, Clifton G, et al. *Management and Prognosis of Severe Traumatic Brain Injury.* New York: Brain Trauma Foundation and American Association of Neurological Surgeons; 2000.
2. Littlejohns LR, Bader MK. Guidelines for the management of severe head injury: Clinical application and changes in practice. *Crit Care Nurse.* 2001;21:48–65.
3. American Association of Neuroscience Nurses. *Guide to the Care of the Patient with Intracranial Pressure Monitoring.* Chicago: AANN; 2005.
4. March K. Technology. In Bader MK, Littlejohns LR. *AANN Core Curriculum for Neuroscience Nursing,* 4th ed. Philadelphia, PA: WB Saunders; 2004:199–227.
5. Alleyne CH Jr, Hassan M, Zabranski JM. The efficacy and cost of prophylactic and periprocedural antibiotics in patients with external ventricular drains. *Neurosurgery.* 2000;47:1124–1129.
6. Bader MK, Littlejohns L, Palmer S. Ventriculostomy and intracranial pressure monitoring: in search of a 0% infection rate. *Heart Lung.* 1995;24:166–172.
7. Coplin WM, Avellino AM, Kim DK, Winn HR, Grady MS. Bacterial meningitis associated with lumbar drains: a retrospective cohort study. *J Neurol Neurosurg Psychiatry.* 1999;67:468–473.
8. Holloway KL, Barnes T, Choi S, et al. Ventriculostomy infection: the effect of monitoring duration and catheter exchange in 584 patients. *J Neurosurg.* 1996;85:419–424.
9. Infection in Neurosurgery Working Party of the British Society for AntiMicrobial Chemotherapy. The management of neurosurgical patients with postoperative bacterial or aseptic meningitis or external ventricular drain-associated ventriculitis. *Br J Neurosurg.* 2000;14:–12.
10. Kaufman AM, Lye T, Redekop G, et al. Infection rates in standard vs. hydrogel coated ventricular catheters. *Can J Neurol Sci.* 2004;31:506–510.
11. Korinek AM, Reina M, Boch AL, et al. Prevention of external ventricular drain-related ventriculitis. *Acta Neurochir.* 2005;147:39–46.
12. Lozier AP, Sciacca RR, Romagnoli MF, Connolly ES Jr. Ventriculostomy-related infections: a critical review of the literature. *Neurosurgery.* 2002;51:170–182.
13. Lyke KE, Obasanjo OO, Williams MA, et al. Ventriculitis complicating use of intraventricular catheters in adult neurosurgical patients. *Clin Infect Dis.* 2001;33:2028–2033.
14. Paramore CG, Turner DA. Relative risks of ventriculostomy infection and morbidity. *Acta Neurochir.* 1994;127:79–84.
15. Pfisterer W, Muhlbauer M, Czech R, Reinprecht A. Early diagnosis of external ventricular drainage infection: results of a prospective study. *J Neurol Neurosurg Psychiatry.* 2003;74:929–932.
16. Rebuck JA, Murry KR, Rhoney DH, Michael DB, Coplin WM. Infection related to intracranial pressure in adults; analysis of risk factors and antibiotic prophylaxis. *J Neurol Neurosurg Psychiatry.* 2000;69:381–384.
17. Sandalcioglu IE, Stolke D. Failure of regular external ventricular drain exchange to reduce cerebrospinal

fluid infection: result of a randomized controlled trial. (letter) *J Neurol Neurosurg Psychiatry.* 2003;74:1598–1599.

18. Schade RP, Schinkel J, Roelandse RWC, et al. Lack of value of routine analysis of cerebrospinal fluid for prediction and diagnosis of external drainage-related bacterial meningitis. *J Neurosurg.* 2006;104:101–108.

19. Sloffer CA, Augspurger L, Wagenbach A, Lanzino G. Antimicrobial-impregnated external ventricular catheters: does the very low infection rate observed in clinical trials apply to daily clinical practice? *Neurosurgery.* 2005;56:1041–1044.

20. Wong GKC, Poon WS, Wai S, et al. Failure of regular external ventricular drain exchange to reduce cerebrospinal fluid infection: result of a randomized controlled trial. *J Neurol Neurosurg Psychiatry.* 2002;73:759–761.

21. Zabramski JM, Whiting D, Darouiche RO, et al. Efficacy of antimicrobial-impregnated external ventricular drain catheters: a prospective, randomized, controlled trial. *J Neurosurg.* 2003;98:725–730.

CLINICAL RECOMMENDATIONS FOR EXTERNAL VENTRICULAR DRAINS

The rating scale for the Level of Recommendation ranges from I to VI, with levels indicated as follows: I, manufacturer's recommendations only; II, theory based, no research data to support recommendations; recommendations from expert consensus group may exist; III, laboratory data only, no clinical data to support recommendations; IV, limited clinical studies to support recommendations; V, clinical studies in more than 1 or 2 different populations and situations to support recommendations; VI, clinical studies in a variety of patient populations and situations to support recommendations.

Period of Use	Recommendation	Rationale for Recommendation	Level of Recommendation	Supporting References	Comments
Patient Selection	EVD is recommended in the following circumstances:				
	Acute hydrocephalus: communicating or noncommunicating.	Acute hydrocephalus is a life-threatening situation that must be treated urgently. Communicating hydrocephalus occurs when the pathways between the ventricles are open and CSF is produced at the normal rate of 18–25 mL/hour, but the CSF cannot be absorbed by the arachnoid villi because they are plugged by blood components or exudate. Noncommunicating hydrocephalus is caused by an obstruction in CSF flow in the brain or spinal cord. An EVD is placed in patients with acute communicating and noncommunicating hydrocephalus.	VI	See Other References: 1–5	Hydrocephalus is a progressive dilation of the ventricles that can be caused by overproduction of CSF or abnormalities in CSF flow or reabsorption. An EVD will treat acute hydrocephalus; however, a ventriculoperitoneal shunt may be required if normal function does not return, fibrotic scarring damages the arachnoid villi, or, for chronic hydrocephalus.
	Subarachnoid hemorrhage, usually due to the rupture of a cerebral aneurysm. The blood spreads through the Sylvian fissures into the basal cisterns. The blood irritates the brain tissues and meninges, raises ICP, and lowers the CPP. The blood may also enter the ventricles, leading to intraventricular hemorrhage (IVH). The symptoms are dependant on the location of the hemorrhage and the resulting ICP.	Following a subarachnoid hemorrhage from a cerebral aneurysm, blood is released into the subarachnoid space and causes an immediate rise in ICP. The patient is also at risk for developing acute hydrocephalus due to obstruction of CSF flow by a blood clot (communicating hydrocephalus; see Other Reference List: 9). The blood components, including red blood cells, white blood cells, and other blood factors, also will cause noncommunicating hydrocephalus when they plug the arachnoid villi and prevent the reabsorption of CSF. An EVD is placed in those patients with a Hunt-Hess grade of 3 or greater to treat increased ICP and acute communicating hydrocephalus.	VI	See Other References: 6–13	The EVD may be placed preoperatively in the emergency department or ICU by a neurosurgeon (or their designee) or during emergent surgery. The duration is dependent on the patient status and return to normal CSF reabsorption through the arachnoid villi, but usually remains between 5 and 10 days.

Period of Use	Recommendation	Rationale for Recommendation	Level of Recommendation	Supporting References	Comments
Patient Selection *(cont.)*	Intracerebral hemorrhage, also known as a hemorrhagic stroke, represents 15% of all strokes and is the result of a rupture of a blood vessel. The patient profile is of a patient with a history of poorly controlled hypertension. The symptoms are dependent on the location of the hemorrhage and the resulting ICP.	The blood mass causes an increase in ICP, physical distortion of the brain, cerebral edema, compromised CPP, and the potential for herniation.	VI	See References: 3, 4 See Other References: 14	Most occur in the basal ganglia or thalamus. A major intracerebral hemorrhage can lead to herniation and death within hours of rupture. Surgery with removal of the blood mass and/or brain tissue may be considered.
	Traumatic brain injury is a broad category that includes contusions, lacerations, epidural hematoma, subdural hematoma, intracerebral hemorrhage, diffuse axonal injury, and penetrating injuries caused by gunshot wounds, stabbing, or impalements. The degree of damage is related to both the primary injury (contact and brain movement) and secondary injury (cascade of cellular events that leads to edema, hemorrhage, increased ICP, mass effect, herniation, ischemic brain damage, and/or death).	Ventriculostomy is the "gold standard" for ICP monitoring. It provides accurate measurement of ICP (when it is used with ICP monitoring equipment) and provides for drainage of CSF. Removing CSF will lower volume in the intracranial cavity volume, thereby lowering ICP.	VI	See References: 1–4 See Annotated Bibliography: 1, 2 See Other References: 15–22	EVDs are used in conjunction with ICP monitoring devices in the traumatic brain injured patient population (please refer to the section on ICP monitoring). The physician will determine the ICP parameters after which CSF will be drained. Nurses should follow their unit or institutional policy for the duration, rate, and limits to the drainage period. The nurse should note the amount and color of the drainage.
	Postoperative craniotomy: depending of the location of a tumor, the surgical approach, or a resulting dural tear, an EVD may be placed to monitor a patient following surgery. EVDs also may be placed for postoperative management following select otolaryngology surgeries.	Increased ICP and/or hydrocephalus can occur postoperatively as a result of cerebral edema or hemorrhage. The location of the tumor may lead to obstructive hydrocephalus. Depending on the surgical approach, penetration of the dura mater may lead to CSF leaks.	VI	See Other References: 23–27	EVDs may be surgically placed intraoperatively in anticipation of postoperative brain swelling or the potential for CSF leakage. A ventriculoperitoneal shunt may be required if normal function does not return or for chronic hydrocephalus.
	CSF infections, particularly bacterial meningitis, may require management with an EVD due to a noncommunicating hydrocephalus. When the neutrophils attack the invading pathogen, the end product is an exudate that plugs the arachnoid villi. This also creates cerebral	The EVD is placed on an urgent basis to treat the hydrocephalus and increased ICP. The ventriculostomy catheter also provides direct access to the ventricle for administration of intrathecal antibiotics.	VI	See References: 4, 9	Ventricular catheters provide a unique opportunity to instill intrathecal antibiotics directly into the ventricular system. It must be administered by a physician or qualified designee (per unit or institutional policy). An EVD will treat acute hydrocephalus; however,

Period of Use	Recommendation	Rationale for Recommendation	Level of Recommendation	Supporting References	Comments
	edema, changes in the blood-brain barrier, and increases ICP levels. Intrathecal antibiotics may be given through the ventriculostomy catheter directly into the ventricles.				a ventriculoperitoneal shunt may be required if normal function does not return, fibrotic scarring damages the arachnoid villi, or for chronic hydrocephalus.
Application of Device and Initial Use	A ventricular catheter can be placed under sterile technique in the emergency department, ICU, or operating room by a neurosurgeon (or other credentialed practitioner) via a burr hole.	The ventriculostomy catheter and EVD system are frequently coupled with ICP monitoring.	VI	See References: 1–4 See Annotated Bibliography: 2 See Other References: 8, 10, 12, 14–16, 22, 23, 28	Due to the number of manufacturers and the variety of products (with and without ICP monitoring), it is essential that the manufacturer's recommendations are followed.
	Review recent laboratory results, particularly the coagulation profile.	The coagulation profile must be reviewed prior to inserting the catheter due to the risk of hemorrhage.		See Other References: 28–30	
	The catheter is inserted into the anterior horn of a lateral ventricle (nondominant side preferred, but not always possible). When using a fluid-coupled system, use strict sterile technique when connecting the catheter to the connecting tubing or pressure tubing/transducer.	The nondominant side is preferred due to the risk of damage to the dominant motor frontal area during the placement of the EVD.			
	Use only preservative-free saline to prime the system.	Preservatives added to medication vials are neurotoxic.			
	Place the transducer (if utilizing ICP monitoring) or drip chamber at the level ordered by the physician or use the unit or institutional protocol. The catheter and EVD system must be secured to prevent inadvertent removal, disruption, or dropping.	The EVD must be leveled for accurate measurement. If the EVD system would suddenly drop, it could drain a large amount of CSF, causing collapsed ventricles, increased negative pressure, torn blood vessels, hemorrhage, and herniation in a very short time span.	IV		
	Apply the dressing per institutional protocol (occlusive clear dressing, gauze pads with tape, or full craniotomy dressing).		IV		
Ongoing Monitoring	The duration of ventriculostomy catheter placement is variable and is dependent on the medical diagnosis, patient	There is no clear limit established for the duration of ventricular catheter placement.	IV	See References: 6, 8–14 See Annotated Bibliography: 3, 4	The potential for complications, especially infection, may increase with the duration of the catheter placement.

Period of Use	Recommendation	Rationale for Recommendation	Level of Recommendation	Supporting References	Comments
Ongoing Monitoring *(cont.)*	response to treatment, and potential for complications. The usual duration is approximately 5 to 10 days.				
	Patient assessment, including neurologic assessment, should be performed every hour per unit or institutional policy.	Observe for a change in the patient's neurologic status.			
	Observe and record ICP and CPP (MAP – ICP = CPP; refer to ICP section).				
	Note the color and amount of CSF drainage.	If the amount of CSF drainage decreases, it may be a sign that CSF is being reabsorbed through the arachnoid villi.			
		Change in the color of the CSF (clear to bloody) may indicate a new hemorrhage or may provide information about an infection (clear to cloudy).			
	Change the CSF collection bag when it is full, every day, or per unit or institutional policy.				
Prevention of Complications	Maintain strict aseptic technique at all times. The dressing should be clean, dry, and occlusive to avoid the potential for infection.	The ventriculostomy catheter provides direct access to the ventricle of the brain and an infection could be devastating.	VI	See References: 6	
	Re-level the system with every patient movement (turning, changing the head of the bed, etc.).	Changing the patient's position necessitates re-leveling the system to maintain accuracy.			It is critical that all healthcare providers are aware of implications of moving the patient (eg, radiology techs may change the head of the bed for an x-ray).
					Due to the number of manufacturers and the variety of products (with and without ICP monitoring), it is essential that the manufacturer's recommendations are followed.
	If the EVD is used with a fluid-coupled system, recalibrate and zero balance the system per unit or institutional guidelines and manufacturer's instructions.	Zero balancing includes opening the transducer to air, recalibrate with the monitor, and then closing the system (refer to ICP section).			

Period of Use	Recommendation	Rationale for Recommendation	Level of Recommendation	Supporting References	Comments
	Using aseptic technique, specimens can be collected from either a port on the tubing (closest to the patient) or from the CSF collection bag per unit or institutional guidelines.	Any break in the closed system increases the potential for infection.			
Quality Control Issues	Routinely assess staff understanding of EVD concepts and practices.	A lack of understanding of how EVD systems function can lead to undesirable consequences.	II		
	Monitor the rate of infection for EVD systems.	This practice should be part of routine infection control monitoring.	VI		Patients with an open injury due to penetrating trauma, depressed skull fracture, etc., are at risk for developing infection.

ANNOTATED BIBLIOGRAPHY FOR EXTERNAL VENTRICULAR DRAINS

1. **Indications for intracranial pressure monitoring. In: Bullock R, Chesnut RM, Clifton G, et al. *Management and Prognosis of Severe Traumatic Brain Injury*. New York: Brain Trauma Foundation and American Association of Neurological Surgeons; 2000.**

Study Sample

This review article established standards or guidelines on indications for ICP monitoring. Sixty-seven articles were reviewed.

Comparison Studied

Three questions related to ICP monitoring of patients with head injury were assessed: Which patients are at high risk for ICP elevation? How do ICP data help in patient management? Does ICP monitoring improve patient outcome?

Study Procedures

The authors conducted a MEDLINE search using the key terms: head injury, ICP, and intracranial hypertension. Only English language articles were reviewed. The final list was limited to those that reported outcome.

Key Results

There were insufficient data to support a treatment standard for this topic. However, 3 guidelines were established: (1) ICP monitoring is appropriate in patients with severe head injury (GCS score of 3–8) with an abnormal CT scan (hematoma, contusion, edema or compressed basal cisterns). (2) ICP monitoring is appropriate in patients with severe head injury and a normal CT scan if two of the following criteria are met: age over 40 years, unilateral or bilateral motor posturing, or systolic BP <90 mm Hg. (3) ICP monitoring is not routinely indicated in patients with mild or moderate head injury.

Study Strengths and Weaknesses

One of the primary strengths is that this review was a joint venture of the Brain Trauma Foundation and American Association of Neurological Surgeons. Studies were critically evaluated and placed in a data class. Limitations are that the article was a review of studies that had a variety of sample sizes, methodologies, etc., and that it was not international.

Clinical Implications

Two distinct patient groups were identified as appropriate candidates for ICP monitoring. This provides direction to the clinicians who care for the patients with traumatic brain injury.

2. **Recommendations for intracranial pressure monitoring technology. In: Bullock R, Chesnut RM, Clifton G, et al. *Management and Prognosis of Severe Traumatic Brain Injury*. New York: Brain Trauma Foundation and American Association of Neurological Surgeons; 2000.**

Study Sample

This review article established standards or guidelines on indications for ICP monitoring. One thousand articles were reviewed.

Comparison Studied

The scientific discussion of ICP monitoring technology was divided into the following sections: ICP monitoring device accuracy and stability, optimal intracranial location of monitor, complications, and cost.

Study Procedures

The authors conducted a MEDLINE search using the key terms: monitor and ICP. Only human studies were reviewed. Case studies were excluded.

Key Results

The assessment of ICP monitoring technology resulted in the following recommendations: the ventricular catheter connected to an external transducer and fluid-coupled system is the most accurate, low-cost, and reliable method of monitoring ICP. Fiberoptic devices provide a similar benefit, but at a higher cost. Parenchymal ICP monitoring with fiberoptic of catheter tip transduction is similar to ventricular ICP monitoring, but has the potential to drift. Subarachnoid, subdural, and epidural monitors are currently less accurate.

Study Strengths and Weaknesses

A primary strength of this review is that it is a joint venture of the Brain Trauma Foundation and American Association of Neurological Surgeons. While the repeat study of this literature might be seen as a weakness, the information in one study as a meta-analysis is useful.

Clinical Implications

One of the most significant findings of this review is that the most reliable product was also the one that has been used the longest and is the least expensive.

3. **Holloway KL, Barnes T, Choi S, et al. Ventriculostomy infection: the effect of monitoring duration and catheter exchange in 584 patients. *J Neurosurg*. 1996;85:419–424.**

Study Sample

This is a retrospective analysis of data on 584 patients with ventriculostomies.

Comparison Studied

Holloway et al. examined data related to ventriculostomy infections and the duration of ICP monitoring. They also evaluated if changing the ventricular catheter at 5 days impacted the infection rate.

Key Results

The study found a relationship of ventriculitis to monitoring duration, but this was not simple or linear. There is a rising risk of infection over the first 10 days, but then it becomes less likely. There was no benefit from catheter exchange.

Study Strengths and Weaknesses

The strength of this study is its size. With data from 584 patients collected from the Traumatic Coma Data Bank and the Medical College of Virginia Neurocore Data Bank, it is the largest study on ventriculostomy infections in the literature. A weakness is the number of diagnoses and variability in management that was provided to these patients.

Clinical Implications

Recommendations from this study are that the ventriculostomy catheters should be removed as quickly as possible to decrease the incidence of infection and that there is no benefit to exchanging the catheters.

4. **Lozier AP, Sciacca RR, Romagnoli MF, Connolly ES Jr. Ventriculostomy-related infections: a critical review of the literature.** *Neurosurgery.* **2002;51:170–182.**

Study Sample

Lozier et al. conducted a MEDLINE search using the key terms: ventriculostomy and infection, and external ventricular drain and ICP monitor. Only human studies were reviewed. Case studies were excluded. Thirty-two original articles from 1941 through 2001 were included.

Comparison Studied

A number of variables were explored, including the definition of a CSF infection, CSF sampling, neurosurgical procedures, catheter manipulation, systemic infection, duration of ventriculostomy, and prophylactic catheter exchange on day 5.

Key Results

Intraventricular hemorrhage, subarachnoid hemorrhage, cranial fractures with CSF leak, craniotomy, systemic infections, and catheter irrigation all predispose patients to the development of ventriculitis. It was also noted that the risk of CNS infections increases over the first 10 days. Prophylactic catheter exchange does not alter the risk of developing an infection; therefore, this procedure is not currently justified.

Study Strengths and Weaknesses

This study was very thorough as it evaluated commonalities between the patients, including bacteriology and sampling techniques. The weakness was that it was a retrospective review, although Lozier et al. do recommend a multicenter, prospective, randomized study.

Clinical Implications

This is the second major study that found that prophylactic catheter exchange did not modify the risk of infection. It was also a reminder that many patients are managed at individual institutions based on historical management rather than evidence-based data.

OTHER REFERENCES FOR EXTERNAL VENTRICULAR DRAINS

1. Bogdahn U, Lau W, Hassel W, et al. Continuous-pressure controlled, external ventricular drainage for treatment of acute hydrocephalus: evaluation of risk factors. *Neurosurgery.* 1992;31:898–904.
2. Hebb AO, Cusimano MD. Idiopathic normal pressure hydrocephalus: a systematic review of diagnosis and outcome. *Neurosurgery.* 2001;49:1166–1186.
3. McGift MJ, Woodworth G, Coon AL, et al. Diagnosis, treatment and analysis of long-term outcomes in idiopathic normal-pressure hydrocephalus. *Neurosurgery.* 2005;57:699–705.
4. Pirouzmand F, Tator DH, Rutka J. Management of hydrocephalus associated with vestibular schwannoma and other cerebellopontine angle tumors. *Neurosurgery.* 2001;48:1246–1254.
5. Roitbert BZ, Khan N, Alp MS, et al. Bedside external ventricular drain placement for the treatment of acute hydrocephalus. *Br J Neurosurg.* 2001;15:324–327.
6. Connolly ES Jr, Kader AA, Frazzini VI, et al. The safety of intraoperative lumbar subarachnoid drainage for acutely ruptured intracranial aneurysm: technical note. *Surg Neurol.* 1997;48:338–344.
7. Fountas KN, Kapsalaki EZ, Machinis T, et al. Review of the literature regarding the relationship of rebleeding and external ventricular drainage in patients with subarachnoid hemorrhage of aneurysmal origin. *Neurosurg Rev.* 2006;29:14–18.
8. Greenberg M. Cerebral Aneurysms. In: M Greenberg, ed. *Handbook of Neurosurgery*, 5th ed. Lakeland, FL: Greenberg Graphics; 2001.

9. Kawai K, Nagashima J, Narita K, et al. Efficacy and risk of ventricular drainage in cases of grade V subarachnoid hemorrhage. *Neurol Res*. 1997;19:649–653.

10. McNair ND. Intracranial pressure monitoring. In Clochesy JM, Breu C, Cardin S, Whittaker AA, Rudy EB, eds. *Critical Care Nursing*, 2nd ed. Philadelphia, PA: WB Saunders; 1996:289–307.

11. Rajshekhar V, Harbaugh RE. Results of routine ventriculostomy with external ventricular drainage for acute hydrocephalus following subarachnoid haemorrhage. *Acta Neurochir*. 1992;115:8–14.

12. Ropper AH, ed. *Neurological and Neurosurgical Intensive Care*, 3rd ed. New York: Raven Press; 1993.

13. Ruijs ACJ, Dirven CMF, Algra A, et al. The risk of rebleeding after external lumbar drainage in patients with untreated ruptured cerebral aneurysms. *Acta Neurochir*. 2005;147(11):1157–1162.

14. Engelhard HH, Andrews CO, Slavin KV, Charbel FT. Current management of intraventricular hemorrhage. *Surg Neurol*. 2003;60:15–21.

15. Critical pathway for the treatment of established intracranial hypertension. In Bullock R, Chesnut RM, Clifton G, et al. *Management and Prognosis of Severe Traumatic Brain Injury*. New York: Brain Trauma Foundation and American Association of Neurological Surgeons; 2000.

16. Updated Cerebral Perfusion Pressure Guidelines. New York: Brain Trauma Foundation and American Association of Neurological Surgeons; March 14, 2003.

17. Adamides AA, Winter CD, Lewis PM, Cooper DJ, Kossman T, Rosenfeld JV. Current controversies in the management of patients with severe traumatic brain injury. *ANZ J Surg*. 2006;76:163–174.

18. Fortune JB, Feustel PJ, Graca L, Hasselbarth J, Kuehler DH. Effect of hyperventilation, mannitol, and ventriculostomy drainage on cerebral blood flow after head injury. *J Trauma*. 1995;39:1091–1099.

19. Kerr ME, Weber BB, Sereika SM, Wilberger J, Marion D. Dose response to cerebrospinal fluid drainage on cerebral perfusion in traumatic brain-injured adults. *Neurosurg Focus*. 2001;11:1–7.

20. Portella GC, Citerio MG. Continuous cerebral compliance monitoring in severe head injury: its relationship with intracranial pressure and cerebral perfusion pressure. *Acta Neurochir*. 2002;81:173–175.

21. Robertson CS. Management of cerebral perfusion pressure after traumatic brain injury. *Anesthesiology*. 2001;95:1513–1517.

22. Vincent JL, Berre J, Dellinger RP. Primer on medical management of severe brain injury. *Crit Care Med*. 2005;33:1392–1399.

23. Pope W. External ventriculostomy: a practical application for the acute care nurse. *J Neurosci Nurs*. 1998;30:185–191.

24. Fishman AJ, Hoffman RA, Roland JT, Lebowitz RA, Cohen NL. Cerebrospinal fluid drainage in the management of CSF leak following acoustic neuroma surgery. *Laryngoscope*. 1996;106:1002–1004.

25. van Aken MO, Feelders RA, de Marie S, et al. Cerebrospinal fluid leakage during transsphenoidal surgery: postoperative external lumbar drainage reduces the risk for meningitis. *Pituitary*. 2004;7:89–93.

26. Moza K, McMenomey SO, Delashaw JB Jr. Indications for cerebrospinal fluid drainage and avoidance of complications. *Otolaryngol Clin N Am*. 2005;38:577–582.

27. Sade B, Mohr G, Frenkiel S. Management of intraoperative cerebrospinal fluid leak in transnasal transsphenoidal pituitary microsurgery: use of postoperative lumbar drain and sellar reconstruction without fat packing. *Acta Neurochir*. 2005;148:13–19.

28. Hoh BL, Nogueira RG, Ledezma CJ, Pryor JC, Ogilvy CS. Safety of heparinization for cerebral aneurysm soon after external ventriculostomy drain placement. *Neurosurgery*. 2005;5:845–849.

29. Ross IB, Gurmeet SD. Ventriculostomy-related cerebral hemorrhages after endovascular aneurysm treatment. *Am J Neuroradiol*. 2003;24:1528–1531.

30. Weisman M, Mayer TE. Intracranial bleeding rates associated with two methods of external ventricular drainage. *J Clin Neurosci*. 2001;8:126–128.

SUGGESTED READINGS

1. Littlejohns LR, Bader MK. Guidelines for the management of severe head injury: clinical application and changes in practice. *Crit Care Nurse*. 2001;21:48–65.

2. American Association of Neuroscience Nurses. *Guide to the Care of the Patient with Intracranial Pressure Monitoring*. Chicago, IL: AANN; 2005.

3. March K. Technology. In Bader MK, Littlejohns LR. *AANN Core Curriculum for Neuroscience Nursing*, 4th ed. Philadelphia, PA: WB Saunders; 2004:199–227.

4. Pope W. External ventriculostomy: a practical application for the acute care nurse. *J Neurosci Nurs*. 1998;30:185–191.

5. Robertson CS. Management of cerebral perfusion pressure after traumatic brain injury. *Anesthesiology*. 2001;95:1513–1517.

LUMBAR DRAINS

CASE STUDY

B.Z., a 45-year-old man, underwent a transsphenoidal hypophysectomy for a pituitary tumor. CSF leakage was noted intraoperatively, thus, following closure of the surgical wound, a catheter was inserted between the 4th and 5th lumbar space. The surgeon prescribed CSF drainage on a continuous basis in order to reduce CSF pressure within the intracranial vault, thereby allowing the dural tear to heal. B.Z. was admitted to the neuro ICU postoperatively. The patient was placed with the head of bed at 45° and the lumbar drainage system was leveled according to the neurosurgeon's orders. The buretrol on the CSF drainage system was leveled to drain at 10 mL/h continuously. B.Z.'s mustache dressing had moderate drainage during the first 12 hours, minimal drainage at 24 hours, and was consistently dry at 48 hours postoperatively.

On post-op day 4, B.Z. suddenly complained of an excruciating headache, which he rated as a 10 out of 10 on the visual analog scale. The nurse checked the position of the drain, noted that the head of bed had been changed and 25 mL of CSF had drained in the previous hour. The CSF was clear in the buretrol, and no leakage of CSF was evident from the nares. The nurse assessed the patient and noted no changes in the clinical exam. She repositioned the drain to the correct level, temporarily clamped the system, and notified the neurosurgeon. Orders were received to decrease the amount of drainage for 2 hours, administer oral pain medication, reassess the patient's headache, and resume drainage of CSF at 10 mL/h if the headache had diminished. Three hours later, the patient's headache was 1 out of 10 and the CSF drainage had returned to the prescribed hourly amount. On post-op day 5, the lumbar drain was removed and no evidence of CSF leakage was evident.

GENERAL DESCRIPTION

Lumbar drains measure the pressure of CSF in the intraspinal subarachnoid space and, when connected to a sterile closed drainage system, allow for drainage of CSF on an intermittent or continuous basis. By introducing a small plastic catheter into the lumbar space (usually between the 4th and 5th vertebral space), CSF can be drained out of the intraspinal subarachnoid space to reduce CSF pressure within the intracranial-spinal compartments. Normal pressure within the intraspinal compartment is between 0 and 15 mm Hg.

There are a number of clinical indications for lumbar CSF drainage, including the treatment of hydrocephalus, traumatic CSF leaks from fractures or operative procedures, and the intraoperative/postoperative monitoring of CSF pressure following craniotomy or thoracolumbar aortic

aneurysm repair (refer to section on thoracic aneurysm lumbar drains). By reducing the pressure in the intracranial and intraspinal CSF compartments, CSF drainage can be used to manage hydrocephalus, prevent spinal cord ischemia, or allow for potential closure of the CSF leak site.

Once the catheter is placed and secured, it is connected to the sterile, closed drainage system. The system allows for drainage of CSF continuously or intermittently. Accurate leveling and frequent monitoring of the CSF drainage system are imperative to avoid potential complications. If the patient is supine, the drain is positioned at the level of the shoulder or at the catheter insertion site. The stopcock on the drainage system is leveled per physician order and drained for a specific volume each hour, usually 8 to 10 mL/h. The patient should be educated not to change the position of the head of the bed if the system is open to drain. In some cases, locking the bed controls or unplugging the electrical controls for the bed is indicated if patient cannot follow commands.

The amount of CSF drainage should be monitored closely to prevent overdrainage of CSF. Typically, 10 mL of CSF is drained per hour. A patient complaint of a sudden or worsening headache should alert the nurse to immediately check for CSF overdrainage. In response to headache symptoms, the practitioners may elect to reduce the amount of CSF drained per hour. Monitor the patient for nausea or vomiting, deterioration in the clinical exam, signs of neck stiffness or photophobia, increasing temperature, changes in blood pressure, pulse, or respiration, changes in motor strength, and/or numbness/paresthesias whenever there is a change in the patient's condition, after position changes or per unit protocol. The physician should be notified immediately for changes in the patient's neurologic status or when signs of infection are observed. Note the characteristics of the CSF and notify the physician immediately if it changes (eg, cloudy, increasing blood, etc.).

ACCURACY

Measurement of CSF pressure is dependent on correct placement of the lumbar drain as well as the correct leveling of the drain to the patient's zero reference point. The amount of CSF drained per hour is recorded by measuring the CSF in the buretrol (part of the closed CSF drainage system).

COMPETENCY

Effective use of lumbar drain monitoring requires knowledge of spinal and intracranial anatomy and physiology; understanding the indications for lumbar drain monitoring; and the implications of nursing, medical, and surgical interventions on CSF drainage. Additional aspects needed for competency verification include the following:

- Identify the clinical indications for lumbar drain placement.
- Identify the correct anatomic location to access CSF drainage from the lumbar space.
- Demonstrate proper assembly of all supplies necessary for lumbar drain placement.
- Demonstrate proper assembly and placement of all monitor and drainage devices used within the patient care area/institution.
- Identify the tasks involved in assisting with the insertion of a lumbar drain.
- Correctly level and calibrate the CSF drainage device.
- Perform maintenance tasks (eg, zero the transducer of a fluid-filled drainage system).
- Demonstrate proper drainage of CSF (per institutional policy).
- Demonstrate collection of CSF specimen for low/normal CSF output, or infected CSF. State how frequently the specimen is collected as well as abnormal CSF analysis values.
- Document amount and color/clarity of drainage every hour, or as ordered, and with changes in the patient's neurologic status.
- Maintain a closed lumbar drain monitoring system and intact dressing or performance of site care per institutional policy.
- Demonstrate/discuss troubleshooting of lumbar drains and when to call the appropriate practitioner.
- Discuss indications for removal of the CSF drainage device.

OCCUPATIONAL HAZARDS

Placement of the system must occur in an aseptic field and anyone placing or assisting with the procedure should wear gloves, gown, cap, mask, and protective eyewear, as necessary. Occupational hazards are predominantly related to exposure to contaminated body fluids in the management of lumbar drainage. Standards were published in 1991 by the Occupational Safety and Health Administration[1] directing practice for healthcare workers who might be exposed to hazardous materials. Universal precautions must be adhered to and healthcare professionals should be aware that CSF is one of the fluids identified as a medium risk fluid for prion disease.[2] Upon removal of the lumbar drainage system, appropriate disposal of the system must occur according to institutional policy.

FUTURE RESEARCH

Areas for future research should relate to the complication rates seen in institutions and the utility of lumbar drainage as a treatment option. Infections, overdrainage, and headache are the most common complications seen in patients treated with CSF drainage.[3] It would be beneficial to healthcare professionals and the public if further information on CSF drainage management was generated. This area of practice currently lacks evidence-based information regarding indications, management and outcomes, thus evidence generated by strong research would enhance care.

REFERENCES

1. US Department of Occupational Safety and Health Administration, Regulations (Standards – 29 CRF) Bloodborne Pathogens 1910.1030. Available at: http://www.osha.gov/pls/oshaweb/owadisp .show_document?p_table=STANDARDS&p_id =10051. Accessed December 18, 2007.
2. World Health Organization Infection Control Guidelines for Transmissible Spongiform Encephalopathies. Report of a WHO Consultation Geneva, Switzerland, 23-26 March 1999. Available at: http://www.who.int /csr/resources/publications/bse/WHO_CDS_CSR _APH_2000_3/en/. Accessed August 17, 2007.
3. Ackbas SC, Akyuz M, Kazan S, Tuncer R. Complications of closed continuous lumbar drainage of cerebrospinal fluid. *Acta Neurochir*. 2002;144:475–480.

CLINICAL RECOMMENDATIONS FOR LUMBAR DRAINS

The rating scale for the Level of Recommendation ranges from I to VI, with levels indicated as follows: I, manufacturer's recommendations only; II, theory based, no research data to support recommendations; recommendations from expert consensus group may exist; III, laboratory data only, no clinical data to support recommendations; IV, limited clinical studies to support recommendations; V, clinical studies in more than 1 or 2 different populations and situations to support recommendations; VI, clinical studies in a variety of patient populations and situations to support recommendations.

Period of Use	Recommendation	Rationale for Recommendation	Level of Recommendation	Supporting References	Comments
Patient Selection	Continuous lumbar CSF drainage is recommended in the following circumstances:				
	Interim action to treat communicating hydrocephalus	Acute hydrocephalus is a life-threatening situation that must be treated urgently. Communicating hydrocephalus occurs when the pathways between the ventricles are open and CSF is produced at the normal rate of 18 to 25 mL/h, but the CSF cannot be absorbed by the arachnoid villi because they are plugged by blood components or exudate.	VI	See Other References: 1–4	Hydrocephalus is a progressive dilation of the ventricles that can be caused by overproduction of CSF or abnormalities in CSF flow or reabsorption. A lumbar drain will treat acute hydrocephalus. This is usually treated with placement of a ventriculostomy; however, a ventricle-peritoneal shunt may be required if normal function does not return; fibrotic scarring damages the arachnoid villi, or, for chronic hydrocephalus. The duration is dependent on the patient status and return to normal CSF reabsorption through the arachnoid villi, but usually remains between 5 and 10 days.
	Assess a shunt in patients with normal pressure hydrocephalus, pseudotumor cerebri, or ventriculomegaly for various etiologies.	If the patient's neurologic and functional status improves following placement of a lumbar drain, the patient may be a candidate for placement of a shunt to consistently divert CSF.	IV	See Annotated Bibliography: 2 See Other References: 1, 3–10	Ventriculoperitoneal shunts are the most common method of shunting. Other options include ventriculoatrial shunts, ventriculopleural shunts, or lumbar peritoneal shunts.
	To deflect CSF away from the site of dural tears, CSF leaks, and/or fistulas. CSF leak may be spontaneous, the result of a traumatic injury, or a consequence of cranial, spinal, or otolaryngologic surgery.	Diverting the CSF from the site of the leak or fistula will allow the dura to heal. If this is successful, the patient will not require surgical intervention.	VI	See Annotated Bibliography: 1, 4 See Other References: 1, 3, 4, 11–21	The physician will determine the level of the drainage/collection system (external auditory meatus, shoulder height, or the level of catheter insertion). Nurses should follow their unit or institutional policy for the duration, rate, and limits to the drainage period. The nurse should note the amount and color

Period of Use	Recommendation	Rationale for Recommendation	Level of Recommendation	Supporting References	Comments
Patient Selection *(cont.)*					of the drainage. If the patient has a CSF leak, the nurse also should observe for continued signs of rhinorrhea or otorrhea. This drainage should be tested for glucose per unit or institutional policies.
	For postoperative craniotomy patients: depending on the location of a tumor, the surgical approach, or a resulting dural tear, a lumbar drain may be placed to monitor a patient following surgery. Lumbar drains also may be placed for postoperative management following select otolaryngology surgeries.	Increased ICP and/or hydrocephalus can occur postoperatively as a result of cerebral edema or hemorrhage. The location of the tumor also may lead to obstructive hydrocephalus. Depending on the surgical approach, penetration of the dura mater may lead to CSF leaks.	VI	See Annotated Bibliography: 4 See Other References: 1–4, 12, 14, 16–21	Lumbar drains may be placed in the operating room in anticipation of postoperative brain swelling or the potential for CSF leakage. A shunt may be required if normal function does not return or for chronic hydrocephalus.
	To manage shunt infection or CSF infections, particularly bacterial meningitis, may require management with a lumbar drain. When the neutrophils attack the invading pathogen, the end product is an exudate that plugs the arachnoid villi. This also creates cerebral edema, changes in the blood-brain barrier, and increases ICP. Intrathecal antibiotics may be given through the catheter directly into the subarachnoid space.	If there is a suspected shunt infection, a lumbar drain is a method of obtaining serial specimens for laboratory diagnosis. If the patient has a change in level of consciousness or other neurologic changes that may be related to shunt malfunction, diverting the CSF via a lumbar drain will assist in the diagnosis of a shunt malfunction.	VI	See Other References: 1, 3, 4, 22	Specimens are obtained using aseptic technique and following manufacturers' guidelines and unit or institutional policies. Lumbar catheters provide a unique opportunity to instill intrathecal antibiotics directly into the subarachnoid system. It must be administered by a physician or qualified designee (per unit or institutional policy).
	Subarachnoid hemorrhage, usually due to the rupture of a cerebral aneurysm. The blood spreads through the Sylvian fissures into the basal cisterns. The blood irritates the brain tissues, raises ICP, and lowers the CPP. The blood also may enter the ventricles, leading to an intraventricular hemorrhage. Symptoms are dependent on the location of the hemorrhage and the resulting ICP.	Following a subarachnoid hemorrhage from a cerebral aneurysm, blood is released into the subarachnoid space and causes an immediate rise in ICP. The patient is also at risk for developing acute hydrocephalus due to obstruction of CSF flow by a blood clot (communicating hydrocephalus). The blood components, including red blood cells, white blood cells, and other blood factors, will cause noncommunicating hydrocephalus when they plug the arachnoid villi and prevent the reabsorption of CSF.	V	See Other References: 1, 3, 4, 23–25	The lumbar catheter may be placed preoperatively in the emergency department or ICU by a neurosurgeon (or his or her designee), or during emergent surgery. The duration is dependent on the patient status and return to normal CSF reabsorption through the arachnoid villi, but usually remains between 5 and 10 days.

Period of Use	Recommendation	Rationale for Recommendation	Level of Recommendation	Supporting References	Comments
	Continuous lumbar CSF drainage may be a substitute to ventriculostomy for patients who require CSF drainage or may be an option to control increased ICP.	If it is preferred to place a lumbar drain instead of an EVD, place in those patients with a Hunt-Hess grade of ≥3 to treat increased ICP and acute communicating hydrocephalus.	V	See Other References: 1, 3, 4, 26, 27	The physician will determine the bounds after which CSF will be drained. Nurses should follow their unit or institutional policy for the duration, rate, and limits to the drainage period. The nurse should note the amount and color of the drainage.
Application of Device and Initial Use	The lumbar drain may be placed using aseptic technique in the emergency department, OR, or at the bedside in the ICU or general unit by a neurosurgeon or his or her designee. A lumbar puncture is performed using a large-bore Tuohy needle at L4-L5. A catheter is advanced into the subarachnoid space and CSF flow is confirmation that the catheter has been placed correctly. The catheter is connected to a sterile, closed drainage system and/or collection bag. The duration is dependent on the patient status and return to normal CSF reabsorption through the arachnoid villi, but usually remains between 5 and 10 days.	A lumbar drain provides for drainage of CSF. Removing CSF will lower brain volume, thereby lowering ICP. The lumbar catheter may be inserted on an urgent basis to treat hydrocephalus and increased ICP. It may also be placed in a controlled setting for a CSF leak, shunt infection, etc. The catheter provides access to the subarachnoid space for administration of intrathecal antibiotics.	VI	See Annotated Bibliography: 4 See Other References: 1, 3, 4, 19, 20, 28–30	Due to the number of manufacturers and the variety of products (with and without ICP monitoring), it is essential that the manufacturers' recommendations are followed. Lumbar drainage will treat acute hydrocephalus; however, a shunt may be required if normal function does not return, fibrotic scarring damages the arachnoid villi, or for chronic hydrocephalus.
	Review recent laboratory results, particularly the coagulation profile.	The coagulation profile must be reviewed prior to inserting the catheter due to the risk of hemorrhage.			
	Use strict sterile technique when connecting the catheter to the connecting tubing or collection bag.				
	Place external drainage system and/or collection bag at the predetermined level (as ordered by the physician or using the unit or institutional protocol). This is usually the external auditory meatus, shoulder height, or the level of the catheter insertion. The catheter and collection	The lumbar drain must be leveled for accurate measurement. If the lumbar drainage system would suddenly drop, it could drain a large amount of CSF, causing collapsed ventricles and increased negative pressure. The collapsed ventricles can cause rupture of bridging	V	See References: 3 See Other References: 1, 3, 4, 19, 31–34	Overdrainage of the CSF may result in complications including headache, tension pneumocranium, central herniation, or subdural hematoma.

Period of Use	Recommendation	Rationale for Recommendation	Level of Recommendation	Supporting References	Comments
	system must be secured to prevent inadvertent removal, disruption, or dropping.	veins in the dura, initiating a cascade that causes a subdural hematoma and herniation if not clinically observed and treated.			
	Apply the dressing per unit or institutional protocol (occlusive clear dressings, gauze pads with tape).		II	See Other References: 1, 3, 4, 19	
Ongoing Monitoring	The duration of lumbar catheter placement is variable and depends on the medical diagnosis, patient response to treatment, and potential for complications. The usual duration is approximately 5 to 10 days.	There is no clear limit established for the duration of lumbar catheter placement.	III	See References: 3 See Other References: 1, 3, 4, 11–14, 16–21, 23, 33	
	Patient assessment, including neurologic assessment should be performed every hour, or per unit or institutional policy.	Observe for a change in the patient's neurologic status.			
	Note the color, clarity, and amount of CSF drainage. Change the CSF collection bag when it is full, every day, or per unit or institutional policy.	If the amount of CSF drainage decreases, it may be a sign that CSF is being reabsorbed through the arachnoid villi. The lumbar catheter provides direct access to the subarachnoid space and an infection could be neurologically devastating and potentially life-threatening.	VI	See Annotated Bibliography: 3 See Other References: 1, 3, 4, 19, 35–38	The potential for complications, especially infection, may increase with manipulation of the system, duration of the catheter placement, open or penetrating trauma, CSF leakage, or other systemic infection.
Prevention of Complications	Maintain strict aseptic technique at all times. The dressing should be clean, dry, and occlusive to avoid the potential for infection. Using aseptic technique, specimens can be collected from either a port on the tubing (closest to the patient) or from the CSF collection bag per unit or institutional policies, and/or manufacturers' recommendations.	Any break in the closed system increases the potential for infection.	VI	See Annotated Bibliography: 3 See Other References: 1, 3, 4, 19, 35–38	Due to the number of manufacturers and the variety of products, it is essential that the manufacturers' recommendations are followed.

Period of Use	Recommendation	Rationale for Recommendation	Level of Recommendation	Supporting References	Comments
	Re-level the system with every patient movement (turning, changing the head of the bed, etc.). Initiate special precautions for patients who may be confused and may attempt to get out of bed without assistance	Changing the patient's position necessitates re-leveling the system to maintain accuracy.	VI	See References: 3 See Other References: 1, 3, 4, 19, 31–34	It is critical that all healthcare providers are aware of implications of moving the patient (eg, radiology techs may change the head of the bed for an x-ray).
Quality Control Issues	Routinely assess staff understanding of lumbar drainage concepts and practices.	A lack of understanding of how lumbar drains function can lead to undesirable or even fatal consequences.	VI	See References: 3 See Other References: 1, 3, 4, 19, 31–38	
	Monitor the rate of infection for lumbar drainage systems.	This practice should be part of routine infection control monitoring.	VI	See References: 3 See Other References: 1, 3, 4, 19, 31–34	

ANNOTATED BIBLIOGRAPHY FOR LUMBAR DRAINS

1. Bell RB, Dierks EJ, Homer L, Potter BE. Management of cerebrospinal fluid leak associated with craniomaxillofacial trauma. *J Oral Maxillofac Surg.* **2004;62:676–684.**

Study Sample

This is a retrospective study of the records of all patients with basilar skull fractures and/or severe facial trauma who were evaluated at a Level 1 trauma center from 1991 to 2001. A total of 735 patients met the criteria for inclusion, with 35 patients diagnosed with a CSF leak (4.6% incidence).

Comparison Studied

The purpose of the study was to establish the incidence of CSF leakage and evaluate the outcome of the patients who received either nonsurgical or surgical treatment.

Study Procedures

Bell et al. reviewed the information included in the hospital Trauma Registry and then completed chart reviews to validate inclusion in the study. Fifteen clinical indicators were abstracted to identify patients who were at risk for CSF leaks. Exclusions were patients who died, received a ventriculostomy, or whose diagnosis was not corroborated by radiographic or laboratory confirmation.

Key Results

The incidence of CSF leak was 4.6% with 73.5% (n = 25) presenting with otorrhea and 26.5% (n = 9) with rhinorrhea. Clinical, laboratory, or radiographic evidence confirmed the CSF leaks. The leak resolved using bedrest and observation (no treatment) in 2 to 10 days in 84.6% of the patients. Five of the remaining 6 patients were treated with CSF diversion via lumbar drainage for 5 to 7 days. The CSF leak resolved for 2 of these patients and the remaining 4 required surgical intervention to resolve the CSF leak. The patients were not prescribed prophylactic antibiotics, and none developed meningitis.

Study Strengths and Weaknesses

One of the primary strengths of this study is that the patients followed an algorithm for the treatment of CSF leaks that began with the diagnosis of CSF leak, continued to conservative treatment, then lumbar drainage, and finally surgical repair (with the exception of 1 patient who underwent surgery without receiving lumbar drainage). The chief limitation is that the sample group is small and limited to 1 hospital.

Clinical Implications

At this time, clinical guidelines have not been published for CSF leaks. The authors propose a management algorithm for CSF otorrhea and rhinorrhea that begins with diagnosis, proceeds to treatment with bedrest and observation for 7 days, followed by lumbar drainage for 5 to 7 days, then operative procedures. Use of this algorithm would provide direction to the clinicians who care for these patients.

2. Marmarou A, Bergsneider M, Klinge P. The value of supplemental prognostic tests for the preoperative assessment of idiopathic normal-pressure hydrocephalus. *Neurosurgery.* **2005;57(Suppl 2):S17–S18.**

Study Sample

This review article establishes evidenced-based guidelines for using supplementary tests in the preoperative assessment of idiopathic normal-pressure hydrocephalus. A total of 242 articles were reviewed.

Comparison Studied

Several procedures or tests may be performed prior to the insertion of a shunt for normal-pressure hydrocephalus that may predict the response to the surgical procedure. These include: radionuclide cisternography, ICP monitoring, CSF removal via high-volume spinal taps (tap test), external lumbar drainage, measurement of the impedance of CSF flow/absorption pathways, and measurement of aqueductal CSF flow velocities.

Study Procedures

Marmarou et al. conducted a MEDLINE search using the key terms: NPH (normal-pressure hydrocephalus), lumbar drain, CSF tap test, and external CSF drainage. Only human studies of a large number of shunted patients were reviewed; case studies were excluded.

Key Results

Marmarou et al. determined that there were insufficient data to support clinical management standards for the use of preoperative testing for predictive purposes for idiopathic normal-pressure hydrocephalus. However, they report that a positive response to a tap test had low sensitivity (26%–61%), CSF outflow resistance testing had higher sensitivity (57%–100%) and a predictive value of 75% to 92%, and external lumbar drainage carried a high sensitivity (50%–100%) with a high predictive value (80%–100%).

Study Strengths and Weaknesses

This article critically evaluated the current literature and placed each study in a data class. The limitation is that it was a review of studies with a variety of sample sizes, methodologies, etc.

Clinical Implications

Although this study did not support a clinical management standard, it reported a hierarchy of supplemental tests. The use of external lumbar drainage was noted to have high sensitivity (50%–100%) with a high predictive value (80%–100%) for a successful response to shunting for patients with idiopathic normal-pressure hydrocephalus.

3. Schade RP, Schinkel J, Roelandse RWC, et al. Lack of value of routine analysis of cerebrospinal fluid for prediction and diagnosis of external drainage-related bacterial meningitis. *J Neurosurg*. 2006;104:101–108.

Study Sample

This is a cohort study of 230 consecutive patients with external CSF drains.

Comparison Studied

CSF samples were collected daily and analyzed for the presence of: bacteria, leukocyte count, protein and glucose concentration, ratio of CSF glucose to serum glucose, and concentration of interleukin-6. Schade et al. compared the samples of the patients who developed bacterial meningitis with the samples of the patients who did not develop bacterial meningitis.

Key Results

There were no significant differences in the analysis of samples in leukocyte count, protein concentration, glucose concentration, or CSF/serum glucose ratio for the group of patients who developed bacterial meningitis against the group of patients who did not develop bacterial meningitis during the first 3 days preceding the infection or the first 3 days of the infection. CSF interleukin-6 concentrations were similar for the 3 days preceding the infections. Using absolute values, ratios, and differences between the current and previous day's values, none of the parameters had predictive or diagnostic value. Gram stain had a high specificity (99.9%) but low sensitivity (18% on the first day), which had limited predictive or diagnostic value.

Study Strengths and Weaknesses

This study sought to validate the use of daily CSF sampling to predict and, hopefully, avert the development of bacterial meningitis. One of its strengths is the size of the sample with 230 consecutive patients. Its weakness is that the patients had external CSF drainage for a variety of brain injuries and neurologic surgeries. Schade et al. concluded that the value of routine CSF analysis is limited in patients with severe disturbances in their CSF levels.

Clinical Implications

The use of daily CSF sampling to predict the development of bacterial meningitis is limited. Gram stain of CSF also is limited in screening for bacterial meningitis in patients with external CSF drainage related to a low sensitivity of 18% on the first day of infection.

4. van Aken ML, Feelders RA, de Marie S, et al. Cerebrospinal fluid leakage during transsphenoidal surgery: postoperative external lumbar drainage reduces the risk for meningitis. *Pituitary*. 2004;7:89–93.

Study Sample

Van Aken et al. evaluated the development of meningitis in patients who underwent transsphenoidal operations with intraoperative CSF leakage. They compared a group of 278 consecutive transsphenoidal operations to a previous group of 228 transsphenoidal operations. The surgeries were performed at 1 hospital, and 3 neurosurgeons participated in the study.

Comparison Studied

This study compared a group of 278 consecutive transsphenoidal operations, 70 (25.2%) with intraoperative CSF leakage, to a previous group of 228, 22 (9.6%) with intraoperative CSF leakage. Two primary differences between the two groups existed: preoperative patients with radiographic evidence of sinusitis were treated until the infection was resolved, and an external lumbar drain was inserted immediately postoperatively in patients with an identified intraoperative CSF leak.

Key Results

The incidence of meningitis in patients with identified intraoperative CSF leaks decreased to 1 of 70 (1.4%) cases compared to 3 of 22 (13.6%) in the previous series. A second patient without an identified intraoperative CSF leak developed a CSF leak on the third postoperative day, was treated with external lumbar drainage, and developed meningitis. This incidence of postoperative meningitis of 2 per 278 cases (0.7%) compared to the previous study with 7 per 228 (3.1%) argues for the implementation of preoperative diagnosis and treatment of sinusitis and the use of external lumbar drainage in patients with identified CSF leakage during transsphenoidal surgery.

Study Strengths and Weaknesses

This study had both the benefit of consistent surgical treatment through the surgical techniques of 3 neurosurgeons operating within 1 hospital and the limitations of the same. All patients received antibiotics the day prior to surgery, the morning of surgery, and following surgery to the 6th postoperative day. Because there were actually two changes in protocol—preoperative diagnosis and treatment of sinusitis as well as the insertion of an external lumbar drain with CSF leakage—it cannot be concluded that the decrease in the incidence of meningitis was related with either one, but rather to both.

Clinical Implications

Implementation of each of these measures, diagnosis and treatment of sinusitis and the use of external lumbar drainage following intraoperative CSF leakage, should be studied separately. Each or both could be easily put into practice within the clinical setting.

OTHER REFERENCES FOR LUMBAR DRAINS

1. March K. Technology. In Bader MK, Littlejohns LR. *AANN Core Curriculum for Neuroscience Nursing*, 4th ed. Philadelphia: WB Saunders; 2004:199–227.

2. Pirouzmand F, Tator DH, Rutka J. Management of hydrocephalus associated with vestibular schwannoma and other cerebellopontine angle tumors. *Neurosurgery.* 2001;48:1246–1254.

3. Thompson HJ. Managing patients with lumbar drainage devices. *Crit Care Nurse.* 2000;20:59–68.

4. Thompson HJ. *American Association of Neuroscience Nurses Clinical Guideline Series: Lumbar Drain Management.* Chicago: American Association of Neuroscience Nurses; 1998.

5. Chen IH, Huang CI, Liu HC, Chen KK. Effectiveness of shunting in patients with normal pressure hydrocephalus predicted by temporary, controlled-resistance, continuous lumbar drainage: a case-control study. *J Neurol Neurosurg Psychiatry.* 1994; 57:1430–1432.

6. Hebb AO, Cusimano MD. Idiopathic normal pressure hydrocephalus: a systematic review of diagnosis and outcome. *Neurosurgery.* 2001;49:1166–1186.

7. Marmarou A, Bergsneider M, Klinge P. The value of supplemental prognostic tests for the preoperative assessment of idiopathic normal-pressure hydrocephalus. *Neurosurgery.* 2005;57(Suppl 2):S17–S18.

8. McGirt MJ, Woodworth GBS, Coon AL, et al. Diagnosis, treatment, and analysis of long-term outcomes in idiopathic normal-pressure hydrocephalus. *Neurosurgery.* 2005;57:699–705.

9. Walchenbach R, Geiger E, Thomeer RT, et al. The value of temporary external lumbar CSF drainage in predicting the outcome of shunting on normal pressure hydrocephalus. *J Neurol Neurosurg Psychiatry.* 2002;72:503–506.

10. Williams MA, Razumovsky AY, Hanley DF. Comparison of Pcsf monitoring and controlled CSF drainage diagnosis normal pressure hydrocephalus. *Acta Neurochir Suppl (Wein).* 1998;71:328–330.

11. Bell RB, Dierks EJ, Homer L, Potter BE. Management of cerebrospinal fluid leak associated with cra-niomaxillofacial trauma. *J Oral Maxillofac Surg.* 2004;62:676–684.

12. Fishman AJ, Hoffman RA, Roland JT, Lebowitz RA, Cohen NL. Cerebrospinal fluid drainage in the management of CSF leak following acoustic neuroma surgery. *Laryngoscope.* 1996;106:1002–1004.

13. Fountas KN, Kapsalaki EZ, Johnston KW. Cerebrospinal fluid fistula secondary to dural tear in anterior cervical discectomy and fusion. *Spine.* 2005;30:e277–e280.

14. Lindstrom DR, Toohill RJ, Loehrl TA, Smith TL. Management of cerebrospinal fluid rhinorrhea: the medical college of Wisconsin experience. *Laryngoscope.* 2004;114:969–974.

15. McCormack BM, Taylor SL, Heath S, Scanlon J. Pseudomeningocele/CSF fistula in a patient with lumbar spinal implants treated with epidural blood patch and a brief course of closed subarachnoid drainage: a case report. *Spine.* 1996;21:2273–2276.

16. Moza K, McMenomey SO, Delashaw JB. Indications for cerebrospinal fluid drainage and avoidance of complications. *Otolaryngol Clin North Am.* 2005;38:577–582.

17. Sade B, Mohr G, Frenkiel S. Management of intraoperative cerebrospinal fluid leak in transnasal transsphenoidal pituitary microsurgery: use of postoperative lumbar drain and sellar reconstruction without fat packing. *Acta Neurochir.* 2005;148:13–19.

18. Savva A, Taylor MJ, Beatty CW. Management of cerebrospinal fluid leaks involving the temporal bone: report on 92 patients. *Laryngoscope.* 2003;113:50–56.

19. Shapiro SA, Scully T. Closed continuous drainage of cerebrospinal fluid via a lumbar subarachnoid catheter for treatment of prevention of cranial/spinal cerebrospinal fluid fistula. *Neurosurgery.* 1992; 30:241–245.

20. van Aken ML, Feelders RA, de Marie S, et al. Cerebrospinal fluid leakage during transsphenoidal surgery: postoperative external lumbar drainage reduces the risk for meningitis. *Pituitary.* 2004;7:89–93.

21. Yilmazlar S, Arslan E, Kocaeli H, et al. Cerebrospinal fluid leakage complicating skull base fractures: analysis of 81 cases. *Neurosurg Rev.* 2006; 29:64–71.

22. Macsween KF, Bicanic T, Brouwer AE, et al. Lumbar drainage for control of raised cerebrospinal fluid pressure in cryptococcal meningitis: case report and review. *J Infect.* 2005;51:e211–e224.

23. Connolly ES Jr, Kader AA, Frazzini VI, et al. The safety of intraoperative lumbar subarachnoid drainage for acutely ruptured intracranial aneurysm: technical note. *Surg Neurol.* 1997;48:338–344.

24. Klimo P, Kestle JF, MacDonald JD, Schmidt RH. Marked reduction of cerebral vasospasm with lumbar

drainage of cerebrospinal fluid after subarachnoid hemorrhage. *J Neurosurg.* 2004;100:215–224.

25. Ruijs ACJ, Dirven CMF, Algra A, et al. The risk of rebleeding after external lumbar drainage in patients with untreated ruptured cerebral aneurysms. *Acta Neurochir.* 2005;147:1157–1162.

26. Munch EC, Bauhuf C, Horn P, et al. Therapy of malignant intracranial hypertension by controlled lumbar cerebrospinal fluid drainage. *Crit Care Med.* 2001;29:976–981.

27. Tomosvari A, Mencser Z, Futo J, Hortobagyi A, et al. Preliminary experience with controlled lumbar drainage in medically refractory intracranial hypertension. *Orv Hetil.* 2005;146:159–164.

28. Hahn M, Murali R, Couldwell WT. Tunneled lumbar drain: technical note. *J Neurosurg.* 2002;96: 1130–1131.

29. Houle PJ, Vender JR, Fountas K, et al. Pump-regulated lumbar subarachnoid drainage. *Neurosurgery.* 2000;46:929–932.

30. Overstreet M. How do I manage a lumbar drain? *Nursing.* 2003;33:74–75.

31. Grady RD, Horlocker TT, Brown RD. Neurologic complications after placement of cerebrospinal fluid drainage catheters and needles in anesthetized patients: implications for regional anesthesia. *Anesth Analg.* 1999;88:388–392.

32. Mcleod ADM, Hirsch NP, Scrutton MJL. Neurologic complications of cerebrospinal fluid drainage catheters (letter). *Anesth Analg.* 2000;90:228.

33. Roland PS, Marple BF, Meyerhoff WL, Mickey B. Complications of lumbar spinal fluid drainage. *Otolaryngol Head Neck Surg.* 1992;107:564–569.

34. Samadani U, Huang JH, Baranov D, et al. Intracranial hypotension after intraoperative lumbar cerebrospinal fluid drainage. *Neurosurgery.* 2003;52: 148–152.

35. Coplin WM, Avellino AM, Kim DK, Winn HR, Grady MS. Bacterial meningitis associated with lumbar drains: a retrospective cohort study. *J Neurol Neurosurg Psychiatry.* 1999;67:468–473.

36. Roca B, Pesudo JV, Gonzalez-Darder JM. Meningitis caused by *Enterococcus galinarum* after lumbar drainage of cerebrospinal fluid. *Eur J Intern Med.* 2006;17:298–299.

37. Schade RP, Schinkel J, Roelandse RWC, et al. Lack of value of routine analysis of cerebrospinal fluid for prediction and diagnosis of external drainage-related bacterial meningitis. *J Neurosurg.* 2006;104: 101–108.

38. Schade, RP, Schinkel J, Visser LG, et al. Bacterial meningitis caused by the use of ventricular or lumbar cerebrospinal fluid catheters. *J Neurosurg.* 2005; 102:220–234.

THORACOABDOMINAL AORTIC ANEURYSM

GENERAL DESCRIPTION

Thoracoabdominal aortic aneurysms are classified according to the extent and involvement of the aorta. These classifications were first proposed by Crawford in 1986.[1] Type I thoracoabdominal aortic aneurysms involve most of the descending aorta extending from just below the left subclavian artery to above the superior mesenteric and renal arteries. Type II aneurysms extend from the left subclavian artery down to the bifurcation of the aorta. Type III involves the distal thoracic aorta from the sixth intercostal space down to the bifurcation of the aorta. Lastly, Type IV extends from just below the diaphragm down to the aortic bifurcation (Figure 3-1).[1] Type II and type I aneurysms have been reported to be associated with the highest incidence of paraplegia at 21% and 8%, respectively.

Blood flow to the spinal cord is divided between two levels. The upper portion is perfused mostly from the vertebral arteries (Figure 3-2) and a small portion from the deep cervical arteries. The lower portion of the spinal cord is perfused by branches of the anterior radicular arteries and the intercostal arteries. The artery of Adamkiewicz, located between T8 and L1, is one of the anterior radicular arteries and is an important vessel perfusing the thoracic and lumbar areas of the spinal cord (Figure 3-3). When this vessel or the intercostal arteries are occluded, the result may be spinal cord infarction.[1,3,4]

During surgical repair of a thoracoabdominal aortic aneurysm, the aorta is cross-clamped while the aneurysm is being repaired. During aortic cross clamping, blood flow to the spinal cord is interrupted for 30 to 40 minutes and sometimes longer. When the clamps are removed, reactive hyperemia of the spinal cord occurs in response to the restored blood flow, which results in tissue swelling. Research has demonstrated the use of several protective strategies perioperatively has contributed to reduction of paralysis. These strategies include the use of hypothermia, maintaining a MAP greater than 80 mm Hg, and drainage of CSF. Perioperative pharmacologic interventions include the administration of nalaoxone, steroids, and mannitol. Postoperatively, the patient is still at risk to develop neurologic impairment (motor or sensory). CSF drainage has been shown to reduce the incidence of this complication.[1]

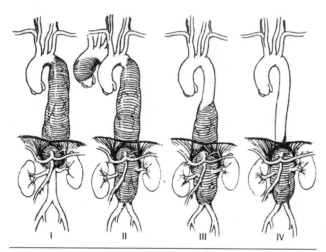

Figure 3-1   Classification of thoracoabdominal aortic aneurysms.

Source: Reprinted from Crawford ES, Svenson LG, Hess KR, et al. A prospective randomized study of CSF drainage to prevent paraplegia after high risk surgery on the thoracoabdominal aorta. *J Vasc Surg.* 1990;13:36–46. Reprinted with permission from Elsevier.

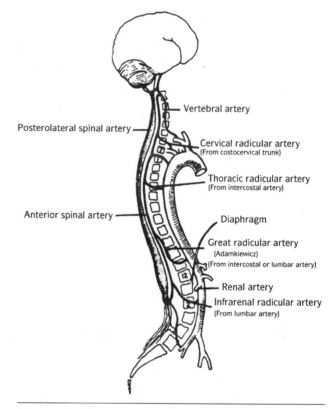

Figure 3-2   Blood supply to the spinal cord.

Source: Reprinted from Szilagyi DE, Hageman JH, Smith RF, Elliot JP. Spinal cord damage in surgery of the abdominal aorta. *Surgery.* 1978;83:38–56. Reprinted with permission from Elsevier.

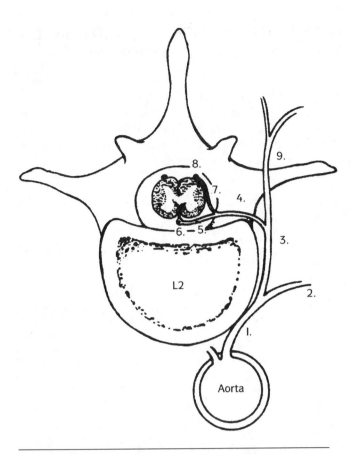

REFERENCES

1. Iacono LA. Naloxone infusion and drainage of cerebrospinal fluid as adjuncts to postoperative care after repair of thoracoabdominal aneurysms. *Crit Care Nurse.* 1999;19:37–47.
2. Crawford ES, Svenson LG, Hess KR, et al. A prospective randomized study of CSF drainage to prevent paraplegia after high risk surgery on the thoracoabdominal aorta. *J Vasc Surg.* 1990;13:36–46.
3. Bigliolo P, Spirito R, Roberto M, et al. The anterior spinal artery: the main arterial supply of the human spinal cord—a preliminary anatomic study. *J Thorac Cardiovasc Surg.* 2000;119:376–379.
4. Metzler MH. Spinal cord injury: are there grounds for new hope? *Current Surgery.* 2000;57:6.

Figure 3-3   Details of the proximal and intermediate divisions of blood supply to the spinal cord.

1. Lumbar (intercostal) artery
2. Anterior ramus lumbar (intercostal) artery
3. Posterior ramus lumbar (intercostal) artery
4. Spinal artery
5. Anterior radicular artery
6. Anterior spinal artery
7. Posterior radicular artery
8. Posterolateral spinal artery
9. Muscular branches

Source: Metzler MH. Spinal cord injury: are there grounds for new hope? *Current Surgery.* 2000;57:37–47. Reprinted with permission from Elsevier.

CLINICAL RECOMMENDATIONS FOR SPINAL PRESSURE MONITORING AND SPINAL DRAINAGE FOR PATIENTS UNDERGOING REPAIR OF A THORACOABDOMINAL AORTIC ANEURYSM

The rating scale for the Level of Recommendation ranges from I to VI, with levels indicated as follows: I, manufacturer's recommendations only; II, theory based, no research data to support recommendations; recommendations from expert consensus group may exist; III, laboratory data only, no clinical data to support recommendations; IV, limited clinical studies to support recommendations; V, clinical studies in more than 1 or 2 different populations and situations to support recommendations; VI, clinical studies in a variety of patient populations and situations to support recommendations.

Period of Use	Recommendation	Rationale for Recommendation	Level of Recommendation	Supporting References	Comments
Patient Selection	Spinal pressure monitoring is recommended in patients undergoing thoracoabdominal aneurysm repair during the perioperative period and postoperative period. Patients are at risk for early (immediately after surgery) or late (>12 h after surgery) neurologic impairment including motor and sensory deficits.	CSF drainage has been shown to reduce the incidence of neurologic impairment (paralysis) following surgery by decreasing CSF pressure, which allows greater spinal cord perfusion. During the operative procedure, the aorta is cross-clamped, resulting in reduced arterial blood flow to the spinal cord. Spinal artery pressure decreases and CSF pressure increases. The spinal cord tissue becomes ischemic with resultant tissue swelling.	V		Spinal cord perfusion pressure (SPP) is the difference between the mean distal aortic perfusion pressure and the CSF pressure. Long aortic cross clamp times greater than 30 minutes are associated with increased incidence of neurologic injury. Prevention has been demonstrated by maintaining SPP to less than 8 mm Hg. CSF drainage helps to accomplish this goal.
Application of Device and Initial Use	The catheter is introduced into the intravertebral space between L4 and L5 prior to the onset of the surgical procedure. The catheter is connected to an external CSF drainage system using sterile isotonic, preservative-free saline. On arrival to the ICU, the pressure monitoring system is referenced to the level of entry (spinal cord) and zeroed.	The reference level should be at the level where the catheter is inserted into the intravertebral space, horizontal to the posterior chest wall (patient's back).	II		There are anecdotal comments in the literature regarding referencing, ie, the level of entry into the intravertebral space or following the physician order for another reference point.
	CSF is drained to maintain a CSF pressure of 10 mm Hg or less.	Normal CSF pressure is 1–10 mm Hg. Draining the excess fluid reduces spinal cord compression, thereby enhancing perfusion of the tissue.	V	See References: 1–3 See Annotated Bibliography: 1, 2 See Other References: 1–3, 8	
Ongoing Monitoring	Monitor CSF pressure continuously, maintaining a closed system at all times. When the pressure exceeds 10 mm Hg, turn the stopcock on the drainage system allowing	Continuous monitoring allows for identifying upward trends in the CSF pressure. Rechecking the CSF pressure during drainage prevents draining	II	See References: 1 See Other References: 3	

Period of Use	Recommendation	Rationale for Recommendation	Level of Recommendation	Supporting References	Comments
Ongoing Monitoring *(cont.)*	for CSF drainage. Recheck the CSF pressure every 15 minutes until the pressure is ≤10 mm Hg. Document the volume of CSF drained as well as the color and turbidity of the fluid.	too much CSF, which can cause complications.			
	Maintain MAP at ≥80 mm Hg.	MAP of 80 mm Hg has been associated with improved perfusion of the spinal cord. Strategies to support a MAP of ≥80 mm Hg should be implemented.	V	See Annotated Bibliography: 4, 5	
Prevention of Complications	Monitor the volume and color of CSF drainage.	Excessive CSF drainage can be dangerous, especially if drainage exceeds 20 mL/h.	II	See Other References: 2, 3, 5	Excessive CSF drainage has been reported to be associated with stretching and tearing of the dural veins, causing a subdural hematoma.
	Clarify activity orders with the physician. Getting the patient out of bed may result in dislocation or removal of the catheter.				
	Do not flush the system.	Flushing the system will introduce fluid into the intravertebral space, causing a marked increase in CSF pressure.			
Quality Control Issues	Appropriate reference.	The reference when zeroing must be consistent. Every 1 inch the system is off will result in a 2 mm Hg under- or overestimation of the pressure measurement.	V	See Other References: 6	
	Continuous monitoring of CSF pressure.	The CSF pressure can rise quickly, which results in neurologic deficit. Continuous monitoring allows for rapid identification of the increasing pressure. Generally, the system is removed 48 to 72 hours following surgery.			

ANNOTATED BIBLIOGRAPHY FOR THORACOABDOMINAL AORTIC ANEURYSM

1. Safi HJ, Hess KR, Randel M, et al. Cerebrospinal fluid and distal aortic perfusion: reducing neurologic complications in repair of thoracoabdominal aortic aneurysm types I and II. *J Vasc Surg*. 1996;23:223–229.

Study Sample

The sample included 94 patients undergoing thoracoabdominal aortic aneurysm (TAAA) repair between September 1992 and December 1994. All patients had spinal fluid drainage and distal aortic perfusion (DAP) perioperatively.

Comparison Studied

The purpose of the study was to evaluate the role of CSF drainage and DAP in the prevention of complications for patients who had undergone TAAA repair.

Study Procedures

The control group consisted of 42 patients who underwent TAAA repair with aortic cross clamping but without DAP and CSF drainage. Traditional procedures for surgical repair in both groups were performed, with the investigational group having DAP and CSF drainage.

Key Results

All patients in the study group survived the surgical procedure. Five patients (5%) had early neurologic deficits and 3% experienced late neurologic deficits. Mean CSF drainage was 45 mL during the surgical procedure and 94 mL postoperatively. When both groups were compared, 9% of the study group experienced neurologic complications while 19% of the control group experienced neurologic complications ($P = 0.090$). Those patients in both groups who had longer aortic cross clamp times (longer than 25 minutes) had higher risks of paraplegia.

Study Strengths and Weaknesses

This study demonstrated the value of CSF drainage and DAP in lowering the incidence of neurologic complications associated with TAAA repair. Previous studies had indicated the incidence ranging from 28% to 31% but this study lowered the rate to 9%. A limitation of this study was that it did not look at the effect of spinal fluid drainage alone.

Clinical Implications

These investigators demonstrated that CSF drainage and DAP contributed to a significant reduction of the incidence of neurologic complications following TAAA repair.

2. Ling E, Arellano R. Systematic review of the evidence supporting the use of cerebrospinal fluid drainage in thoracoabdominal aneurysm surgery for prevention of paraplegia. *Anesthesiology*. 2000;93:1115–1122.

Study Sample

Ling and Arellano conducted a computerized MEDLINE search from 1966 through March 1999 using the terms aortic aneurysm and thoracic surgery alone and combined with paraplegia and CSF. Additionally the "Thoracic Aorta" chapters in the *Yearbook in Vascular Surgery* series were reviewed from 1992 through 1998 for related articles. A total of 13 articles met the inclusion criteria and were reviewed.

Comparison Studied

The study's purpose was to provide a systematic review of the literature regarding the use of CSF drainage in patients undergoing surgical repair of thoracoabdominal aortic aneurysms.

Study Procedures

A blind review of the articles was conducted independently by two observers. Inclusion criteria were: (1) patients undergoing elective or emergent TAAA repair, (2) with intraoperative CSF drainage for spinal cord protection, (3) with postoperative neurologic deficits as outcomes, and (4) studies were designed as randomized controlled trials, nonrandomized trials with concurrent controls, nonrandomized trials with historical controls, and case series. Each article was assessed critically for these criteria by the reviewers; 13 were identified for review. Analysis of agreement between authors for inclusion was calculated using weighted κ statistics and was found to be 0.70. They were considered in good agreement if the κ score was between 0.6 and 0.8.

Key Results

Two randomized control trials were reviewed. One study, though well designed, failed to show CSF drainage would prevent paraplegia primarily because the CSF drainage was limited to 50 mL. The second study combined CSF drainage with intrathecal papaverine. That study was terminated early because of a statistically significant difference in the rate of postoperative neurologic deficits. The reviewer concluded that there was probably an error in the statistical calculations; therefore, there was no conclusion regarding the effects of CSF drainage on paraplegia. The other studies that were reviewed did not clearly demonstrate improved neurologic outcomes following TAAA repair.

Study Strengths and Weaknesses

A strength of this article was that the reviewers demonstrated the difficulty they experienced during this time frame while establishing the effects of CSF drainage on postoperative neurologic deficits. At the time of publication, CSF drainage was emerging as a potentially protective strategy for the spinal cord and there were few clinical trials in humans.

Clinical Implications

Ling and Arellano concluded that there was no strong evidence to support the use of CSF drainage for the prevention of spinal cord ischemia

3. **Estera AL, Miller CC, Huynh TTT, Porat E, Safi HJ. Neurologic outcome after thoracic and thoracoabdominal aortic aneurysm repair.** *Ann Thorac Surg.* 2001;72:1225–1231.

Study Sample

The sample included 654 patients who underwent TAAA repair or thoracic aneurysm repair between February 1991 and March 2000. Patient demographics included 420 males (64%) and 234 females (36%) with a mean age of 67 years (range 8–88 years).

Comparison Studied

The purpose of the study was to review one institution's experience with repair of thoracic and thoracoabdominal aortic aneurysms. A secondary purpose was to determine the effect of combined support of distal aortic perfusion and CSF drainage on neurologic outcome. Standard surgical repair was performed. Postoperatively, the MAP was maintained at 80 to 100 mm Hg. CSF was drained to maintain a CSF pressure of <10 mm Hg for 3 days. If a late neurologic symptom appeared after the drain was removed, the drain was immediately reinserted.

Key Results

The in-hospital mortality was 16% and incidence of neurologic deficits for all patients was 5.0% (33 of 654). Preoperative factors predicting neurologic deficits included a history of cerebrovascular disease and the extent of the aneurysm. The incidence of neurologic deficit for all aneurysm types was 3.3% when CSF drainage and distal aortic perfusion were combined. These were found to be protective against neurologic deficit ($P = 0.0001$). Delayed neurologic deficits occurred in 16 of 754 patients (2.4%). CSF drainage was used in 14 of the patients and resulted in improved neurologic status in 9 of the 16 patients (56%).

Study Strengths and Weaknesses

An improved neurologic outcome was associated with the use of CSF drainage. Limitations of the study include the fact that CSF drainage was not used alone during the perioperative period and, therefore, the full effect of CSF drainage on reducing neurologic deficits remained unknown. The positive effect of implementing CSF drainage immediately in those patients who developed late neurologic impairment was demonstrated; however, the number was small. The investigators noted another limitation in that the study was retrospective and additional factors related to surgical technique were not controlled.

Clinical Implications

This study supports the utilization of CSF drainage in this high risk group of surgical patients. Additionally, maintaining the MAP greater than 80 mm Hg as well as draining CSF to maintain spinal fluid pressures below 10 mm Hg were demonstrated to positively impact outcomes.

4. **Ackerman LL, Traynelis VC. Treatment of delayed-onset neurological deficit after aortic surgery with lumbar cerebrospinal fluid drainage.** *Neurosurgery.* 2002;51:1414–1422.

Study Sample

The sample included 6 patients who had TAAA repair without immediate postoperative neurologic deficits (motor or sensory). Their neurologic deficits presented between 12 and 40 hours postoperatively.

Comparison Studied

Six patients underwent surgical repair of TAAA. None of the 6 patients had signs or symptoms of any motor or sensory deficits preoperatively and in the immediate postoperative period. Five patients began demonstrating deficits between 12 and 40 hours postoperatively. All 5 experienced a hypotensive episode prior to the onset of the neurologic deficit. Following volume administration and initiation of vasoactive medications to achieve a MAP greater than 70 mm Hg, lumbar CSF drainage was begun. The sixth patient experienced the acute onset of back pain and was found to have a thrombus in the aorta.

Key Results

Two of the 5 patients had CSF drainage for several hours and did not improve while 3 of the 5 did have improvement in their neurologic deficit. The time of CSF drainage was from 15 to 72 hours. The CSF pressure was targeted to be kept <10 mm Hg. Ackerman and Traynelis concluded that CSF drainage may increase perfusion of the spinal cord. They suggested that rapid initiation of CSF drainage, when accompanied with measures to support blood pressure, may result in neurologic improvement in some patients.

Clinical Implications

These anecdotal cases demonstrate the need for patients undergoing surgical repair to have full neurologic assessments in the postoperative period. Additionally, in these cases, postoperative hypotension appeared to have a relationship to the onset of the deficits. Therefore, hypotensive events should be avoided if possible or treated aggressively when they occur. Of interest is that Ackerman and Traynelis reported that CSF drainage was the common denominator as successful treatment of delayed onset deficits in this group of patients. Based on these cases, a standard protocol was implemented to continue CSF drainage maintaining a spinal fluid pressure of <10 mm Hg for 2 days when treating delayed-onset neurologic deficits.

5. **Coselli JS, LeMaire SZ, Koksoy C, Schmittling ZC, Curling PE. Cerebrospinal fluid drainage reduces paraplegia after thoracoabdominal aortic aneurysm repair: results of a randomized clinical trial. *J Vasc Surg*. 2002;35: 631–639.**

Study Sample

After randomization, 145 patients (mean age 65.5 years) underwent thoracoabdominal aortic aneurysm repair.

Comparison Studied

The purpose of the randomized clinical trial was to evaluate the impact of cerebrospinal fluid drainage (CSFD) on the incidence of spinal cord injury after extensive thoracoabdominal aortic aneurysm repair.

Study Procedures

Initially, 156 patients met study criteria and were randomized following informed consent to either the control (74 patients, 47.4%) or the study (CSFD; 82 patients, 52.6%) group. All patients went through standardized operative techniques for this procedure and were consistent for spinal cord protection including hypothermia, heparinization, and aggressive reattachment of available critical intercostal and lumbar arteries. Additionally, the control group had CSFD. Patients in the control group had a 5F catheter introduced into the subarachnoid space at L3 or L4 intervertebral space. Following insertion, the catheter was connected to a pressure transducer and a drainage set. The "zero" reference point was leveled with the patient's spine. CSF was monitored continuously during the intraoperative and postoperative periods. CSF was permitted to drain freely whenever the CSF pressure exceeded 10 mm Hg. The CSF pressure was maintained at ≤10 mm Hg. The drain was removed on the second postoperative day in patients who did not have a neurologic injury. The drain was left in place for a longer period of time in patients with a neurologic deficit. Each patient's neurologic status was assessed daily, focusing on lower extremity motor functioning with respect to the ability of the patient to lift each leg off of the bed or observing ambulation (later in the recovery phase).

Key Results

Neurologic deficits (paralysis or paraparesis) occurred in 12.1% (9 of 74) of patients in the control group and 2.7% (2 of 84) patients in the CSFD group, which was an 80% reduction in the relative risk of paraplegia or paraparesis. Additionally, logistic regression curves indicated that the longer the spinal cord ischemic time, the greater the benefit derived from CSFD. In-hospital mortality rates were similar for both groups. The CSFD group had a mean of 64.1 mL ±42.9 mL CSF drained during surgery and 260.9 mL ±190.5 mL drained in the postoperative period. There was no difference in the volume of CSF drained during surgery between patients with and without neurologic injury. Two patients experienced occlusion of the spinal catheter during surgery and another patient's catheter became dislodged during transport to the ICU; these were not replaced. There were no other complications associated with the CSFD. The mean duration of CSFD was approximately 77 hours in those patients with neurologic injury and 42 hours in those patients without any neurologic deficits. These data indicate the rationale for CSFD during thoracoabdominal aortic aneurysm repair is based on the fact that CSF pressure increases during aortic clamping and reduction of CSF pressure is associated with improvement of spinal fluid pressure.

Study Strengths and Weaknesses

The strength of this study is that it focused solely on CSFD and the impact on neurologic deficits. Both groups were well matched with respect to risk for paralysis and all other perioperative interventions were used consistently. There were no limitations on the amount of CSF that could be drained to obtain a CSF pressure of ≤10 mm Hg. Interim analysis of study results after enrolling 156 patients indicated significant differences resulting in termination of the study.

This study had several limitations. The surgical team was not blinded to the treatment group primarily because CSFD requires active management. Those conducting the neurologic assessment postoperatively also were not blinded. The investigators suggest insertion of a spinal catheter without draining might have provided a more pure control group. CSF pressures were not collected during aortic clamping and other interventions which might have increased the understanding between surgical procedures and the effect on spinal pressures. Lastly, the study population was too small to determine if CSFD improves survival rates. A larger study would be required to make this determination.

OTHER REFERENCES FOR THORACOABDOMINAL AORTIC ANEURYSM

1. Azzizzadeh A, Huynh TTT, Miller CC, Safi HJ. Reversal of twice-delayed neurologic deficits with

cerebrospinal fluid drainage after thoracoabdominal aortic aneurysm repair: a case report and plea for national database collection. *J Vasc Surg.* 2000;31: 592–598.

2. Basauri LT, Conch-Julio E, Selman JM, et al. Cerebrospinal fluid spinal lumbar drainage: indications, technical tips, and pitfalls. *Crit Rev Neurosurg.* 1999;9:21–27.

3. Bethal SA. Use of lumbar cerebrospinal fluid drainage in thoracoabdominal aortic aneurysm repairs. *J Vasc Nurs.* 1999;17:53–58.

4. Coselli JS, LeMaire SA, Miller CC, et al. Mortality and paraplegia after thoracoabdominal aortic aneurysm repair: a risk factor analysis. *Ann Thorac Surg.* 2000;69:409–414.

5. Dardik A, Perler BA, Roseborough GS, Williams GM. Subdural hematoma after thoracoabdominal aortic aneurysm repair: an underreported complication of spinal fluid drainage. *J Vasc Surg.* 2002;36:47–50.

6. Darovic G. *Hemodynamic Monitoring: Invasive and Noninvasive Clinical Application*, 3rd ed. Philadelphia: WB Saunders; 2002.

7. Grabitz K, Sandamann W, Stumeier K, et al. The risk of ischemic spinal cord injury in patients undergoing graft replacements for thoracoabdominal aortic aneurysms. *J Vasc Surg.* 1996;23:230–240.

8. Guerit JM, Dion RA. State-of-the-art of neuromonitoring for prevention of immediate and delayed paraplegia in thoracic and thoracoabdominal aorta surgery. *Ann Thorac Surg.* 2002;74:S1867–S1869.

9. Huynh TTT, Miller CC, Estera AL, et al. Determinants of hospital length of stay after thoracoabdominal aortic aneurysm repair. *J Vasc Surg.* 2002; 35:648–653.

10. LeMaire SA, Miller CC, Conklin LD, Schmittling ZC, Coselli JS. Estimating group mortality and paraplegia rates after thoracoabdominal aortic aneurysm repair. *Ann Thorac Surg.* 2003;75:508–513.

11. Makkad B, Pilling S. Management of thoracic aneurysm. *Semin Cardiothorac Vasc Anesth.* 2005; 9:227–240.

12. Safi HJ, Winnerkvist A, Miller CC, et al. Effect of cross clamp time during thoracoabdominal aortic aneurysm repair. *Ann Thorac Surg.* 1998;66: 1204–1209.

13. Wada T, Yao H, Miyamoto S, Mukai, Yamamura M. Prevention and detection of spinal cord injury during thoracic and thoracoabdominal aortic repairs. *Ann Thorac Surg.* 2001;72:80–85.

Brain Oxygen Monitoring

Patricia A. Blissitt, RN, PhD, CCRN, CNRN, CCM, APRN, BC

CEREBRAL OXYGENATION

CASE STUDY

Mr J. is a 22-year-old man involved in a motor vehicle crash. His initial Glasgow Coma Scale (GCS) score was 7 (Eye Opening 2, Verbal Response 1, Motor Response 4). His pupils were 3 mm bilaterally and sluggishly reactive to light. He was intubated in the field. Computed tomography (CT) of the head revealed a left frontal lobe contusion. Systemic hemodynamic monitoring and multimodality cerebral monitoring were initiated upon arrival to the neuroscience intensive care unit (NICU). A triple bolt system with catheters to monitor intracranial pressure (ICP), cerebral perfusion pressure (CPP), brain tissue oxygen ($Pbto_2$), and brain temperature was placed in the left frontal lobe adjacent to the contusion. The $Pbto_2$ catheter was placed adjacent to the contusion as a monitor of regional cerebral oxygenation. His initial ICP and CPP values were 16 mm Hg and 72 mm Hg, respectively. His initial $Pbto_2$ stabilized at 24 mm Hg about 1.5 hours after insertion. A catheter was placed in the right jugular bulb as a monitor of global cerebral oxygenation. His initial jugular venous oxygen saturation ($Sjvo_2$) was 65%, with arteriojugular venous oxygen content difference ($AjvDo_2$) of 6 mL/dL, and cerebral extraction of oxygen (CEo_2) of 35%. Transcranial oximeter near infrared spectroscopy (NIRS) sensors were placed bilaterally on his forehead. The baseline regional oxygen saturation (rSo_2) indices were 66% on the right and 62% on the left.

Approximately 24 hours after admission, his ICP increased to 25 mm Hg and his CPP decreased to 64 mm Hg. The GCS score was 6 (Eye Opening 1, Verbal Response 1T, and Motor Response 4). Mannitol (25 g IV) was given, and continuous propofol (Diprivan; AstraZeneca, London, UK) was initiated for sedation. The ICP decreased to 12 mm Hg. However, CPP fell to 55 mm Hg; the $Pbto_2$ fell to 18 mm Hg; and the left rSo_2 decreased to 56% while the right rSo_2 was stable at 65%. The $Sjvo_2$ decreased to 60%; $AjvDo_2$ increased to 7 mL/dL; and the CEo_2 increased to 38%. The central venous pressure (CVP) was 5 mm Hg. A 250 mL bolus of 5% albumin and 500 mL bolus of normal saline were given and the maintenance IV was increased from 100 to 125 mL/h. His $Pbto_2$ increased to 22 mm Hg along with a rise in the CVP to 8 mm Hg. The CPP increased to 65 mm Hg. His intracranial dynamics were stable and within acceptable limits over the next 16 hours.

About 48 hours after the injury, Mr J.'s GCS score decreased to 5 (Eye Opening 1, Verbal Response 1T, Motor Response 3) and the ICP was refractory to mannitol and propofol and only temporarily decreased following several 30 mL boluses of 23.4% hypertonic saline. Pupils were 5 mm and nonreactive to light. His serum osmolality reached 322 mOsm and his serum sodium increased to 160 mg/dL. The $Sjvo_2$ was 82% with an $AjvDo_2$ of 3 mL/dL; CEo_2 decreased to 22%, and the $Pbto_2$ was 20 mm Hg. The right rSo_2 was 64% and left rSo_2 was 55%. CT revealed increased cerebral edema with midline shift but without evidence of hemorrhage or infarction. A diagnosis of hyperemia was supported by the $Sjvo_2$ data. The ventilator rate was increased from 12 to 16 breaths per minute, maintaining a partial pressure of oxygen (pO_2) of 100 to 110 mm Hg but decreasing partial pressure of carbon dioxide (pCO_2) from 35 to 30 mm Hg. His $Sjvo_2$ declined to 65%, $AjvDo_2$ increased to 5 mL/dL, ICP fell to 18 mm Hg, $Pbto_2$ increased to 24 mm Hg, and his left rSo_2

increased to 60%. The right rSo_2 remained stable at 63% to 65%. The pCO_2 was maintained at 30 to 32 mm Hg for the next 24 hours with a corresponding end-tidal CO_2 ranging between 29 and 33 mm Hg. The patient's intracranial dynamics stabilized over the next 24 hours, and mechanical ventilation rate was returned to 12 breaths per minute.

Over the next 2 days, Mr J.'s GCS score improved to 9 (Eye Opening 3, Verbal Response 1T, and Motor Response 5) and his pupils returned to 3 mm bilaterally and reactive to light. Over the next couple of weeks, Mr J. continued to improve and left the NICU with only minimal language deficits and a slightly weak right arm.

GENERAL DESCRIPTION

Three cerebral oxygen monitors are currently in use. Two devices, the $Pbto_2$ monitor and the transcranial cerebral oximeter (rSo_2), measure regional cerebral oxygenation. The third device, the $Sjvo_2$ monitor, is a measure of global cerebral oxygenation. While they may be used together, as in the case study presented earlier, each are described separately. Many research studies on transcranial cerebral oximetry (using NIRS) have been published. However, only the transcranial cerebral oximeter that is currently U.S. Food and Drug Administration-approved and commercially available is included in this discussion.

Brain Tissue Oxygen Monitoring

Brain tissue oxygen catheters provide a continuous quantitative measurement of local tissue oxygen partial pressure ($Pbto_2$).[1,2] Brain tissue extracts oxygen from the arterial blood. Oxygen is released from the hemoglobin into the brain tissue and measured as partial pressure. The highest brain tissue oxygen is in neuron-rich areas close to penetrating blood vessels such as the cortex and hippocampus.[3] The lowest $Pbto_2$ is in the white matter or axons. Until recently, 2 $Pbto_2$ monitoring systems were commercially available: the Licox (Integra NeuroSciences, Plainsboro, NJ) and the Neurotrend (Johnson and Shurtleff, Rayham, MA). The Neurotrend monitoring system is no longer manufactured.[4]

The Licox monitoring system uses a polarographic Clark-type electrode on the tip of a flexible microcatheter, 0.8 mm in diameter.[5,6] Oxygen diffuses from the brain tissue through the polyethylene-coated catheter wall. After diffusing through the catheter wall, the oxygen passes into an inner electrolyte chamber where the partial pressure of oxygen (Pao_2) is converted to a current between a cathode and an anode (Figure 4-1).[2,7,8] The amount of current is proportional to the $Pbto_2$ and is displayed in mm Hg (Figure 4-2). The catheter detects tissue oxygen in a surface area of 18 mm^2 on the probe.[8] The Licox catheter also monitors brain tissue temperature.[8]

In contrast, the Neurotrend monitoring system used an optical luminescence microcatheter.[5] The optical sensor on the fiberoptic catheter had dye embedded on a plastic matrix. Depending on the partial pressure of the surrounding brain tissue, the dye changed its light transmission and reflectance properties to quantify the brain tissue oxygen tension.[2] The Pao_2 values of the Neurotrend catheter were also displayed in mm Hg. The Neurotrend catheter was multiparameteric, monitoring the partial pressure of brain tissue carbon dioxide ($Pbtco_2$), brain tissue pH, and temperature as well as $Pbto_2$.[1,2] The catheter was 0.5 mm in diameter. The Neurotrend monitoring system was developed from the Paratrend monitoring system, which was originally used for continuous arterial blood gas monitoring.[4]

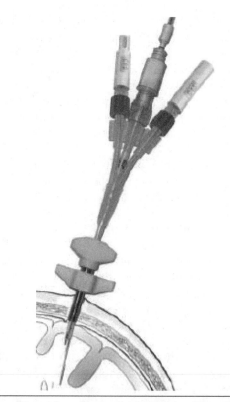

Figure 4-2   Licox brain tissue oxygen ($Pbto_2$) catheter inserted into white matter of the brain.

Source: © Integra LifeSciences Corporation 2006. Compliments of Integra LifeSciences.

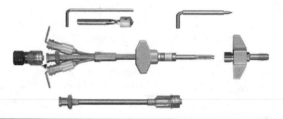

Figure 4-1   Licox brain tissue oxygen ($Pbto_2$) catheter through triple bolt.

Source: © Integra LifeSciences Corporation 2006. Compliments of Integra LifeSciences.

Because the Licox and Neurotrend monitoring systems employed different technologies, ischemic thresholds were not the same. Using xenon-CT as the standard by which the Neurotrend catheter was compared, an ischemic threshold of 18 mL/100 g/min of cerebral blood flow (CBF) by xenon-CT had been found to correlate with a Neurotrend Pbto$_2$ of 22 mm Hg.[5,9] In contrast, the ischemic threshold for jugular venous oxygenation saturation (Sjvo$_2$) of 50% was found to correspond with a Licox Pbto$_2$ of 8.5 mm Hg.[5,9] Investigators disagreed in regard to ischemic thresholds for each catheter.[5,10] Normal brain tissue oxygen values for the 2 systems differed as well. Normal Pbto$_2$ using the Licox monitoring system is 20 to 35 mm Hg and was 35 to 50 mm Hg for the Neurotrend monitoring system.[4,11]

Because of the heterogeneity of CBF and metabolism within the brain, normal values depend on the location of the probe as well. Recommendation for placement of the Licox catheter is in the frontal white matter, 2 to 3 cm below the dura.[8] A CT scan is recommended to verify correct placement. The Licox catheter must be stored in a cool temperature between 2°C and 10°C.[8] The Licox catheter is also precalibrated. Each Licox probe has its own calibration "smart" card that includes data for use with that particular catheter only (Figure 4-3).[8]

The Pbto$_2$ sensor on the Neurotrend catheter was not on the tip of the catheter, but 2.5 mm from the distal end, which meant the depth of insertion had to be greater for correct placement in the white matter.[6] Like the Licox catheter, the Neurotrend catheter was inserted into the brain through a bolt that was screwed into the skull. The triple bolt system for the Licox catheter also may include an ICP catheter, a separate temperature probe, and a microdialysis catheter. A more recent version of the Licox can be tunneled through the scalp and does not require a bolt.

ACCURACY

Both the Licox and Neurotrend monitoring systems have been deemed accurate and reliable when the manufacturers' instructions are followed. In one study, the Licox monitoring system was found to be more accurate during low Pbto$_2$ values and exhibited less drift. No catheter or monitoring system malfunctions occurred. The Neurotrend monitoring system was found to have a faster response time in regard to change in Pbto$_2$ following an intervention. However the Neurotrend system was found to malfunction more.[6] The Licox system requires an equilibration period of 20 minutes to 2 hours before values are considered accurate.[12] The time of good quality data has been found to be 99.2%.[2]

Both monitoring systems were found to be safe based on recent research. The complication rate has been 0% to 3%. Microhemorrhages and edema may occur with placement

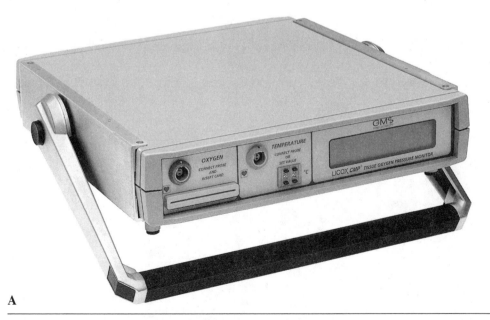
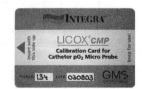

A   **B**

Figure 4-3   (A) Licox brain tissue oxygen (Pbto$_2$) monitor. (B) Calibration "smart" card.

Source: © Integra LifeSciences Corporation 2006. Compliments of Integra LifeSciences.

but do not require treatment and do not alter $Pbto_2$ results.[13] A contraindication to the insertion of the probe is systemic coagulopathy. Accidental removal and broken catheters and cables are the most frequent technical issues, but another potential concern is infection. However, the infection rate has repeatedly been reported as 0%.[4]

COMPETENCY

Competent monitoring of $Pbto_2$ requires knowledge of neuroanatomy and physiology, intracranial dynamics, and pathophysiology of neurologic injury. In addition, the critical care nurse must be able to correlate the $Pbto_2$ data with neurologic assessment and other physiologic parameters to develop a comprehensive approach to the care of the critically ill neuroscience patient.

ETHICAL CONSIDERATIONS

Ethical considerations include utilizing current research findings and any available consensus statements to maximize the benefit to risk ratio for a particular patient. $Pbto_2$ monitoring may not be an ethical option for every brain-injured patient with a poor prognosis. Other concomitant injuries and diagnoses must be considered. Placement in neurologically intact patients also presents an ethical dilemma. Though considered safe, introduction of the bolt and catheter causes local brain and skull trauma and places the patient at risk for infection.

OCCUPATIONAL HAZARDS

Other than a risk of exposure to body fluids and the usual electrical hazards present with all critical care technology, $Pbto_2$ monitoring does not have any associated occupational hazards. Insertion of the catheter requires sterile technique, so those performing or assisting with insertion should be wearing a gown, gloves, face mask, and eyeglasses or goggles.

FUTURE RESEARCH

Multicenter prospective randomized controlled trials are needed to establish the optimal location, goal parameters, and ischemic thresholds for the different monitoring systems and specific patient populations. Duration of ischemia must be considered as well. One potential area of research already underway is the role of hyperoxia in the management of cerebral ischemia, beneficial or harmful.[14] Additional research in the area of $Pbto_2$ monitoring includes optimal monitoring of acute ischemic stroke, triple H therapy in the management of aneurysmal subarachnoid hemorrhage vasospasm, and correlation with microdialysis. Other biomarkers in acute brain injury are needed as well.

JUGULAR VENOUS OXYGEN SATURATION MONITORING

DESCRIPTION

Jugular venous oxygen saturation is a measurement of global cerebral oxygen supply and demand. $Sjvo_2$ may be measured intermittently by withdrawing blood from a central venous catheter positioned in the bulb of the jugular vein and sending it to a lab for co-oximetric analysis. However, continuous monitoring of the jugular bulb is also available through in vivo reflectance oximetry using a fiberoptic catheter. This technology is analogous to systemic mixed venous oxygen saturation monitoring from the pulmonary artery.[15] The $Sjvo_2$ catheter is positioned in the bulb of the jugular vein, at the base of the skull medial to the mastoid process above the interspace between C1 and C2 (Figure 4-4).[15]

Two monitoring systems have been used, the Edslab Sat II (Baxter Edwards Critical Care Division, Irvine, CA) and the Abbott Labs Oximetrix III (Abbott Park, IL). In both instances, the technology is based on oxyhemoglobin's unique light absorption spectrum.[15–17] The Edslab system uses 2 wavelengths of light and the Abbott Critical Care system uses 3 wavelengths of light. Both catheters have a cable that directs fiberoptic light to the blood, which is reflected back to the second fiberoptic cable. The light is then transferred to a photosensor that measures the absorp-

tion of the reflected light at various waveforms. $Sjvo_2$ is expressed as the percentage of the oxygenated hemoglobin to the percentage of total hemoglobin. Fiberoptic jugular venous oxygen catheters containing 2 waveforms require manual entry of the hemoglobin into the monitor for the $Sjvo_2$ to be valid. Fiberoptic jugular venous oxygen catheters with a third wavelength automatically determines the hemoglobin from the absorption spectrum.[16,18]

Normal $Sjvo_2$ values are 55% to 70%. A *decrease* in $Sjvo_2$ is the result of an increase in oxygen extraction or a decrease in delivery of oxygen to the cerebral tissues. An *increase* in $Sjvo_2$ is the result of a decrease in oxygen extraction or an increase in delivery of oxygen to the cerebral tissues.[5,7] A derived parameter, the $AjvDo_2$ is an indirect measure of CBF.[12] Normal $AjvDo_2$ ranges from 4 to 8 mL/dL.[19] If the $AjvDo_2$ is less than 4 mL/dL, the delivery is greater than the extraction of oxygen. If the $AjvDo_2$ is greater than 8 mL/dL, the extraction of oxygen is greater than the delivery. An elevated $Sjvo_2$ and a low $AjvDo_2$ may be the result of hyperemia. A low $Sjvo_2$ and high $AjvDo_2$ may be an indication of ischemia. The ischemic threshold is approximately 50%.[16,20] Subtracting the $Sjvo_2$ from the oxygen saturation (Sao_2) provides an estimate of the CEo_2 with normal ranging from 24% to 42%.[12,21] A CEo_2 less than 24% is indicative of hyperemia while a CEo_2 greater than 42% suggests ischemia.[5]

ACCURACY

$Sjvo_2$ is considered an accurate measure of global cerebral oxygenation. However, a number of factors may affect values. Correlation between the cerebral oximetry catheter and jugular bulb blood specimen analysis by co-oximetry has been found to be poor.[5,16,19] Two factors that can affect accuracy include the position of the catheter and the rate of blood withdrawal from the catheter. The signal quality intensity may be poor if the catheter is against the wall of the blood vessel or extracerebral contamination may occur if the catheter is out from the jugular bulb as little as 2 cm.[15] Withdrawal of blood from the catheter at a rate faster than 2 mL/min may result in extracerebral contamination and a 3% or greater inaccuracy in the value.[22] Recalibration of the oximetry catheter is frequently necessary. Side of placement of the catheter is controversial.[15]

Though considered relatively safe, a number of complications are associated with jugular bulb catheterization, including: carotid artery injury, infection, nerve injury, pneumothorax, and jugular thrombosis.[3] Routine ultrasound of the neck veins after discontinuation of $Sjvo_2$ monitoring is recommended to minimize complications.[23] The risk of infection increases with duration of monitoring, particularly beyond 5 to 7 days. The complication rate is reported at 1% to 3%.[16,20] If carotid artery puncture occurs, pressure at the site for 10 minutes is generally sufficient. Contraindications to $Sjvo_2$ monitoring include cervical spine injury,

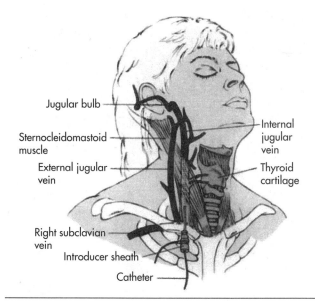

Figure 4-4 Jugular venous oxygen saturation ($Sjvo_2$) catheter in bulb of internal jugular vein.

Source: Schell RM, Cole DJ. Cerebral monitoring: jugular venous oximetry. *Anesth Analg.* 2000;90:559–566. Used with permission from Elsevier.

coagulopathy, neck trauma, impairment of cerebral venous drainage, and tracheostomy. Care must be taken during insertion to minimize increases in ICP with neck manipulation.[3]

COMPETENCY

Competent monitoring of $Sjvo_2$ monitoring requires knowledge of neuroanatomy and physiology, intracranial dynamics, and pathophysiology of neurologic injury. In addition, the critical care nurse must be able to correlate the $Sjvo_2$ data with neurologic assessment and other physiologic parameters to develop a comprehensive approach to the care of the critically ill neuroscience patient.

ETHICAL CONSIDERATIONS

Ethical considerations include utilizing current research findings and any available consensus statements to determine the benefit/risk ratio for a particular patient. $Sjvo_2$ monitoring may not be an ethical option for the patient with a poor prognosis. Concomitant illness and injury must be considered. $Sjvo_2$ monitoring has been used intraoperatively during neurosurgical and cardiac procedures to monitor for cerebral ischemia in neurologically intact patients. Placement in neurologically intact patients also presents an ethical dilemma. Insertion of a jugular bulb catheter is not without potential risks and these risks must be considered.

OCCUPATIONAL HAZARDS

Other than a risk of exposure to body fluids and the usual electrical hazards present with all critical care technology, $Sjvo_2$ monitoring does not have any occupational hazards associated with it. Insertion of the catheter requires a sterile technique, so those performing or assisting with insertion should wear a gown, gloves, face mask, and eyeglasses or goggles. Universal precautions to minimize risk of blood exposure should be followed as well when jugular blood specimens are drawn for calibration or comparison or when the catheter is discontinued.

FUTURE RESEARCH

Areas for future research in regard to jugular venous saturation monitoring include large well-designed prospective randomized controlled trials in regard to side of placement when $Sjvo_2$ monitoring is used alone or in conjunction with $Pbto_2$ or rSo_2, and correlation with other neurophysiologic monitoring. A study focusing on the importance of duration of desaturation in the presence of normal brain and various neurologic illnesses or injuries is warranted also.[12] A safety and efficacy study of controlled hyperventilation to manage refractory increased ICP utilizing $Sjvo_2$ monitoring or simultaneous $Sjvo_2$ and $Pbto_2$ monitoring is also needed.

TRANSCRANIAL CEREBRAL OXIMETRY MONITORING

GENERAL DESCRIPTION

Transcranial cerebral oximetry, also known as transcranial NIRS, is based on the general principle that as near infrared light penetrates brain tissue, it is absorbed differently by oxygenated and deoxygenated hemoglobin.[24] Transcranial NIRS monitors use different technology and algorithms and are therefore not comparable. In the United States only the INVOS (IN Vivo Optical Spectroscopy) cerebral oximeter (Somanetics, Inc, Troy MI) is U.S. Food and Drug Administration-approved and commercially available.[12,24]

The INVOS cerebral monitor transmits light in fiberoptic bundles (optodes) through the skull and into the frontal cerebral cortex. A proximal electrode detects light absorbed by hemoglobin in extracranial tissue and a distal electrode detects light absorbed by hemoglobin in both extracranial and intracranial tissue. The monitor subtracts the difference between the extracranial tissue and the combined extracranial and intracranial tissue to determine the intracranial tissue light absorption (Figure 4-5). The monitor determines the ratio of oxygenated hemoglobin to the total hemoglobin to display a numerical value, the rSo_2 index (Figure 4-6). The range of rSo_2 detectable by the monitor is from 15% to 95%.[25] Several models of the INVOS monitor have been developed, the earlier ones with only one sensor. The 5100 model has bilateral adhesive sensors that are attached to the right and left of the midline of the forehead (Figure 4-7). Sensors are available for children (0 to 40 kg) and adults;[24] they are not interchangeable, as children have thinner skulls and different extracranial tissues than adults and the algorithm for detecting the pediatric rSo_2 is different.[25] Unlike systemic oxygen saturation monitors that also use NIRS technology, transcranial NIRS does not rely on a pulsatile signal. Therefore, it can be used during extracorporeal circulation (cardiopulmonary bypass) and extracorporeal membrane life support (eg, ECLS and ECMO).[24]

ACCURACY

Much has been written about the questionable accuracy of transcranial NIRS and its value as a cerebral oxygenation monitor continues to be studied.[5,12,24,26–28] A number of factors must be kept in mind when using transcranial NIRS. It is a trends monitor so assessment and management of cerebral oxygenation must be based on changes from the patient's baseline not on an absolute range of normal value. However, a change in rSo_2 from 20% to 30% from the baseline or by 12 to 20 points (%) has been correlated with neurologic deterioration. An rSo_2 (index) of <50% has been associated with a poor outcome.[24,25,27,29]

Though the contribution of venous (deoxygenated hemoglobin) to arterial blood (oxygenated hemoglobin) has been found to be a 75%:25% ratio, variation as much as 85%:15% has been found.[27] NIRS can only assess cerebral tissue 2 to 3 cm beyond the cortex and, therefore, may not detect intraparenchymal ischemia in the posterior aspect of the frontal lobes or the other lobes of the cerebrum. Interfering factors such as extracranial blood, extra-axial hematomas, and cerebral infarction may limit its efficacy to detect cerebral ischemia. The use of CT scan to aid in placement of the sensor is recommended.[26,30]

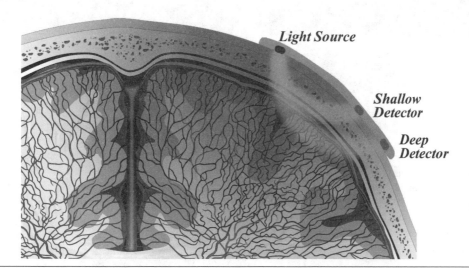

Light Source

Shallow Detector

Deep Detector

Figure 4-5   Extracranial (shallow) and intracranial (deep) detection of infrared light absorption with INVOS NIRS transcranial cerebral oxygen (rSo_2) monitor. The INVOS cerebral monitor determines the intracranial tissue light absorption by subtracting the extracranial tissue and combined extracranial and intracranial tissue light absorption.

Source: Used with permission of Somanetics Corporation, Troy, MI.

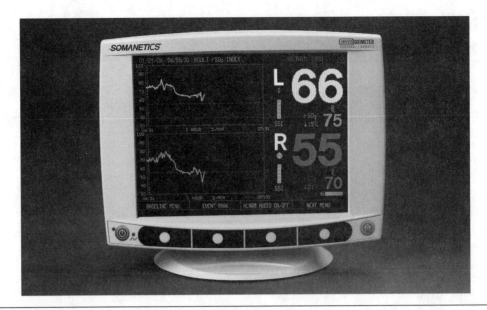

Figure 4-6   INVOS NIRS transcranial cerebral oxygen (rSo₂) monitor.
The ratio of oxygenated hemoglobin to total hemoglobin is displayed as the rSo₂ index on the right, while it is tracked over time on the left.

Source: Used with permission of Somanetics Corporation, Troy, MI.

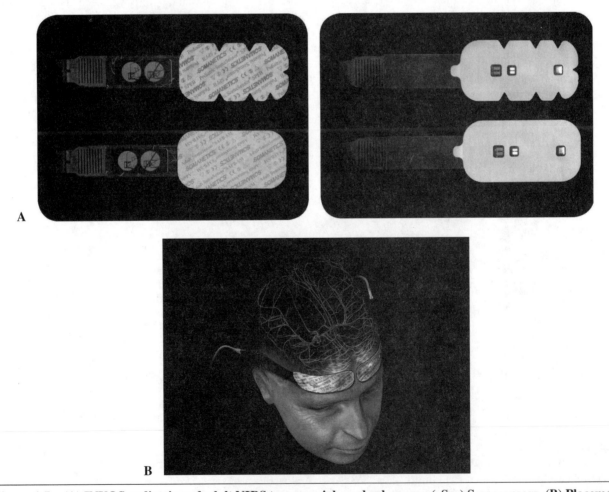

Figure 4-7   (A) INVOS pediatric and adult NIRS transcranial cerebral oxygen (rSo₂) Somasensors. (B) Placement of Somasensors.

Source: Used with permission of Somanetics Corporation, Troy, MI.

COMPETENCY

Competent monitoring of transcranial near infrared spectroscopy requires knowledge of neuroanatomy and physiology, intracranial dynamics, and pathophysiology of neurologic injury. In addition, the critical care nurse must be able to correlate the transcranial cerebral oximetry data with neurologic assessment and other physiologic parameters to develop a comprehensive approach to the care of the critically ill neuroscience patient.

ETHICAL CONSIDERATIONS

Current research findings and any available consensus statements should be used to determine the benefit for a particular patient. Though the technology has few potential adverse effects, its accuracy has been repeatedly questioned. Until definitive research is completed, the clinician must be cautious when using transcranial cerebral oximetry to assess and manage a neurologically intact or neurologically injured patient. Data from transcranial cerebral oximetry must be considered in conjunction with other assessment modalities.

OCCUPATIONAL HAZARDS

Other than the usual electrical hazards present with all critical care technology, transcranial cerebral oximetry monitoring does not have any additional associated occupational hazards.

FUTURE RESEARCH

Because transcranial NIRS is a trends monitor and an absolute range of normal values for all patients cannot be used to assess and guide therapy, additional research is warranted regarding the detection of critical rSo_2, percentage from baseline, and duration of those values indicative of ischemia for the individual patient with and without a neurologic injury. One particular area of research where NIRS might be promising would be in the detection of cerebral vasospasm following aneurysmal subarachnoid hemorrhage. A cerebral blood volume index can be calculated by the INVOS cerebral oximeter for research purposes but is not currently approved for standard care.

Indocyanine green dye can be intravenously injected as a tracer to assist in determining an estimate of CBF using transcranial NIRS.[31,32] Further development of the technology, such as multiple channels for monitoring the temporal, parietal, and occipital lobes, might provide more insight into the value of this technology.

REFERENCES

1. Rose JC, Neill TA, Hemphill JC. Continuous monitoring of the microcirculation in neurocritical care: an update on brain tissue oxygenation. *Curr Opin Crit Care.* 2006;12:97–102.
2. Mulvey JM, Dorsch NWC, Mudaliar Y, Lang EW. Multimodality monitoring in severe traumatic brain injury. The role of brain tissue oxygenation monitoring. *Neurocrit Care.* 2004;1:391–402.
3. Sarrafzadeh A, Kiening KL, Unterberg AW. Neuromonitoring: brain oxygenation and microdialysis. *Curr Neurol Neurosci Rep.* 2003;3:517–523.
4. Nortje J, Gupta AK. The role of tissue oxygen monitoring in patients with acute brain injury. *Br J Anaesth.* 2006;97:95–106.
5. DeGeorgia M, Deogaonkar A. Multimodal monitoring in the neurological intensive care unit. *Neurologist.* 2005;11:45–54.
6. Smythe PR, Samra SK. Monitors of cerebral oxygenation. *Anesthesiol Clin North Am.* 2002;20: 293–313.
7. Dunn, IF, Ellegala, DB, Kim DH, et al. Neuromonitoring in neurological critical care. *Neurocrit Care.* 2006;4:83–92.
8. Integra Neurosciences. Licox IMC Directions for Use. Plainsboro NJ: Integra NeuroSciences; 2004.
9. Doppenberg EM, Zauner A, Bullock R, et al. Correlations between brain tissue oxygen tension, carbon dioxide tension, pH, and cerebral blood flow: a better way of monitoring the severely injured brain. *Surg Neurol.* 1998;49;650–654.
10. Kiening KL, Unterberg AW, Bardt TF, et al. Monitoring of cerebral oxygenation in patients with severe head injuries: brain tissue pO_2 versus jugular vein oxygen saturation. *J Neurosurg.* 1996;85:751–757.
11. Hoffman WE, Charbel FT, Edelman G, et al. Thiopental and desflurane treatment for brain protection. *Neurosurgery.* 1998;43:1050–1053.
12. Springborg JB, Friedericksen H-J, Eskesen V, et al. Trends in monitoring patients with aneurysmal subarachnoid hemorrhage. *Br J Anesth.* 2005;94:259–270.
13. Hemphill JC, Morabito D, Farrant M, et al. Brain tissue oxygen monitoring in intracerebral hemorrhage. *Neurocrit Care.* 2005;3:260–270.
14. Magnoni S, Ghisoni L, Locatelli M, et al. Lack of improvement in cerebral metabolism after hyperoxia in severe head injury: a microdialysis study. *J Neurosurg.* 2003;98:952–958.
15. Schell RM, Cole DJ. Cerebral monitoring: jugular venous oximetry. *Anesth Analg.* 2000;90:559–566.

16. Feldman Z, Robertson CS. Monitoring of cerebral hemodynamics with jugular bulb catheters. *Crit Care Clin.* 1997;13:51–77.

17. White H, Baker A. Continuous jugular venous oximetry in the neurointensive care unit—a brief review. *Can J Anaesth.* 2002;49:623–629.

18. Gopinath SO, Valadka A, Uzura M, et al. Comparison of jugular venous oxygen saturation and brain tissue pO_2 as monitors of cerebral ischemia after head injury. *Crit Care Med.* 1999;27:2337–2345.

19. De Deyne C, Van Aken J, Decruyenaere J, et al. Jugular bulb oximetry: review on a cerebral monitoring technique. *Acta Anaesthesiol Belg.* 1998;49: 21–31.

20. Mayberg TS, Lam AM. Jugular bulb oximetry for the monitoring of cerebral blood flow and metabolism. *Neurosurg Clin North Am.* 1996;7:755–765.

21. Cruz J. Relationship between early patterns of cerebral extraction of oxygen and outcome from severe acute traumatic brain swelling: cerebral ischemia or cerebral viability. *Crit Care Med.* 1996;24:953–956.

22. Matta BF, Lam AM. The rate of blood withdrawal affects the accuracy of jugular venous bulb: oxygen saturation measurements. *Anesthesiology.* 1997;86: 806–808.

23. Coplin WM, O'Keefe GE, Grady MS, et al. Thrombotic, infectious, and procedural complications of the jugular bulb catheter in the intensive care unit. *Neurosurgery.* 1997;41:101–107.

24. Tobias JD. Cerebral oxygenation monitoring: near-infrared spectroscopy. *Expert Rev Med Devices.* 2006; 3:235–243.

25. Somanetics. Principles of Operation, INVOS Frequently Asked Questions, and Clinical Center. Troy, MI: Somanetics; 2006. Available at: http://www .somanetics.com. Accessed August 20, 2007.

26. Andrews RJ. Monitoring for neuroprotection. New technologies for the new millennium. *Ann NY Acad Sci.* 2001;939:101–113.

27. Fraser CD, Andropoulos D. Neurologic monitoring for special cardiopulmonary bypass techniques. *Semin Thorac Cardiovasc Surg Pediatr Card Surg Annu.* 2004;7:125–132.

28. Taillefer MC, Denault AY. Cerebral near-infrared spectroscopy in adult heart surgery: systematic review of its clinical efficacy. *Can J Anaesth.* 2005;52: 79–87.

29. Robson MJA, Alston RP, Deary IJ, et al. Jugular bulb oxyhemoglobin desaturation, S100B, and neurologic and cognitive outcomes after coronary artery surgery. *Anesth Analg.* 2001;93:839–845.

30. Nemoto EM, Yonas H, Kassam A. Clinical experiences with cerebral oximetry in stroke and cardiac arrest. *Crit Care Med.* 2000;28:1052–1054.

31. Hongo K, Kobayashi S, Okudera H, et al. Noninvasive cerebral optical spectroscopy: depth-resolved measurements of cerebral haemodynamics using indocyanine green. *Neurol Res.* 1997;17:89–93.

32. Keller E, Ishihara H, Nadler A, et al. Evaluation of brain toxicity following near infrared light exposure after indocyanine green dye injection. *J Neurosci Meth.* 2002;117:23–31.

CLINICAL RECOMMENDATIONS FOR BRAIN TISSUE OXYGENATION MONITORING

The rating scales for the Level of Recommendation column range from I to VI, with levels indicated as follows: I, manufacturer's recommendation only; II, theory based, no research data to support recommendations; recommendations from expert consensus group may exist; III, laboratory data only, no clinical data to support recommendations; IV, limited clinical studies to support recommendations; V, clinical studies in more than 1 or 2 different populations and situations to support recommendations; VI, clinical studies in a variety of patient populations and situations to support recommendations.

Period of Use	Recommendation	Rationale for Recommendation	Level of Recommendation	Supporting References	Comments
Patient Selection	Recommended in patients with the following neurologic diagnoses:		IV		
	Patients at risk for regional cerebral hypoxia including those with:	Following neurologic insult, the patient is at risk for secondary neuronal injury related to ischemia. Loss of adequate blood flow results in hypoxia. Cerebral hypoxia leads to an influx of intracellular calcium, increased release of glutamate, formation of free radicals, and other molecular disturbances that may permanently injure or destroy neurons. $Pbto_2$ monitoring may detect regional hypoxia and guide interventions to improve oxygenation before permanent injury or neuronal death occurs.			
	1. Acute severe traumatic brain injury (GCS score ≤8).			See References: 1–7 See Other References: 112 See Annotated Bibliography: 2, 8–10, 13, 17, 19–21, 30, 32, 33, 35	
	2. Aneurysmal subarachnoid hemorrhage.			See References: 1–3, 5, 6, 12 See Other References: 6, 10, 13–15 See Annotated Bibliography: 9, 26, 28, 31	
	3. Brain tumor.			See Other References: 16	
	4. Spontaneous intracerebral hemorrhage.			See References: 13	
	5. Normal pressure hydrocephalus.			See References: 1	
	$Pbto_2$ monitoring also may be used to detect regional hypoxia and guide and monitor the efficacy of therapy in the following clinical situations:				
	1. Children with severe traumatic brain injury.	Following severe traumatic brain injury, both children and adults may experience regional	IV	See Annotated Bibliography: 22, 33, 35	

Period of Use	Recommendation	Rationale for Recommendation	Level of Recommendation	Supporting References	Comments
Patient Selection (cont.)		cerebral hypoxia. Pediatric cerebral hypoxia may respond to similar interventions used in adults, including ventilator management (increasing fraction of inspired oxygen [F_{IO_2}]), inotrope administration, and blood transfusion.			
	2. Intraoperatively during craniotomy for brain tumor, ruptured and nonruptured cerebral aneurysm, and during temporary clipping of the parent vessel during resection of an arteriovenous malformation or aneurysm.	The pharmacologic effects of anesthesia on: cerebral metabolism and CBF, systemic oxygenation, and alterations in blood pressure in association with blood loss and manipulation of brain tissue and blood vessels during surgical procedures may result in cerebral hypoxia.	IV	See References: 5, 6, 11, 12 See Other References: 17, 18	
	3. Assist with the determination of brain death.	Absence of cerebral blood flow in brain death results in cerebral anoxia.	IV	See Annotated Bibliography: 23	
	4. During cardiopulmonary resuscitation (CPR) in patients being monitored prior to CPR.	Brain tissue oxygen monitoring during CPR may indicate adequacy of cerebral perfusion.	IV	See Other References: 3	
	$Pbto_2$ may be used to monitor the effects of the following interventions on regional cerebral oxygenation:				
	1. Cerebral perfusion management (manipulation of mean arterial pressure [MAP] and/or ICP)	While $Pbto_2$ and cerebral perfusion monitoring do not measure the same parameters, increasing CPP and MAP may increase blood flow, particularly in impaired autoregulation. With impaired cerebral autoregulation, increasing the MAP or decreasing the ICP, an increase in CBF may passively follow resulting in an increase in $Pbto_2$.	IV	See References: 1, 2, 6 See Other References: 1, 4, 19 See Annotated Bibliography: 32	Neurologic injury results in varying degrees of impaired autoregulation. Autoregulation is also impaired in chronic hypertension, a major risk factor for stroke.
	2. Increase F_{IO_2}	Increasing the F_{IO_2} will supply much needed oxygen to damaged brain tissue.	IV	See References: 1, 2 See Other References: 7, 19 See Annotated Bibliography: 21, 22	
	3. Controlled hyperventilation in the management of increased ICP.	A decrease in the partial pressure of systemic carbon dioxide results in cerebral vasoconstriction, which decreases intracranial blood	IV	See Other References: 20 See Annotated Bibliography: 8, 9, 35	Brain tissue oxygenation monitoring is recommended as an option rather than a standard or guideline

Period of Use	Recommendation	Rationale for Recommendation	Level of Recommendation	Supporting References	Comments
Patient Selection *(cont.)*		volume. A decrease in cerebral blood volume will decrease ICP and increase CPP. However, this vasoconstriction also may result in cerebral hypoxia.			(based on Class III evidence with I being the highest degree of certainty and III being the lowest) in the *Management and Prognosis of Severe Traumatic Brain Injury* (See Other References: 20).
	4. Red blood cell transfusion.	Increasing the hematocrit/hemoglobin, increases the blood's oxygen-carrying capacity, which may increase $Pbto_2$.	IV	See Other References: 19 See Annotated Bibliography: 26	
	5. Decompressive hemicraniectomy for refractory increased ICP.	Decreasing the ICP increases the CPP and the CBF which results in an increased $Pbto_2$.	IV	See Annotated Bibliography: 29	
	6. Controlled hypothermia.	Brain temperature has been demonstrated to inversely correlate with $Pbto_2$. Hypothermia decreases cerebral metabolic demand.	IV	See References: 1 See Other References: 11	
	$Pbto_2$ monitoring may be used to detect regional hypoxia and guide and monitor the effectiveness of the following therapies in cerebral vasospasm following aneurysmal subarachnoid hemorrhage:				
	1. Hypertensive hypervolemic hemodilution therapy.	Increasing the MAP or CPP may improve CBF through constricted blood vessels.	IV	See References: 1, 12	
	2. Nimodipine administration.	Despite evidence to support improved outcomes with nimodipine, it is associated with a decrease in $Pbto_2$ independent of blood pressure.	IV	See References: 1 See Annotated Bibliography: 28	
	3. Angioplasty.	Dilation of vasospastic cerebral vessels improves regional oxygen delivery.	IV	See References: 5	
	4. Intra-arterial administration of papaverine.	While intra-arterial papaverine is an arterial vasodilator, a decrease in $Pbto_2$ may occur in other vessels related to the increase in CBF to the vessel receiving papaverine.	IV	See Annotated Bibliography: 31	

Period of Use	Recommendation	Rationale for Recommendation	Level of Recommendation	Supporting References	Comments
Insertion of Device and Initial Use	The brain tissue oxygen monitor may be placed on: 1. The side of the pathology but in viable tissue. 2. The side of the greater injury as a measure of regional cerebral hypoxia. 3. Either side in diffuse injury. 4. The uninjured side as measure of cerebral oxygenation in healthy tissue.	Regional measurement of $Pbto_2$ in areas of potential ischemia may provide early detection and prompt intervention for ischemia before infarction occurs. Neuronal death is irreversible, and insertion in infarcted tissue will not guide therapy for viable tissue. Regional measurement of oxygenation on the uninjured side may provide an indication of the effect of interventions on healthy tissue and prevent additional harm.	IV	See References: 1, 6, 8 See Annotated Bibliography: 13, 25 See Other References: 19	 Use of the $Pbto_2$ monitor as representative of the uninjured portion of brain is controversial as the $Pbto_2$ catheter only measures cerebral oxygen in a small area.
	Place the $Pbto_2$ monitor in the frontal white matter.	The greater cerebral metabolic rate and blood flow of the cortex will result in a higher $Pbto_2$.	IV	See References: 1–3	
	Verify placement of the oxygen monitor by noncontrast brain CT.	CT scan verifies that the $Pbto_2$ catheter is in the white matter rather than gray matter. Depth of insertion varies by manufacturer. The oxygen sensor is on the tip of the Licox catheter; the oxygen sensor is more proximal on the Neurotrend catheter.	IV	See Annotated Bibliography: 8, 9	
	Allow a time period of approximately 20 minutes to 2 hours after insertion for accurate values.	During insertion, the brain tissue surrounding the catheter is traumatized sufficiently to provide inaccurate results.	IV	See Other References: 6, 8 See Annotated Bibliography: 8, 9	
Ongoing Monitoring	Attain and maintain parameters specific to the type of $Pbto_2$ catheter in use. Normal values for the Licox catheter range between 20 and 35 mm Hg and normal value for the Neurotrend/Paratrend 7 catheter is approximately 40 mm Hg.	Until recently, only 2 different $Pbto_2$ catheters—the Neurotrend and the Licox—were available, but now only the Licox catheter is available. They used different technologies and were different in regard to normal values and ischemic thresholds. The critical threshold value below which the brain tissue is considered ischemic depends on the manufacturer of the $Pbto_2$ catheter. Range: Licox: 8.5–15 mm Hg, Neurotrend: <35 mm Hg.	IV	See References: 2, 3, 5, 9 See Other References: 4, 13, 21 See Annotated Bibliography: 8–10, 20, 22	Exact goal parameters vary from study to study, even in regard to the same catheter.

Period of Use	Recommendation	Rationale for Recommendation	Level of Recommendation	Supporting References	Comments
	Do not use $Pbto_2$ interchangeably with $Sjvo_2$ monitoring.	$Pbto_2$ monitoring is a measure of regional cerebral oxygenation. $Sjvo_2$ monitoring is a measure of global cerebral oxygenation.	IV	See References: 2, 18 See Annotated Bibliography: 13, 17	
Prevention of Complications	Consider removing or changing $Pbto_2$ monitor after 5 to 7 days to minimize risk of infection.	The infection rate for intraparenchymal brain tissue oxygen monitoring is 0%. However, the longer the invasive device remains in place, the more likely infection will occur.	I, IV	See References: 1, 2, 6 See Annotated Bibliography: 9	
	Do not insert the $Pbto_2$ monitor in the presence of systemic coagulopathy.	The bolt that holds the catheter in position and the $Pbto_2$ catheter traumatize tissue as they are inserted.	II	See References: 6 See Other References: 12	
	Support and protect the patient's head and the $Pbto_2$ catheter when moving and positioning the patient.	The most common complications associated with the $Pbto_2$ catheter are dislodgement and breakage (up to 13% in 1 study).	IV	See References: 2, 6 See Other References: 12 See Annotated Bibliography: 9	
Quality Control Issues	Remove/change $Pbto_2$ catheter after 5 days to maintain accuracy.	Both the Neurotrend and Licox catheters exhibit acceptable drift the first 5 days. After 5 days, readings may be less accurate.	IV	See References: 2, 6, 8 See Other References: 1–3, 22, 23 See Annotated Bibliography: 2, 8, 9	
	Utilize a particular brand of $Pbto_2$ catheter with knowledge of the advantages and features of that specific brand.	Both the Licox and Neurotrend catheters are accurate and reliable. The Licox catheter has demonstrated greater accuracy at lower $Pbto_2$, less drift, and less malfunction. The Neurotrend catheter had a faster $Pbto_2$ response time. The Neurotrend catheter also accurately measured pH and pCO_2, which has been found to inversely correlate. The Neurotrend catheter provided information regarding cerebral metabolism.	IV	See References: 2, 6, 8 See Other References: 18, 21 See Annotated Bibliography: 15, 25	
	Interpret $Pbto_2$ values in the context of the neurologic assessment and other cerebral and systemic parameters. Monitor and document $Pbto_2$ hourly.	$Pbto_2$ monitoring is only 1 of many assessment tools in the care of the critically ill neuroscience patient. Low sustained $Pbto_2$ is associated with poor outcomes. However, interpretation of the data derived from this device must be correlated with other data and the underlying pathology for appropriate use.	IV	See References: 2, 3, 5–7, 12 See Other References: 8, 18, 21–23 See Annotated Bibliography: 2	

CLINICAL RECOMMENDATIONS FOR JUGULAR VENOUS OXYGEN SATURATION MONITORING

The rating scales for the Level of Recommendation column range from I to VI, with levels indicated as follows: I, manufacturer's recommendation only; II, theory based, no research data to support recommendations; recommendations from expert consensus group may exist; III, laboratory data only, no clinical data to support recommendations; IV, limited clinical studies to support recommendations; V, clinical studies in more than 1 or 2 different populations and situations to support recommendations; VI, clinical studies in a variety of patient populations and situations to support recommendations.

Period of Use	Recommendation	Rationale for Recommendation	Level of Recommendation	Supporting References	Comments
Patient Selection	Recommended in the following diagnoses and clinical situations:		VI		
	1. In patients at risk for global cerebral hypoxia including: a. Adults and children with acute severe traumatic brain injury (GCS score ≤8). b. Aneurysmal subarachnoid hemorrhage.	Following severe traumatic brain injury and aneurysmal subarachnoid hemorrhage, the patient is at risk for secondary neuronal injury related to ischemia. Loss of adequate blood flow results in hypoxia. Cerebral hypoxia leads to an influx of intracellular calcium, increased release of glutamate, formation of free radicals and other molecular disturbances that may permanently injure or destroy neurons. $Sjvo_2$ monitoring may detect global hypoxia and guide interventions to improve oxygenation before permanent injury or neuronal death occurs.		See References: 3, 6, 15–17 See Other References: 24–29 See Annotated Bibliography: 4, 6, 11, 13, 17, 18, 24 See References: 17 See Other References: 30 See Annotated Bibliography: 5, 11, 14	
	2. Intraoperative monitoring during craniotomy for tumor, abscess, aneurysm, arteriovenous malformation, and spontaneous intracerebral hemorrhage and carotid endarterectomy for carotid stenosis.	The pharmacologic effects of anesthesia on: CBF and cerebral metabolism, systemic oxygenation, and alterations in blood pressure place the patient undergoing neurosurgical procedures at risk for global cerebral hypoxia. Blood loss, trauma, and manipulation of cerebral tissue and vasculature further increase the risk of global cerebral hypoxia.		See References: 15, 22 See Other References: 30, 31 See Annotated Bibliography: 11, 12	
	3. Intraoperative monitoring during cardiac surgery, especially hypothermic cardiopulmonary bypass and rewarming.	Pharmacologic effects of anesthesia on: cerebral metabolism, systemic oxygenation, and alterations in blood pressure place the patient undergoing neurosurgical procedures at risk for global cerebral hypoxia. While hypothermia provides neuroprotection, cerebral metabolic demand during rewarming may not be coupled with adequate CBF.		See References: 6, 15–17 See Other References: 32–39	

Period of Use	Recommendation	Rationale for Recommendation	Level of Recommendation	Supporting References	Comments
Patient Selection *(cont.)*	4. Patients successfully resuscitated.	During cardiopulmonary arrest, the patient is at risk for global cerebral hypoxia. A high $Sjvo_2$ after successful resuscitation indicates the inability of ischemic or infarcted neurons to utilize available oxygen.	IV	See References: 17 See Other References: 40	
	$Sjvo_2$ monitoring may be used to detect global hypoxia and guide and monitor the efficacy of therapy in the following situations:				
	1. ICP/CPP management.	Following traumatic brain injury, patients may experience global ischemia related to increased ICP, decreased CPP and MAP, and impaired autoregulation or hyperemia related to impaired autoregulation that may contribute to increased ICP and decreased CPP.	IV	See References: 15, 16, 21 See Other References: 25, 26, 28 See Annotated Bibliography: 4, 13, 17	
	2. Controlled hyperventilation for increased ICP.	Monitoring the $Sjvo_2$ during controlled hyperventilation may effectively decrease ICP while minimizing the risk of ischemia. Decreasing pCO_2 constricts cerebral arteries.	IV	See References: 3, 15, 16 See Other References: 20, 41 See Annotated Bibliography: 17	$Sjvo_2$ monitoring is recommended as an option rather than a standard or guideline during controlled hyperventilation (based on Class III evidence with I being the highest degree of certainty and III being the lowest) in the *Management and Prognosis of Severe Traumatic Brain Injury* (See Other References: 20).
	3. Barbiturate therapy for refractory ICP.	Barbiturates decrease cerebral metabolic rate and CBF with a concomitant decrease in $Sjvo_2$.	IV	See References: 15, 17, 21	
	4. Cerebral vasospasm following aneurysmal or traumatic subarachnoid hemorrhage.	$Sjvo_2$ monitoring in conjunction with transcranial Doppler ultrasonography may differentiate hyperdynamic flow from vasospasm.	IV	See References: 15, 16 See Annotated Bibliography: 14	
Insertion of Device and Initial Use	The $Sjvo_2$ catheter may be inserted in: 1. The dominant jugular bulb as a monitor of global cerebral oxygenation or in diffuse injury.		IV	See References: 3, 6, 15–17, 19 See Other References: 25, 27, 29–31, 33	Placement side of the $Sjvo_2$ catheter is controversial.

Period of Use	Recommendation	Rationale for Recommendation	Level of Recommendation	Supporting References	Comments
Patient Selection *(cont.)*	2. The jugular bulb ipsilateral to the focal injury.				
	3. Bilateral jugular bulbs to monitor global and regional Sjvo$_2$.				
	Determine jugular dominance with: 1. Manual compression of internal jugular and observe increase in ICP; compression of dominant jugular results in greater increase in ICP. 2. CT scan of internal jugular veins, the dominant vein being larger. 3. Ultrasound of internal jugular veins. 4. Angiogram.	Placement of Sjvo$_2$ catheter in the dominant jugular will more likely result in a measure of global cerebral oxygenation.	IV	See References: 15, 16 See Annotated Bibliography: 11, 18	
	Verify placement in jugular bulb by: 1. Lateral skull/cervical spine film. 2. CT scan. 3. Ultrasound. 4. Co-oximetry using jugular blood samples.	Placement in the jugular bulb will be visualized at the mastoid process and above the C1-C2 interspace.	IV	See References: 15–17, 19, 22 See Other References: 38, 39, 42–45 See Annotated Bibliography: 4–6, 14	
	Use co-oximetry jugular blood sample results after insertion (in vivo) to validate values.	The gold standard by which continuous Sjvo$_2$ monitoring is compared is a jugular bulb blood sample drawn from the jugular catheter and sent to the lab for co-oximetry analysis.	IV	See Other References: 33, 34, 36–39, 44, 45 See Annotated Bibliography: 6, 18.	
	Jugular bulb blood specimens, from the catheter, must be drawn slowly, 2 mL/min or slower to calibrate accurately.	Blood specimens drawn faster than 2 mL/min from the jugular bulb catheter result in erroneously high Sjvo$_2$ values.	IV	See References: 6, 15, 19, 22 See Other References: 29, 36 See Annotated Bibliography: 6	
Ongoing Monitoring	Attain and maintain a normal Sjvo$_2$ of 55% to 70%.	Normal Sjvo$_2$ is 55% to 70%; ischemia is <55%; hyperemia or ischemic/ infarcted tissue metabolically unable to use oxygen supply is >70%. A threshold for ischemia has been reported at 50%.	IV	See References: 7, 15–17, 19 See Other References: 44, 45 See Annotated Bibliography: 6, 24	

Period of Use	Recommendation	Rationale for Recommendation	Level of Recommendation	Supporting References	Comments
Ongoing Monitoring (*cont.*)	Obtain derived parameters to provide additional information regarding cerebral oxygenation/metabolism: 1. $AjvDo_2$: hyperemia versus ischemia (normal $AjvDo_2$ is 4–8 mL/dL; ischemia is >8 mL/dL with low $Sjvo_2$; hyperemia or greater than demand is <4 mL/dL with high $Sjvo_2$). 2. Cerebral extraction of oxygen ($CEO_2 = Sao_2 - Sjvo_2$) normal range is 24%–42% with >42% and high $AjvDo_2$ indicating ischemia and <24% and low $AjvDo_2$ indicating hyperemia.	Additional derived parameters provide additional information in regard to cerebral blood flow and metabolism.	IV	See References: 15, 16, 21 See Other References: 25, 26, 29, 34, 36, 37, 44–47 See Annotated Bibliography: 4, 14, 24	
	Maintain $Sjvo_2$ with pressurized saline bag with continuous flush.	Lack of continuous flush may result in inaccurate values and promote thrombosis.	IV	See References: 22 See Other References: 27, 39, 44, 45 See Annotated Bibliography: 6, 11	
	Use signal quality intensity indicator, x-ray, and jugular blood specimens for co-oximetry analysis to verify optimal placement in jugular bulb.	Failure to maintain $Sjvo_2$ in the jugular bulb may result in extracerebral contamination and inaccurate values.	IV	See References: 6, 19 See Other References: 36, 37, 39, 44, 45, 48	
	Recalibrate in vivo using co-oximetry jugular blood sample results every 24 hours and whenever $Sjvo_2$ desaturations or elevations detected by continuous monitoring are of questionable accuracy.	Continuous $Sjvo_2$ is more prone to inaccuracy than jugular bulb blood samples. The gold standard by which continuous $Sjvo_2$ monitoring is compared is a jugular bulb blood sample co-oximetry analysis.	IV	See References: 2, 3, 6, 15, 16 See Other References: 27, 33, 35, 36, 38, 39 See Annotated Bibliography: 4–6, 13	
	Do not use $Sjvo_2$ interchangeably with $Pbto_2$ or rSo_2 monitoring.	$Sjvo_2$ monitoring is a measure of global oxygenation. $Pbto_2$ and rSo_2 monitoring are measures of rSo_2. They are complementary and not redundant.	IV	See References: 6, 15, 16, 18 See Other References: 37, 44, 49, 50 See Annotated Bibliography: 12, 17	

Period of Use	Recommendation	Rationale for Recommendation	Level of Recommendation	Supporting References	Comments
Prevention of Complications	Monitor for possible complications at insertion: 1. Carotid artery puncture. 2. Nerve injury. 3. Pneumothorax. After insertion: 1. Infection. 2. Thrombosis. Consider changing catheter every 5 to 7 days.	The jugular vein is adjacent to the carotid artery and several nerves. An invasive monitoring device in the jugular vein may result in infection and/or thrombosis, particularly if maintained over a prolonged period or if sterile technique is not maintained.	IV	See References: 3, 15, 16 See Other References: 44, 45 See Annotated Bibliography: 11	
Quality Control Issues	Ascertain that $Sjvo_2$ catheter is properly positioned and properly calibrated before basing interventions on values.	$Sjvo_2$ is most valid and reliable when (1) positioned in jugular bulb, (2) routinely calibrated at least every 24 hours, and (3) slow blood draws (2 mL/min or slower) to avoid extracerebral contamination.	IV	See References: 2, 3, 6, 15, 16, 18 See Other References: 27, 29, 33, 35, 38, 39, 44, 45, 48 See Annotated Bibliography: 4, 5, 13, 24	
	Interpret $Sjvo_2$ values in the context of other cerebral and systemic parameters. Monitor and document $Sjvo_2$ hourly.	Brain tissue oxygen monitoring is only 1 of many assessment tools in the care of the critically ill neuroscience patient. Low sustained $Sjvo_2$ is associated with poor outcomes. However, interpretation of the data derived from this device must be correlated with other data and the underlying pathology for appropriate use.	IV	See References: 12, 15, 18 See Other References: 44, 45, 48 See Annotated Bibliography: 4, 5, 13, 24	

CLINICAL RECOMMENDATIONS FOR TRANSCRANIAL CEREBRAL OXIMETRY MONITORING (NEAR INFRARED SPECTROSCOPY)

The rating scales for the Level of Recommendation column range from I to VI, with levels indicated as follows: I, manufacturer's recommendation only; II, theory based, no research data to support recommendations; recommendations from expert consensus group may exist; III, laboratory data only, no clinical data to support recommendations; IV, limited clinical studies to support recommendations; V, clinical studies in more than 1 or 2 different populations and situations to support recommendations; VI, clinical studies in a variety of patient populations and situations to support recommendations.

Period of Use	Recommendation	Rationale for Recommendation	Level of Recommendation	Supporting References	Comments
Patient Selection	Recommended in the following diagnoses and clinical conditions:				
	1. In patients at risk for regional cerebral hypoxia including those with acute severe traumatic brain injury (GCS score ≤8).	Following severe traumatic brain injury, aneurysmal subarachnoid hemorrhage, and stroke, the patient is at risk for secondary neuronal injury related to ischemia. Loss of adequate blood flow results in hypoxia. Cerebral hypoxia leads to an influx of intracellular calcium, increased release of glutamate, formation of free radicals, and other molecular disturbances that may permanently injure or destroy neurons. Pbto$_2$ monitoring may detect regional hypoxia and guide interventions to improve oxygenation before permanent injury or neuronal death occurs.	VI	See References: 12, 24 See Other References: 9, 51 See Annotated Bibliography: 3	
	2. Subarachnoid hemorrhage.			See References: 6, 12 See Other References: 9 See Annotated Bibliography: 3	
	3. Acute ischemic stroke.			See References: 26 See Other References: 49 See Annotated Bibliography: 7	
	4. Adult and pediatric cardiac surgery, including cardiopulmonary bypass with hypothermia.	Patients undergoing cardiac surgery are at risk for regional cerebral ischemia related to the effects of anesthesia, rewarming, and blood loss based on cerebral metabolism and CBF, systemic oxygenation, and blood pressure.		See References: 24, 27 See Other References: 52 See Annotated Bibliography: 1	
	5. Carotid endarterectomy or angioplasty with stenting.	Trauma and manipulation of cerebral vasculature (eg, cross-clamping) put the patient at risk for regional cerebral hypoxia.		See References: 6, 25 See Other References: 51, 53, 54 See Annotated Bibliography: 12, 16	
	6. Seizures.	Changes in regional cerebral oxygenation during seizures may differentiate type and have been found to correlate with electroencephalogram and single photon emission computed tomography changes.		See Other References: 51 See Annotated Bibliography: 27	

Period of Use	Recommendation	Rationale for Recommendation	Level of Recommendation	Supporting References	Comments
Patient Selection (*cont.*)	7. Following successful cardiopulmonary resuscitation.	During cardiopulmonary resuscitation, the patient is at risk for regional cerebral ischemia.		See References: 30 See Other References: 49, 55	
	8. Pediatric extracorporeal life support and extracorporeal membrane oxygenation.	During cannulation for extracorporeal life support, the patient is at risk for ischemia.		See Other References: 56	
	9. Caesarean section with spinal anesthesia.	Spinal anesthesia is associated with systemic hypotension, which may result in cerebral hypoxia.		See Other References: 57	
	10. Hemorrhage and transfusion.	During hemorrhage, the oxygen-carrying capacity of the blood decreases. As a result cerebral oxygenation decreases. During transfusion, the oxygen-carrying capacity of the blood increases. As a result, cerebral oxygenation improves.		See Other References: 58 See Annotated Bibliography: 36	
Application and Initial Use	Place on frontal temporal area of forehead to left and right of midline; do not place on scalp. Avoid subdural hematoma, epidural hematoma, subgaleal hematomas, or cerebral infarction.		IV	See References: 25, 30	See quality control section for placement options.
	Use appropriate sensors: pediatric (0–40 kg) and adult.	Pediatric and adult sensors are not interchangeable as they are based on anatomic and physiologic variation in CBF and are skull-specific to each age group.	I	See References: 25	
	Note baseline and follow rSo_2 trends rather than absolute numbers.	Individual variation exists with regards to venous and arterial contribution (75%–85% arterial vs. 15%–25% venous). A change of 20% to 30% from baseline or 12 to 20 points (%) from baseline is associated with neurologic deterioration. An rSo_2 of less than 50% is associated with a poor outcome.	IV	See References: 24, 25, 27	
Ongoing Monitoring	Only use sensor once.	When the INVOS sensor has been used and removed, it has a layer of skin cells on the adhesive that may impair the oximeter's ability to detect changes in rSo_2 accurately when reapplied. A reused sensor is also more likely to allow ambient light	I	See References: 25	

Period of Use	Recommendation	Rationale for Recommendation	Level of Recommendation	Supporting References	Comments
		and perspiration to interfere with accurate rSo_2 determination.			
Quality Control Issues	Utilize CT scan to position sensors over viable brain tissue.	Placement over hematomas, air, or infarcted tissue will result in inaccurate results.	IV	See References: 25, 30 See Other References: 53, 54 See Annotated Bibliography: 3	
	Recognize conditions in which baseline rSo_2 is: (1) artificially high, such as with an increased bilirubin; (2) low; or (3) may not register (ie, with polycythemia).		IV	See References: 12, 24 See Other References: 24	
	Recognize conditions that may alter rSo_2 values within the adult population (ie, cerebral atrophy).		IV	See References: 25	
	Do not use rSo_2 monitoring in place of ICP or CBF/blood flow velocity (transcranial Doppler) monitoring.		IV	See References: 2, 6, 24 See Other References: 59	Correlation has not been substantiated with other intracranial monitoring devices.
	Do not use rSo_2 monitoring in brain death.	In the absence of CBF or in very low flow states, venous blood pooled in the capillaries will result in erroneous values.	IV	See References: 12, 24 See Other References: 55	
	Do not use rSo_2 monitoring during craniotomy.	During a craniotomy, rSo_2 monitoring may not be accurate as the brain falls away from the skull and sensors.	I	See References: 25	
	Do not use rSo_2 interchangeably with $Sjvo_2$ monitoring.	rSo_2 monitoring is a measure of regional cerebral oxygenation and not global cerebral oxygenation.	IV	See References: 2, 6, 24 See Other References: 49, 50	
	rSo_2 may be useful in detecting change in $Pbto_2$.	Both $Pbto_2$ and rSo_2 are measures of regional cerebral oxygenation.	IV	See Other References: 9 See Annotated Bibliography: 3	
	Interpret rSo_2 values in the context of other cerebral and systemic parameters. Monitor and document rSo_2 hourly.	A number of studies involving rSo_2 monitoring have had controversial results. rSo_2 monitoring is only 1 of many assessment tools in the care of the critically ill neuroscience patient. Interpretation of the data derived from this device must be correlated with other data and the underlying pathology for appropriate use.		See References: 6 See Other References: 60	

ANNOTATED BIBLIOGRAPHY

1. Austin EH, Edmonds HL, Auden SM, et al. Benefit of neurophysiologic monitoring for pediatric cardiac surgery. *J Thorac Cardiovas Surg.* **1997;114:707–717.**

Study Sample

Two hundred fifty pediatric cardiac patients were included in this study. All were undergoing repair of congenital cardiac abnormalities. Ages ranged from less than 7 days to greater than 5 years.

Study Procedures

An INVOS transcranial cerebral oximeter 3100A (Somanetics Corporation, Troy, MI) was used to monitor rSo_2. The sensor was affixed to the left side of the head. Transcranial Doppler (TCD) of the middle cerebral artery and electroencephalogram (EEG) were monitored as well.

Key Results

Desaturations detected by the transcranial cerebral oximeter were by far the most common indicator of change. Fifty-eight percent of the indications for change were a result of rSo_2 desaturations of greater than 20%. Most of the time, EEG slowing accompanied the desaturations afterwards. TCD and NIRS were associated with cardiopulmonary bypass changes in pump flow or perfusion pressure. The rSo_2 desaturations were associated with airway obstruction, low hemoglobin, low Fio_2, low carbon dioxide, low arterial pressure or pump flow, cerebral hypermetabolism with rewarming, and low cardiac output. Ninety-seven of 171 interventions occurred as a result of a desaturation.

Study Strengths and Weaknesses

Statistical analyses of correlation or association of rSo_2 with EEG and TCD changes were not included. Postoperative neurologic outcome was not discussed specific to rSo_2 desaturations.

Clinical Implications

NIRS monitoring during pediatric cardiac surgery may detect cerebral oxygen desaturations and prompt early intervention.

2. Bardt TF, Unterberg AW, Härtl R, Kiening KL, Schneider GH, Canksch WR. Monitoring of brain tissue pO_2 in traumatic brain injury: effect of cerebral hypoxia on outcome. *Acta Neurochir Suppl.* **1998;71:153–156.**

Study Sample

Thirty-five patients with severe head injury, GCS score less than 8, with a mean age of 33.2 (±11.3) years were included in this study. Two-thirds had mass lesions that were evacuated.

Study Procedures

Continuous $Pbto_2$ monitoring with the Licox catheter (GMS MBH, Kiel, Germany) was conducted over a mean of 119.3 (±65.7) hours. It was placed into the frontal lobe white matter within 8 to 125 hours after injury. Position was verified by CT scan. The $Pbto_2$ catheter was assessed for accuracy after monitoring. ICP and CPP monitoring was conducted as well. Outcome was assessed at time of discharge and 6 months after injury. CPP was maintained over 70 mm Hg.

Key Results

Over half (56%) of the patients with a $Pbto_2$ of less than 10 mm Hg for more than 5 hours died and another 22% had poor outcomes, defined as severe disability or vegetative state. Twenty-two percent had good outcomes defined as good recovery or moderate disability despite a $Pbto_2$ of less than 10 mm Hg. When the $Pbto_2$ was less than 10 mm Hg, an end-tidal CO_2 of less than 28 mm Hg was present 48% of the time. The etiology of the cerebral hypoxia was not known in 45% of the patients.

Study Strengths and Weaknesses

The total number of patients with a $Pbto_2$ less than 10 mm Hg for greater than 5 hours was not stated. Outcome was associated with $Pbto_2$. However, the investigators were unable to explain the association of low end-tidal CO_2 and low $Pbto_2$. The low end-tidal CO_2 may be related to the use of hyperventilation in an unsuccessful attempt to increase $Pbto_2$. Furthermore, no explanation was given why 22% of the patients with a $Pbto_2$ of less than 10 mm Hg had good outcomes.

Clinical Implications

Brain tissue oxygen values may be predictive of outcome in some head injury patients.

3. Buchner K, Meixensberger J, Dings J, Roosen K. Near infrared spectroscopy: not useful to monitor cerebral oxygenation after severe brain injury. *Zentralbl Neurochir.* **2000;61: 69–73.**

Study Sample

Thirty-one patients with subarachnoid hemorrhage (SAH; n = 12) or severe traumatic brain injury (TBI; n = 19) were included in this study.

Comparison Studied

Transcranial cerebral oximetry (rSo_2) and $Pbto_2$ were compared in patients with severe TBI and SAH.

Study Procedures

Regional oxygen saturation was continuously monitored using an INVOS 3100 monitor (Somanetics, Detroit, MI) in 23 patients. Another NIRS monitor was used as well (but is no longer commercially available in the United States) in 8 patients. ICP, CPP, and $Pbto_2$ were monitored as well. $Pbto_2$ was monitored using a Licox (GMS, Kiel-Mielkendorf, Germany). The NIRS sensor and $Pbto_2$ catheter were both placed on the side of the injury. In diffuse injury, both the $Pbto_2$ probe and the rSo_2 sensor were placed on the right side.

Key Results

INVOS NIRS monitoring resulted in good data quality, without artifact, in 79.6% of performed measurements while the $Pbto_2$ catheter produced quality data 100% of the time. Technical issues with the INVOS included moisture between the sensor and skin, ambient light interference, galeal hematomas, and subdural air after craniotomy. Increasing the Fio_2 to 100% showed a moderate to strong correlation between $Pbto_2$ and rSo_2 (0.67, $P < 0.01$). $Pbto_2$ and rSo_2 did not correlate after changes in pCO_2 or mannitol administration.

Study Strengths and Weaknesses

The rSo_2 values were not monitored bilaterally. Bilateral monitoring might have provided additional information regarding accuracy. The investigator made an assumption that $Pbto_2$ is the gold standard and 100% accurate.

Clinical Implications

NIRS may not correlate with $Pbto_2$ after mannitol administration or an increase in pCO_2. Technical issues complicate transcranial cerebral oximetry use.

4. **Chan K-H, Dearden NM, Miller JD, Andrews P, Midgley S. Multimodality monitoring as a guide to treatment of intracranial hypertension after severe head injury.** *Neurosurgery.* 1993; 32:547–553.

Study Sample

Twenty-two patients with severe brain injury were included in the study, 13 with focal injuries and 9 with diffuse injuries. Their mean age was 29 and the age ranged from 9 to 59 years.

Study Procedures

In addition to ICP/CPP monitoring, continuous bilateral middle cerebral artery (MCA) TCD and $Sjvo_2$ monitoring was performed. The $Sjvo_2$ catheter was placed on the side of greatest venous drainage. Position was verified by x-ray. The Oximetrics 3 system (Abbott Laboratories, Chicago, IL) was calibrated in vivo every 2 hours. Cerebral arteriovenous oxygen content difference ($AjvDo_2$) was calculated as well using the formula ($Sao_2 - Sjvo_2$) × (hemoglobin × 1.3)/100. Global ischemia was defined as $Sjvo_2$ less than 40% and $AjvDo_2$ greater than 9 mL/dL; global hyperemia was defined as $Sjvo_2$ greater than 75% and $AjvDo_2$ less than 4 mL/dL. ICP/CPP goals were less then 20 mm Hg and greater than 60 mm Hg, respectively. All patients were mechanically ventilated and chemically paralyzed. Management of ICP/CPP included administration of mannitol or thiopentone, drainage of CSF, or elevation of MAP. $Sjvo_2$ was monitored during 35 treatments which included 20 of the 22 patients.

Key Results

Successful treatment of ICP/CPP was associated with a rise in $Sjvo_2$ and an $AjvDo_2$ decrease only when the CPP was less than 60 mm Hg before treatment. Increasing the CPP beyond 70 mm Hg did not increase cerebral oxygen delivery. Administration of hypnotic drugs decreased ICP but also decreased MAP, CPP, and $Sjvo_2$, and increased $AjvDo_2$.

Study Strengths and Weaknesses

This study looked at the $AjvDo_2$ as well as $Sjvo_2$. The procedure for determining the cerebral hemisphere with the greatest venous drainage was not explained but was referenced. Samples of blood from the $Sjvo_2$ catheter were not obtained prior to and after treatment for comparison with the continuous $Sjvo_2$ monitor.

Clinical Implications

Successful treatment of ICP/CPP may result in a rise in $Sjvo_2$ and a decrease in $AjvDo_2$ following head injury. Treatment of ICP/CPP to an ICP of less than 20 mm Hg and a CPP between 60 and 70 mm Hg improves oxygen delivery to the brain. Hypnotic agents to decrease ICP may negatively impact CPP, $Sjvo_2$, and $AjvDo_2$.

5. **Citerio G, Cormio M, Portella G, Vascotto E, Galli D, Gaini SM. Jugular saturation ($SjvO_2$) monitoring in subarachnoid hemorrhage (SAH).** *Acta Neurochir Suppl.* 1998;71:316–319.

Study Sample

Twenty-six patients with aneurysmal subarachnoid hemorrhage were included in the study. Ages ranged from 20 to 80 years. Sixteen were women and 10 were men. Seven were Hunt-Hess Grade I–II; 6 were Hunt-Hess Grade III; and 13 were Hunt-Hess Grade IV–V.

Study Procedures

$Sjvo_2$ catheters were placed on the side of the aneurysm in 78% of the study participants and on the dominant side with bilateral or midline lesions. Correct position was verified by x-ray. $Sjvo_2$ was monitored up to 12 days with a total of 354 samples drawn every 6 hours. ICP and CPP were monitored as well.

Key Results

The mean $Sjvo_2$ for all samples was 0.66 ± 0.07 with a range of 0.43 to 0.89 and a median of 0.67. Thirty-seven of the 354 jugular bulb samples (approximately 10%) revealed desaturation episodes. The critical threshold of $Sjvo_2$ was set at 0.55. The ICP was noted to be higher during lower $Sjvo_2$ episodes ($P = 0.008$). Lower CPP was also associated with decreases in $Sjvo_2$. Blood greater than 25 mL was noted to be associated with lower $Sjvo_2$ at the time of the first CT scan and then higher $Sjvo_2$ with the second CT on days 7 to 9.

Study Strengths and Weaknesses

This study looked at the association of high ICP, low CPP, and low $Sjvo_2$. This retrospective study did not include continuous data or data at the time deterioration was noted at the bedside. The continuous data with the fiberoptic $Sjvo_2$ catheter were noted to be of poor quality. $Sjvo_2$ blood samples were collected routinely every 6 hours. Vasospasm and $AjvDo_2$ were not discussed in this study.

Clinical Implications

Decreases in $Sjvo_2$ may alert the clinician to high ICP and low CPP episodes that result in ischemia following aneurysmal SAH.

6. Coplin WM, O'Keefe GE, Grady MS, Grant GA, March KS, Winn HR, Lam AM. Accuracy of continuous jugular bulb oximetry in the intensive care unit. *Neurosurgery.* 1998;42: 533–540.

Study Sample

Thirty-one patients with acute TBI were included in this study. All patients were on mechanical ventilation with a median GCS score of 5 after resuscitation. All but 3 were severe TBI.

Sample Procedures

A 4 French $Sjvo_2$ oximetry catheter (Baxter-Edwards, Santa Ana, CA) was placed ipsilateral to the intracranial lesion or on the right side for bilateral or diffuse injuries. Correct placement was confirmed by x-ray. The catheter was attached to a pressurized continuous flush bag to maintain patency and the $Sjvo_2$ was continuously monitored using an oximetric monitor. In vivo calibration was performed upon insertion and every 24 hours, simultaneously withdrawing arterial and $Sjvo_2$ blood samples over 1 to 2 minutes. The total number of samples obtained was 195 over 1 to 6 days. $Sjvo_2$ desaturations, defined as less than 50% for 10 min-

utes, were examined in the context of changes in clinical condition as well.

Key Results

The correlation between in vivo continuous $Sjvo_2$ monitoring and in blood samples from the $Sjvo_2$ was strong at 0.80. Sensitivity for detection of jugular bulb desaturation from continuous bedside monitoring was 45% to 50%. The specificity for continuous $Sjvo_2$ monitoring to detect jugular bulb desaturations was 98% to 100%.

Study Strengths and Weaknesses

The continuous $Sjvo_2$ monitoring was assessed using the gold standard, blood sampling from the $Sjvo_2$ catheter. Blood samples were withdrawn slowly over 1 to 2 minutes. Only 3 major desaturations of $Sjvo_2$ occurred with the $Sjvo_2$ being less than 46%. Monitor drift was not assessed. Recalibration of the $Sjvo_2$ to reflect changes in hemoglobin was not performed.

Clinical Implications

While continuous monitoring may not detect up to 50% of all jugular bulb desaturations, when a decrease is detected by the continuous monitoring, it corresponds to a decrease in $Sjvo_2$ from blood sampling.

7. Demet G, Talip A, Nevzat U, Serhat O, Gazi O. The evaluation of cerebral oxygenation by oximetry in patients with ischaemic stroke. *J Postgrad Med.* 2000;46:70–74.

Study Sample

Twenty-four patients with ischemic stroke in the middle cerebral artery were included in this study.

Study Procedures

The transcranial cerebral oximeter, INVOS 3100-DS (Somanetics), was used to measure rSo_2 bilaterally on the 1st, 3rd, 7th, and 15th days after the stroke. Sensors were placed 1 cm above the eyebrow to avoid the frontal sinuses. Blood pressure, oxygen saturation (So_2), arterial blood gases, and GCS score were noted as well.

Key Results

The rSo_2 values varied significantly as the number of days from the stroke increased. Values of the rSo_2 increased significantly throughout the chronic phase. The rSo_2 was also higher on the contralateral side than the ipsilateral side in the acute phase, the first 48 hours ($P = 0.0034$). The relationship between GCS score and rSo_2 was not statistically significant.

Study Strengths and Weaknesses

Regional So_2 was not measured continuously. Intermittent measurements were obtained.

Clinical Implications

Measurement of rSo_2 by NIRS may indicate improvement in cerebral oxygenation as the number of days after the stroke increases.

8. Dings J, Meixensberger J, Amschler J, Roosen K. Continuous monitoring of brain tissue pO_2: a new tool to minimize the risk of ischemia caused by hyperventilation therapy. *Zentralbl Neurochir.* 1996;57:177–183.

Study Sample

Twenty-one patients with severe TBI, GCS score 3–8, and 1 patient with a GCS score of 12 (with an epidural hematoma) were included in this study.

Study Procedures

A Licox brain tissue oxygen catheter (GMS Kiel-Mielkendorf, Germany) was placed in the frontal white matter, away from contusion or hypodensity. A CT scan was performed to assure placement. Upon removal, the drift in air ($<10\%$) and at the zero point (mean 1.5 ± 1.5 mm Hg) was performed. Patients were monitored for 7.4 ± 2.5 days. Seventy hyperventilation tests were performed from days 0 to 9 after the injury. ICP was monitored as well. CO_2 reactivity was assessed by TCD. Patients were placed in 2 groups depending on their baseline $Pbto_2$ of $>$ or <15 mm Hg.

Key Results

In the group with a baseline $Pbto_2$ <15 mm Hg, hyperventilation aggravated ischemia while for baseline $Pbto_2$ >15 mm Hg, no ischemia occurred. Six of 22 patients had at least 1 episode of ischemia when hyperventilated. CO_2 reactivity was not significantly different for either group.

Study Strengths and Weaknesses

The area of tissue sampled by the $Pbto_2$ catheter is small and some areas of ischemia may have been undetected.

Clinical Implications

Hyperventilation may cause cerebral hypoxia by inducing ischemia in healthy tissue. The $Pbto_2$ catheter may detect regional areas of cerebral hypoxia as a result of hyperventilation.

9. Dings J, Meixensberger J, Jager A, Roosen K. Clinical experience with 118 brain tissue oxygen partial pressure catheter probes. *Neurosurgery.* 1998;43:1082–1095.

Study Sample

The partial $Pbto_2$ was measured in 101 patients using 118 Licox polarographic $Pbto_2$ catheter probes (Medical Sys-tems, Corporation, Greenvale, NY). The study participants included: 57 with severe head injury, defined as a GCS score less than 9; 43 Hunt-Hess Grade IV–V SAH patients or SAH patients with vasospasm-related clinical deterioration; and 1 brain tumor patient after surgery.

Study Purpose

The purpose of the study was to determine the safety and reliability of brain tissue oxygen catheters in patients with severe traumatic brain injury, poor grade subarachnoid hemorrhage, or clinical deterioration from vasospasm.

Study Procedures

The $Pbto_2$ probes were placed in the white matter of frontal lobes of 101 patients at 22 to 27 mm below the dura level. The side of the brain with greater injury was monitored. The initial time for the catheters to provide reliable signals was noted. In 27 patients, the catheters were removed in 3 increments of 5 mm each and the $Pbto_2$ was noted at each level. Complications were noted also. After their removal, the used catheters' $Pbto_2$ drift was determined and compared with unused $Pbto_2$ catheter probes. A flow chart to determine artificial readings after insertion was used during the study and is included in the publication.

Key Results

$Pbto_2$ monitoring 17 to 27 mm below the dura in white matter is safe and reliable. The average adaptation/equilibration time was 79.0 ± 51.7 minutes. The following complications and associated rates among patients were as follows: (1) small iatrogenic hematoma in 1.7%; (2) 0% infection rate after 6.7 ± 3.9 days; and (3) a dislocation or defect rate in 13.6%. $Pbto_2$ increased as the catheters were moved from the white to the gray matter. This is thought to be related to the higher CBF and metabolism of the gray matter. Older catheter probes had the highest drift values during the first 4 days of monitoring.

Study Strengths and Weaknesses

The major strength of this study is that this was a large in vivo prospective study to determine the reliability of the $Pbto_2$ catheter with consideration for location, adaptation time, drift, and associated complications. Used and unused catheters were compared for drift in vitro. However, not all of the 118 brain tissue oxygenation probes were available for testing of $Pbto_2$ for drift. Seventeen of the probes had electrical defects or were not returned to humid protection chambers upon removal; the first 8 catheters were destroyed prior to checking for drift. Also, simultaneous monitoring of $Pbto_2$ at the various depths was not performed. Information regarding the catheters' detection of the patients' clinical deterioration or improvement was not noted.

Clinical Implications

The Licox Pbto₂ catheter reliably reflects the partial pressure of brain tissue oxygen in severe brain injury, aneurysmal subarachnoid hemorrhage, and related vasospasm. Data are reliable when the probe is placed 17 to 22 mm below the dura and an adaptation time of approximately 30 minutes to 2.5 hours is allowed. The greatest complication of its use is dislocation or technical defect. Older catheter probes are associated with greater drift.

10. **Doppenberg EM, Zauner A, Bullock R, Ward JD, Fatouros PP, Young HF. Correlations between brain tissue oxygen tension, carbon dioxide tension, pH, and cerebral blood flow: a better way of monitoring the severely injured brain?** *Surg Neurol.* **1998;49:650–654.**

Study Sample

Twenty-five patients with severe traumatic brain injury (GCS score ≤8) were included in this study. All were greater than 16 years.

Study Procedures

This study compared the Pbto₂ catheter with xenon-CT. A Paratrend 7 (Biomedical Sensors, Malvern, PA) Pbto₂ catheter was inserted in the right frontal cortex to measure Pbto₂, Pbtco₂, and pH. Prior to insertion, the sensor was calibrated by bubbling gases in sequence through the tonometer. Data from the Paratrend monitor were averaged 1 hour before and 1 hour after the xenon-CT. A Pbto₂ of ≤18 mm Hg was established as the criteria for ischemia. Xenon-CT was used to measure CBF using 30% xenon, 30% to 50% oxygen and room air. CBF was measured in a 20 to 30 mm² region at the site of the Paratrend sensor. One CBF measurement was taken for each patient. The time between the TBI and the measurement ranged from 3 to 96 hours with a mean of 27 ± 28 hours.

Key Results

Mean Pbto₂ and regional xenon-CT CBF strongly correlated ($r = 0.74$, $P = 0.0001$). Xenon-CT CBF less than 18 mL/100 g/min was associated with a Pbto₂ ≤26 mm Hg. Patients with a Pbto₂ <18 mm Hg died. Brain tissue carbon dioxide and pH did not correlate with CBF. Patients with a CBF of greater than 40 mL/100 g/min had Pbto₂ levels >30 mm Hg. No complications occurred.

Study Strengths and Weaknesses

This study looked at the validity of the Paratrends catheter by comparing it to xenon-CT CBF. Responses to interventions were not reported. Patients were not described in regard to type of injury, or diffuse versus focal (mass lesion). In all patients, regardless of injury, the Paratrend monitor was placed in the right cortex.

Clinical Implications

The brain tissue oxygenation catheter may accurately reflect CBF in traumatic brain injury. Interventions to increase oxygenation to injured brain may be evaluated accurately by monitoring the Pbto₂.

11. **Gemma M, Beretta L, De Vitas A, et al. Complications of internal jugular vein retrograde catheterization.** *Acta Neurochir Suppl.* **1998;71: 320–323.**

Study Sample

The study sample consisted of 126 patients with a variety of neurologic injury, including head injuries, subarachnoid hemorrhage, arteriovenous malformation, brain tumors, spontaneous intracerebral hemorrhage, and cerebral abscess.

Study Procedures

The total number of retrograde internal jugular catheters placed was 172. In 91% of the cannulations, the Sjvo₂ catheter was placed on the right side. The left internal jugular was used if the clinician was unable to insert it into the right internal jugular bulb or the right had already undergone prolonged cannulation. In 37% of the patients, the right internal jugular was identified as the dominant one by CT or angiogram. An Opticatheter was inserted through a 14-gauge introducer in 10%. The remaining 90% had 16- or 18-gauge single lumen catheters. Placement was verified by x-ray. Catheters remained in place from 1 to 13 days. Catheter patency was maintained by pressurized continuous heparinized saline flush. Neck echography (ultrasound) was performed at the time of placement and 1 week later.

Key Results

Internal jugular cannulation was declared safe with a low incidence of serious complications. Approximately 50% of the insertions were associated with complications that included: carotid artery puncture, lymphatic vessel puncture, catheter failure related to difficulty of insertion, catheter misplacement involving catheter looping, paravertebral venous plexus cannulation, extracranial jugular afferent cannulation, placement of the catheter tip in internal jugular lumen or beyond bulb, perivascular hematoma, and jugular venous thrombosis. Misplacement, which occurred in 23% of the complications, was correctable. Only 3 patients developed jugular thrombosis, which was clinically silent but detected on echography. Though catheter tip cultures were positive for bacteria, none of the patients developed catheter-related septicemia.

Study Strengths and Weaknesses

This study included a discussion regarding strategies to minimize the complication rate. Echography was not completed on patients who died or those who had the $Sjvo_2$ catheters in place less than 24 hours. The bacterial colonization of the catheter or thrombosis was not discussed in regard to duration of cannulation or repositioning of the catheter.

Clinical Implications

Complications may occur with retrograde catheterization of the internal jugular vein. Clinicians must be aware of these potential complications.

12. Grubhofer G, Lassnigg A, Manlik F, Marx E, Trubel W, Hiesmayr M. The contributions of extracranial blood oxygenation on near-infrared spectroscopy during carotid thromboendarterectomy. *Anaesthesia*. 1997;52: 116–120. See comments in 1997;52:704–707.

Study Sample

This study included 12 patients aged 43 to 84 years; 8 men and 4 women had greater than 75% stenosis at the bifurcation of the common carotid artery.

Comparison Studied

This is a comparison of $Sjvo_2$ and rSo_2 during carotid endarterectomy.

Study Procedures

Prior to carotid endarterectomy, an $Sjvo_2$ catheter (Opticath, Oximetrix, Mountain View, CA) was inserted into the jugular bulb. Another catheter was placed in the facial vein to determine the contribution of extracerebral contamination in transcranial cerebral oximetry (NIRS) technology. An INVOS 3100 A (Somanetics, USA) monitor was used to measure rSo_2.

Key Results

Significant correlation was seen between rSo_2 and $Sjvo_2$ (0.97, $P = 0.027$). However, rSo_2 had reduced sensitivity to decreases in global cerebral oxygenation. A 10% decrease in $Sjvo_2$ was reflected by a decrease of only 3.6% in rSo_2. The extracerebral blood did not correlate with NIRS.

Study Strengths and Weaknesses

Grubhofer et al. concluded that NIRS is not a reliable measure of global cerebral oxygenation but acknowledged that $Sjvo_2$ is a measure of global oxygenation and not a measure of regional oxygenation.

Clinical Implications

NIRS rSo_2 may be used to determine the trend in regional cerebral oxygenation. However, actual rSo_2 values should not be interpreted as $Sjvo_2$.

13. Gupta AK, Hutchinson PJ, Al-Rawi P, et al. Measuring brain tissue oxygenation compared with jugular venous oxygen saturation for monitoring cerebral oxygenation after traumatic brain injury. *Anesth Analg*. 1999;88: 549–553.

Study Sample

Thirteen patients with severe TBI were studied. Ages ranged from 26 to 78 years and the mean age was 50 years. Their GCS score was less than 8 with a median of 5.

Comparison Studied

$Sjvo_2$ was compared to $Pbto_2$ during hyperventilation. The brain tissue oxygenation catheter was placed in injured brain tissue in 5 patients and in the healthy tissue of 8 patients.

Study Procedures

Jugular bulb oximetry and brain tissue oxygenation were continuously monitored while patients were hyperventilated in stepwise 4 mm Hg increments, decreasing the pCO_2 from 35 to 22 mm Hg. ICP and CPP were monitored as well. A Paratrend (Diametric Medical, High Wycombe, UK) catheter was used to measure $Pbto_2$, $Pbtco_2$, brain pH, and temperature. All patients were sedated and chemically paralyzed. Appropriate placement of the $Pbto_2$ catheter was verified with CT. The $Pbto_2$ catheter was calibrated before insertion and the $Sjvo_2$ and was intermittently calibrated with blood samples.

Key Results

Strong positive correlation was found between changes in $Sjvo_2$ and $Pbto_2$ in areas without focal pathology ($r^2 = 0.69$, $P < 0.0001$). No correlation was demonstrated between changes in $Sjvo_2$ and $Pbto_2$ in areas with focal pathology ($r^2 = 0.07$, $P = 0.23$).

Study Strengths and Weaknesses

The sample size was small. The $Pbto_2$ was not measured in healthy and injured brain tissue in the same patient simultaneously.

Clinical Implications

$Sjvo_2$ and $Pbto_2$ in brain injury provide different information. In healthy tissue, $Sjvo_2$ and $Pbto_2$ may positively correlate. However, in severe TBI, $Sjvo_2$ may more accurately reflect global oxygenation while $Pbto_2$ reflects regional oxygenation in injured tissue.

14. Heran NS, Hentschel SJ, Toyota BD. Jugular bulb oximetry for prediction of vasospasm following subarachnoid hemorrhage. *Can J Neurol Sci*. 2004;31:80–86.

Study Sample

Ten patients with aneurysmal SAH were included in the final data analysis. Their ages ranged from 35 to 72 years. Five were women and 5 were men. Eight were Hunt-Hess II–III and all were Fisher grade 3. Four patients, all women, developed clinical vasospasm and 6 did not.

Study Procedures

Jugular bulb catheters were placed on the side with the most blood on CT scan or on the right side if the blood was evenly dispersed. The $Sjvo_2$ catheter position was verified by x-ray. $AjvDo_2$ and cerebral oxygen extraction (CEo_2, and calculated as $Sao_2 - Sjvo_2$) were determined every 12 hours and correlated with signs and symptoms of neurologic deterioration. Catheters were removed between days 10 to 14 after hemorrhage or when vasospasm was no longer observed to be a problem.

Key Results

The patients with clinical vasospasm had a significant rise in $AjvDo_2$ approximately 1 day before the onset of clinical deficits ($P < 0.0001$). When triple H therapy was started, $AjvDo_2$ improved and symptoms resolved. The 6 patients who did not have clinical vasospasm did not exhibit an increase in $AjvDo_2$.

Study Strengths and Weaknesses

This study looked at CEo_2 and $AjvDo_2$ rather than just $Sjvo_2$. $Sjvo_2$ data were not reported. $Sjvo_2$ reflects a balance between cerebral metabolic rate and CBF. $AjvDo_2$ and CEo_2 are thought to be more closely related to CBF. Three participants were not included in the final data analysis due to inability to maintain a functional $Sjvo_2$ catheter. The sample size was small. t-tests were used to compare $AjvDo_2$ within groups and unpaired t-tests were used between groups. The diagnosis of vasospasm was based on clinical presentation alone and not supported by TCD or angiogram findings.

Clinical Implications

Use of the $Sjvo_2$ catheter for $AjvDo_2$ determination may be useful in predicting and managing SAH vasospasm.

15. Hoelper BM, Alessandri B, Heimann A, Behr R, Kempski O. Brain oxygen monitoring: in-vitro accuracy, long-term drift and response time of Licox and Neurotrend sensors. *Acta Neurochir (Wien)*. 2005;147:767–774.

Comparison Studied

Twelve Licox (Integra NeuroSciences, Hampshire, UK) and 12 Neurotrend (Codman, Rayham, MA) $Pbto_2$ catheters were compared for in vitro accuracy, long-term drift, and response time.

Study Procedures

All of the catheters were equilibrated in a liquid tonometer chamber maintained at $37° \pm 0.2°C$ using 5 different gases with different O_2 and CO_2 concentration. Readings were taken for each gas. Both the Licox and Neurotrend catheters were placed in 3% oxygen and 9% carbon dioxide and drift was assessed at 24, 48, 72, 96, and 120 hours. Response time was tested using 1% to 5% oxygen and pre-equilibrated tonometers.

Key Results

The failure rate of the Neurotrend catheter to calibrate was 14%. The Licox catheter had a 0% failure rate. The Licox probes were more accurate than the Neurotrend sensor. The Neurotrend catheter read lower in 1% oxygen and deviated more at higher oxygen concentrations. Both catheters demonstrated a quicker response time to increases in pO_2 than decreases in pCO_2. The Neurotrend catheter's $Pbto_2$ drift was greater but not sufficiently to impair long-term use. The Neurotrend catheter accurately measures the partial pressure of carbon dioxide and pH.

Study Strengths and Weaknesses

Both catheters were assessed for failure rate, accuracy, response time, and drift over 5 days in vitro. The sample size was small. Data regarding in vivo performance were not included in this study.

Clinical Implications

The Licox catheter demonstrated a lower failure rate and less drift. This may be an important consideration when choosing between the 2 $Pbto_2$ catheters. The Neurotrend catheter provides additional information regarding $Pbtco_2$ and pH.

16. Horie N, Kitagawa N, Morikawa M, Kaminogo M, Nagata I. Monitoring of regional cerebral oxygenation by near-infrared spectroscopy in carotid artery stenting: preliminary study. *Neuroradiology*. 2005;47:375–379.

Study Sample

Twenty-four patients undergoing carotid artery stenting were included in this study.

Study Procedures

The INVOS 3100 transcranial cerebral oximeter (Somanetics, MI) was placed on forehead ipsilateral to the carotid lesion. The baseline rSo_2, the stable rSo_2 during temporary occlusion, and the highest rSo_2 after reperfusion were noted. The change from the second and third rSo_2 determination was calculated as well. A preoperative and postoperative SPECT scan was obtained.

Key Results

The rSo_2 changes correlated with ischemic symptoms and postoperative hyperperfusion demonstrated by SPECT. The rSo_2 also correlated with the asymmetry index and cerebral vasoreactivity demonstrated on the preoperative SPECT.

Study Strengths and Weaknesses

NIRS sensors were only placed on the side of the carotid lesion and stenting. A second sensor might have served as a control.

Clinical Implications

Transcranial cerebral oximetry may be helpful in detecting carotid stenosis and ischemic changes during carotid artery stenting.

17. Imberti R, Bellinzona G, Langer M. Cerebral tissue pO_2 and $SjvO_2$ changes during moderate hyperventilation in patients with severe traumatic brain injury. *J Neurosurg*. 2002;96: 97–102.

Study Sample

Thirty-six patients with severe closed TBI (GCS score <8) ranging from 16 to 75 years were studied a total of 94 times. Twenty-nine of the 36 experienced diffuse injury; 7 had mass lesions.

Comparison Studied

$SjvO_2$ and $Pbto_2$ in patients with severe TBI were compared during 20-minute periods of moderate hyperventilation, defined as a goal pCO_2 of 27 to 32 mm Hg. The $Pbto_2$ catheter was placed in uninjured brain.

Study Procedures

The ventilatory rate was increased while maintaining a constant tidal volume to decrease the pCO_2 between the second and 5th day after the TBI. All patients were chemically paralyzed for the procedure. The study procedure was performed at least 2 hours after the administration of mannitol. ICP, $SjvO_2$, and $Pbto_2$ were monitored. Each patient underwent the study procedure 3 times from days 4 to 9 after the injury. ICP, mean arterial blood pressure, CPP, Licox (GMS, Kiel Germany) $Pbto_2$, and end-tidal CO_2 were continuously monitored. The $SjvO_2$ was monitored by intermittent blood sampling in some patients as well as continuously. Normal $SjvO_2$ and $Pbto_2$ values were defined as greater than 50% and 10 mm Hg. Zero drift of the $Pbto_2$ catheter was 0.5 ± 1.5 mm Hg, and the sensitivity drift was $4.5\% \pm 3.7\%$. $SjvO_2$ catheter drift was not reported.

Key Results

The response of $SjvO_2$ and $Pbto_2$ was unpredictable and variable. After 20 minutes of moderate hyperventilation,

79.8% of the time both $SjvO_2$ and $Pbto_2$ remained greater than 50% and 10 mm Hg, respectively. However, 16.6% of the time, $Pbto_2$ decreased below 10 mm Hg while $SjvO_2$ remained greater than 50%. Patients with $Pbto_2$ below 10 mm Hg were noted to have low $Pbto_2$ and CPP before hyperventilation and higher CO_2 reactivity. Three-fourths of the time hyperventilation resulted in a decrease in both $SjvO_2$ and $Pbto_2$; one-fourth of the time, $SjvO_2$ and $Pbto_2$ trended in opposite directions.

Study Strengths and Weaknesses

Each patient was reportedly studied 3 times which would be 108 total data collections. Only 94 were included in the final data analysis. The $Pbto_2$ catheter was placed in uninjured white matter which would be more likely to correspond to changes in $SjvO_2$ than if it were placed in vulnerable ischemic tissue. This study did not address the use of the $Pbto_2$ catheter as a measure of regional oxygenation in vulnerable tissue.

Clinical Implications

Continuous monitoring of $Pbto_2$ may reflect decreases in regional cerebral oxygenation not detected by $SjvO_2$. Simultaneous monitoring of $Pbto_2$ and $SjvO_2$ is complementary, is not redundant, and may detect ischemia not demonstrated by $SjvO_2$.

18. Lam JM, Chan MS, Poon WS. Cerebral venous oxygen saturation monitoring: is dominant jugular bulb cannulation good enough? *Br J Neurosurg*. 1996;10:357–364.

Study Sample

Thirteen patients with traumatic brain injury were included in the study; 7 had severe head injury (GCS score ≤ 8) and 5 had mass lesions with deterioration.

Study Procedures

Size 6 French gauge angiographic catheters (n = 10) and size 3.5 French gauge Oximetric Opticath catheters (Abbott Laboratories, North Chicago, IL; n = 3) were used. Pressurized continuous heparin flush maintained patency. All catheters were placed in the jugular bulb and confirmed by angiography. The dominant jugular bulb was selected by compressing the jugular vein. The side with the greater rise in ICP was considered the dominant vein. When the bilateral response was similar, the catheter was placed in the right jugular bulb. A catheter also was placed in the confluence of the cerebral sinus (CCS) under angiography for comparison. Blood samples were drawn simultaneously from the jugular bulb and the cerebral sinus at intervals of 15 minutes to 2 hours. The hemoglobin of each sample was also assessed to assure adequate mixing and minimal contamination. Data analysis was conducted on 176 pairs of blood samples.

Key Results

Correspondence between the paired samples was good overall with agreement 80% to 100% within 4% in 9 of the participants. In the remaining 4 patients, the agreement was moderate (50%–57%) in 2 and poor (0%–4%) in the remaining 2. The range of Sjvo$_2$ was 19% to 97.8%. Utilizing the dominant jugular bulb was a strong reflection of global oxygenation in 11 patients, moderate reflection in 2 patients, and poor reflection in 2 patients.

Study Strengths and Weaknesses

The Sjvo$_2$ was compared to the CCS to determine the dominant jugular bulb. The CBF to the CCS reflected blood from the cerebral hemispheres without the extracerebral contamination that can occur during withdrawal of blood from the jugular bulb. This was a small sample size. The side of injury was not taken into consideration. Bilateral imaging of the jugular foramens by CT to determine dominance was not reported. Inadvertent puncture of the carotid artery occurred once during insertion and 2 catheters occluded related to failure of the pressurized flush system. Cannulation of the CCS was determined to be safe when performed by experienced neuroradiologists.

Clinical Implications

The jugular compression test may be an accurate way to determine jugular dominance. Placement of the Sjvo$_2$ catheter in the dominant jugular may more accurately indicate global oxygenation.

19. **Meixensberger J, Renner C, Simanowski R, Schmidtke A, Dings J, Roosen K. Influence of cerebral oxygenation following severe head injury on neuropsychological testing.** *Neurol Res.* **2004;26:414–417.**

Study Sample

This sample consisted of 20 severely TBI patients, 14 men and 6 women; 12 had mass lesions that were evacuated.

Study Procedures

Pbto$_2$ monitoring was performed in all patients from admission until day 10 using Clark type polarographic microcatheter probes (GMS, Kiel Germany). Probes were positioned in the right frontal lobe, on the side of the injury in cases of focal injury. ICP and CPP monitoring were performed as well. The critical value for cerebral hypoxia was defined as 15 mm Hg. Patients underwent neuropsychological testing 2 to 3 years after injury and after rehabilitation. Tests of intelligence, speech, and long- and short-term memory were employed. Patients were divided into 2 groups, group A with less than 20% of their recorded Pbto$_2$ less than 15 mm Hg and Group B with more than 20% of their recorded Pbto$_2$ greater than 15 mm Hg.

Key Results

Patients with more than 20% of their Pbto$_2$ less than 15 mm Hg had lower neuropsychological testing scores in regard to intelligence, selective attention, and short- and long-term memory ($P < 0.05$). Group A had a mean Glasgow Outcome Scale (GOS) score of 4.6 while Group B had a mean GOS score of 4.1, which was not statistically significant.

Study Strengths and Weaknesses

The Pbto$_2$ catheter was placed on the side of the injury when the injury was focal. Initial GCS scores were not included in the report. The investigators did not consider the effects of maintaining a Pbto$_2$ greater than 20 mm Hg in their data analysis. Would it have resulted in even better neuropsychological testing results? Brain tissue oxygenation values were considered without regard to ICP/CPP.

Clinical Implications

Maintaining Pbto$_2$ greater than 15 mm Hg may result in better neuropsychologic outcomes following severe traumatic brain injury. Patients with Pbto$_2$ less than 15 mm Hg 20% or more of the time may have worse neurocognitive outcomes.

20. **Meixensberger J, Vath A, Jaeger M, Kunz E, Dings J, Roosen K. Monitoring of brain tissue oxygenation following severe subarachnoid hemorrhage.** *Neurol Res.* **2003;25:445–450.**

Study Sample

Forty-two patients with an aneurysmal SAH, an initial Hunt-Hess grade IV, or with secondary deterioration to grade IV related to vasospasm were included in this study. Fourteen patients had poor outcome; 28 had moderate to good outcome.

Study Procedures

A Licox Pbto$_2$ catheter (GMS, Kiel-Mielkendorf, Germany) was placed in the vascular territory determined to be at risk for ischemia, usually adjacent to the vessel with the aneurysm. Catheter reactivity to oxygen was assessed and a head CT was performed to rule out bleeding or infarction around the catheter. Fourteen of the patients had bilateral monitoring with the second catheter being placed in normal tissue contralateral to the side with hypodensity. ICP and CPP were monitored as well. Monitoring was continuous. The patients were categorized as survivors and nonsurvivors. Data were analyzed as total monitoring time, total time minus the last 2 days, the second to the last day of monitoring, and the last day of monitoring. Critical values were CPP ≤ 70 mm Hg, ICP > 20 mm Hg, and Pbto$_2$ ≤ 10 mm Hg. The mean duration of monitoring in poor outcome patients was 3.7 (2.7–6.5) days. The mean duration of monitoring in good outcome patients was 7.8 (4.7–10.0) days.

Key Results

A Pbto$_2$ value of ≤10 mm Hg over the entire monitoring period was 3.5 times greater in the nonsurvivor group than in the survivor group. ICP >20 mm Hg and CPP ≤70 mm Hg in nonsurvivors was 8 times and 5 times greater in non-survivors, respectively. Critical values of Pbto$_2$, ICP, and CPP were also more frequent in nonsurvivors during the last monitoring day. However, the good and poor outcome groups did not have any significant differences in CPP and Pbto$_2$ before the last day of monitoring. By the last day of monitoring, cerebral edema, herniation, and brain death were present. Pbto$_2$ monitoring along with ICP and CPP were not early predictors of death in patients with SAH.

Study Strengths and Weaknesses

The last 2 days of monitoring and the last day of monitoring after severe aneurysmal SAH were noted rather than simply looking at the entire time period to avoid skewing the predictive value of Pbto$_2$ catheters. Critical values of ICP were more statistically significant than critical values of Pbto$_2$.

Clinical Implications

Pbto$_2$ catheters may be not be an early predictor of outcome in severe aneurysmal SAH patients.

21. Menzel M, Doppenberg EM, Zauner A, Soukup J, Reinert MM, Bullock R. Increased inspired oxygen concentration as a factor in improved brain tissue oxygenation and tissue lactate levels after severe human head injury. *J Neurosurg.* 1999;91:1–10. Comments in 1999;91:1065–1067; 2000;92:736–738; 2003;98: 223–224, author's reply 98:224–225.

Study Sample

Twenty-two patients with severe traumatic brain injury (TBI) GCS score of ≤8 and were older than 16 years were included in the study.

Study Procedures

Patients were divided into 2 matching cohorts: 12 under-went standard treatment for severe head injury; the other 12 received 6 hours of increased F$_{IO2}$ within the first 24 hours after admission to the hospital to increase the patients' pO$_2$ level. A Paratrend 7/Neurotrend brain tissue oxygenation catheter (Diametric Medical Inc, Roseville, MN) with Pbtco$_2$, pH, and brain temperature monitoring capability was placed after the sensor was calibrated by bubbling sterile precision gases through the tonometer chamber. ICP/CPP and microdialysis were conducted as well in all 24 patients.

Key Results

Mean Pbto$_2$ levels increased in the hyperoxygenated group up to 359% ± 39% above the baseline during the 6-hour study procedure and the lactate levels decreased by 40% (P <0.05). The brain Pbto$_2$ increased in each patient treated with oxygen enhancement. The mean Pbto$_2$ was found to be 82.7 ± 44.1 mm Hg. Not all of the patients' Pbto$_2$ levels increased to the same extent. The control cohort did not demonstate significant variations in Pbto$_2$ or brain lactate.

Study Strengths and Weaknesses

The location of the catheter in relation to the brain injury was not stated. Furthermore, while Pbto$_2$ increased in the area detected by the catheter, the tissue oxygenation beyond the catheter or globally was not specified. Hyperoxygenation without additional monitoring must be used with caution as it may also cause ischemia to healthy brain tissue or induce oxygen toxicity.

Clinical Implications

Increasing the systemic oxygen in severe head injury may increase the Pbto$_2$ and decrease the brain lactate levels. This may represent a shift to aerobic metabolism.

22. Narotam PK, Burjonrappa SC, Raynor SC, Rao M, Taylon C. Cerebral oxygenation in major pediatric trauma: its relevance to trauma severity and outcome. *J Pediatr Surg.* 2006;41:505–513.

Study Sample

Sixteen patients with major trauma and significant head injury were included in this study. The mean age was 14 years with 10 men and 6 women. The mean Injury Severity Score was 36, Revised Trauma Score was 5.4, and the Pediatric Trauma Score (PTS) was 3.

Study Procedures

A triple lumen ICP, Pbto$_2$, and brain temperature monitoring system (Licox, Integra NeuroSciences, Plainsboro, NJ) was placed into the parenchyma of noncontused, noninfarcted brain. Adaptation time was allowed for the Pbto$_2$ catheter. Pbto$_2$ was used to direct therapy.

Key Results

The Revised Trauma Score correlated moderately with Pbto$_2$ and predicted low cerebral oxygenation. In patients with Pbto$_2$ less than 20 mm Hg, the PTS correlated moderately ($r = 0.671$, $P = –0.033$). A mean Pbto$_2$ for 2 hours and the final Pbto$_2$ in survivors were higher than in those who died (21.6 vs. 7.2 mm Hg, $P = 0.009$, and 25 vs. 11 mm Hg, $P = 0.01$). Low Pbto$_2$ responded to ventilator management, administration of inotropes, and blood transfusions. Four of

6 deaths were associated with high ICP, PTS, and sustained 2-hour low $Pbto_2$.

Study Strengths and Weaknesses

Details regarding TBI and placement side of the $Pbto_2$ catheter in relation to the TBI (ipsilateral or contralateral) were not given.

Clinical Implications

Low $Pbto_2$ values of less than 20 mm Hg may be improved with ventilator management, inotrope administration, and blood transfusions. Licox values of less than 20 mm Hg may be indicative of low oxygenation and predictive of poor outcome. Low $Pbto_2$ also may be associated with increased ICP and PTS.

23. Palmer S, Bader MK. Brain tissue oxygenation in brain death. *Neurocrit Care.* 2005;2:217–222.

Study Sample

This study consisted of 11 patients who experienced brain death as a result of severe TBI, aneurysmal SAH, brain tumor, intracerebral hemorrhage, or systemic injury. Ages ranged from 31 to 65 years. The study sample was exclusively men. Nine of the 11 had a GCS score of 3 on admission. Time of brain death from admission varied from 5 hours to 7 days. The study sample was derived from a large sample of 72 patients with intracranial pathology.

Study Procedures

A Licox (Integra NeuroSciences, Plainsboro, NJ) $Pbto_2$ catheter was placed on the side opposite the major intracranial injury in trauma patients and on the same side in SAH patients. ICP and CPP were monitored also. CPP was maintained at 60 to 70 mm Hg initially and then adjusted based on $Pbto_2$ and ICP data. Brain death was confirmed by established guidelines and nuclear medicine cerebral flow studies.

Key Results

$Pbto_2$ fell to 0 mm Hg on 100% of the 11 brain dead patients. None of the other 61 patients with intracranial pathology experienced a $Pbto_2$ of 0 mm Hg. Sensitivity and specificity for $Pbto_2$ to detect brain death were 100%.

Study Strengths and Weaknesses

Multimodality monitoring was used in the management of study sample prior to brain death and continued to be used as an adjunct to the usual clinical determination of brain death, including coma, absence of brainstem reflexes, and apnea. The sample size of 11 is small and additional studies are warranted. The $Pbto_2$ catheter is considered a monitor of regional rather than global oxygenation. Brain death is a global phenomenon.

Clinical Implications

Brain injury may progress to brain death despite aggressive multimodality monitoring and management. Brain tissue oxygenation monitoring may be useful as an adjunct to usual clinical determination of brain death.

24. Robertson CS, Contant CF, Narayan RK, Grossman RG. Cerebral blood flow, $AVDO_2$, and neurologic outcome in head-injured patients. *J Neurotrauma.* 1992;9(Suppl 1): S349–S358.

Study Sample

Thirty-three patients with severe head injury who were admitted in or deteriorated to a coma were included in this study. Eighty-eight percent of the patients were men with a mean age of 35 ± 9 years. Closed head injuries constitute 88% of the patients; gunshot wounds made up the remaining 12%. The GCS score was 9 or less. Three-fourths of this cohort had a poor outcome with severe disability, vegetative state, or death. Three months after injury, one-third were dead.

Study Procedures

$Sjvo_2$ was monitored using a fiberoptic catheter. CBF, cerebral metabolic rate of oxygen and lactate, $AjvDo_2$, and cerebral metabolic rate of oxygen were monitored every 8 hours as well and whenever the $Sjvo_2$ decreased to less than 50%. CBF was categorized as normal, increased, or decreased within 2 standard deviations for the pCO_2.

Key Results

Half of the patients had $Sjvo_2$ desaturations with the $Sjvo_2$ falling below 50%. The $Sjvo_2$ desaturations were associated with decreased CPP (CPP <50 mm Hg), system hypoxia (pO_2 <90%), hypocapnia (pCO_2 <25 mm Hg), vasospasm, or any combination of these clinical conditions. $AjvDo_2$ was the greatest on day 1 and decreased over time. The mortality rate was greatest in patients with decreased CBF. Decreased $Sjvo_2$ occurred in 69% of the patients with decreased CBF and only 29% of the patients with normal CBF and 30% of the patients with elevated CBF. Decreased CBF and high $AjvDo_2$ were associated with poor neurologic outcomes. $Sjvo_2$ decreases were 2 times more likely in patients with decreased CBF.

Study Strengths and Weaknesses

CBF was measured by nitrous oxide saturation method. Clinical conditions were associated with not only $Sjvo_2$ desaturation but an increase in $AjvDo_2$. $Sjvo_2$ desaturations were associated with outcomes. However, the relationship among all of these variables was not 100% and variances could not be explained. These findings were identified as preliminary results.

Clinical Implications

Decreases in Sjvo$_2$ and increases in AjvDo$_2$ are associated with cerebral ischemia in severe brain injury and may be predictive of outcome.

25. Sarrafzadeh AS, Kiening KL, Bardt TF, Schneider GH, Unterberg AW, Lanksch WR. Cerebral oxygenation in contusioned vs. nonlesioned brain tissue: monitoring of ptiO$_2$ with Licox and Paratrend. *Acta Neurochir Suppl.* 1998;71:186–189.

Study Sample

This study included 7 patients aged 22 to 54 years with severe TBI and GCS score <8. All 7 had diffuse injury.

Study Procedures

Two Pbto$_2$ catheters were placed in each patient. One catheter was a Licox brain tissue oxygen catheter (Licox System, GMS, Germany) and the other a Paratrend (Diametrics Medical, UK). In 3 patients, both catheters were inserted in nonlesioned tissue; in another 2 patients, the Paratrend catheter was inserted into nonlesioned tissue and the Licox catheter was inserted into pericontusional tissue; finally, in another 2 patients, both catheters were inserted into contused tissue. CT scan was obtained to verify placement in the white matter and to assess for any hemorrhage around the catheters. Pericontusional tissues were defined as 1–2 cm adjacent to the contused tissue. Upon removal of the catheters they were checked for drift. The catheters remained in place 2.1 to 10.4 days.

Key Results

In the nonlesioned tissue both catheters closely correlated with the Pbto$_2$ within <5 mm Hg after 20 hours of insertion. In the pericontusional tissue, the Pbto$_2$ was decreased compared to nonlesioned tissue by 10.3 mm Hg. In the contused brain, the Pbto$_2$ was always less than 10 mm Hg regardless of the catheter used. The Pbto$_2$ decreased when the MAP decreased below 60 mm Hg. A positive response to increased Fio$_2$ was seen only in percontusional and nonlesioned brain. Brain tissue oxygen monitors recognize cerebral hypoxia or ischemia in percontusional or nonlesioned brain.

Study Strengths and Weaknesses

This was a small sample size and statistical power is lacking. Two different brain tissue oxygen catheters were compared as though their values were equivalent. The technology is different and the critical thresholds are thought to be different.

Clinical Implications

Optimal placement of the Pbto$_2$ catheter is in percontusional or nonlesioned brain to detect regional cerebral hypoxia. The lesioned tissue may not respond to interventions to improved regional cerebral oxygenation.

26. Smith JM, Stiefel MF, Magge S, Gracias V, Le Roux PD. Packed red blood cell transfusion increases local cerebral oxygenation. *Crit Care Med.* 2005;33:1104–1108. Comments in 33:1171–1172, 33:2856.

Study Samples

Thirty-five patients with TBI, closed head injuries or subdural hematomas, or aneurysmal SAH were included in this study. Twenty-three were TBI injuries and 12 were aneurysmal SAH. The median age was 47 years with a range of 14 to 80 years. All were fully resuscitated and without cardiac disease. All patients had a GCS score of ≤8 on admission or within 24 hours of admission.

Study Procedures

All patients had a Licox Pbto$_2$ catheter (Integra Neuro-Sciences, Plainsboro, NJ) and an ICP/CPP monitor. Each patient received at least 1 unit of packed red blood cells. Twenty-eight patients received more than 1 unit. Patients were transfused to a goal hemoglobin of 10 g/dL and a hematocrit of 30%. The age of the red blood cells was noted for each unit. The Pbto$_2$ was continuously monitored before, during, and after transfusion.

Key Results

In 26 of the 35 patients (75%), the transfusion of packed red blood cells (RBCs) was associated with an increase in Pbto$_2$ within an hour after transfusion, regardless of CPP, So$_2$, or Fio$_2$. The mean increase was 5.1 ± 9.4 mm Hg, a 49% increase (P <0.01). However, in 9 patients, the Pbto$_2$ decreased after transfusion. RBC transfusion did not change the Sao$_2$, Fio$_2$, or CPP significantly.

Study Strengths and Weaknesses

Placement of the Pbto$_2$ catheter on the side of the injury or bleed rather than contralateral side was not noted. Though hypothesized to be a significant factor, the relationship of the age of the RBCs and transfusion's effect on Pbto$_2$ was not statistically significant.

Clinical Implications

Transfusion of packed RBCs may increase or decrease Pbto$_2$. The patient must be assessed for changes in Pbto$_2$ during transfusion.

27. Sokol DK, Markand ON, Daly EC, Luerssen TG, Malkoff MD. Near infrared spectroscopy (NIRS) distinguishes seizure types. *Seizure.* 2000;9:323–327.

Study Sample

Eight adult patients with medically refractory temporal lobe epilepsy were included in the study. Four men and 4 women were included in the study.

Study Procedures

The Somanetics 3100A transcranial cerebral oximeter was placed on the patient's forehead to the right or left of the midline, behind electroencephalogram leads F7/F8. Sensors were placed ipsilateral to the epileptogenic focus and were secured to prevent artifact during seizure activity. Simultaneous electroencephalogram monitoring occurred. Mean rSo_2 values were recorded preictal for 5 minutes, 30 seconds during the seizure, and 5 minutes postictal. Minimum and maximum rSo_2 values were used to determine the percentage change from preictal to ictal periods.

Key Results

NIRS transcranial cerebral oximeter differentiated complex partial seizures and secondarily generalized seizures. The rSo_2 levels increased (16.6% change) for all 12 complex partial seizures but decreased with all 4 secondarily generalized seizures (51.1% change). No change in rSo_2 was seen during a subclinical seizure.

Study Strengths and Weaknesses

This was a small sample size. The decrease in rSo_2 may be related to a decrease in systemic Sao_2 rather than an actual reflection of CBF flow patterns.

Clinical Implications

NIRS cerebral oximetry may differentiate seizure types related to CBF flow patterns during seizure activity.

28. Stiefel MF, Heuer GG, Abrahams JM, et al. The effect of nimodipine on cerebral oxygenation in patients with poor-grade subarachnoid hemorrhage. *J Neurosurg.* 2004;101:594–599.

Study Sample

Eleven patients with poor grade aneurysmal SAH, Hunt-Hess IV–V were included in this study and were stable for at least 12 hours. Three men and 8 women were included with a mean age of 64.3 ± 10.9 years. None of these patients demonstrated a decrease in blood pressure after nimodipine administration, and none received a vasopressor to increase their blood pressure. All were within 7 days of their SAH.

Study Procedures

Brain tissue oxygenation using a Licox $Pbto_2$ catheter (Integra NeuroSciences, Plainsboro, NJ) was inserted in the frontal white matter and continuously monitored. ICP and CPP were monitored as well. Nimodipine 60 mg was administered through a nasogastric or small bowel feeding tube every 4 hours. MAP was continuously monitored.

Key Results

The baseline $Pbto_2$ was 38.4 ± 10.9 mm Hg before nimodipine administration. In 7 of 11 patients, the administration of nimodipine resulted in a reduction in $Pbto_2$ without a concomitant decrease in arterial blood pressure. The greatest reduction in $Pbto_2$ occurred about 15 minutes after administration with a mean of 26.9 ± 7.7 mm Hg. The $Pbto_2$ remained decreased at 30 minutes with a mean of 27.5 ± 7.7 mm Hg. The $Pbto_2$ was still decreased at 60 minutes with a mean of 29.7 ± 11.1 mm Hg. $Pbto_2$ values returned to baseline after about 2 hours. All decreases were statistically significant at $P < 0.05$. The presence or absence of vasospasm was not associated with a change in $Pbto_2$.

Study Strengths and Weaknesses

The investigator excluded a decrease in blood pressure as a cause for a decrease in $Pbto_2$. The investigators did not look at the effect of changing the nimodipine administration to 30 mg every 2 hours. Location of the $Pbto_2$ in regard to the side of the injury was not noted. Sample size was small. A larger study, specifically a prospective randomized controlled trial would substantiate or repudiate these findings.

Clinical Implications

Nimodipine administration for aneurysmal SAH may decrease $Pbto_2$ without a concomitant decrease in blood pressure. The nurse must monitor for associated decreases in $Pbto_2$ and intervene as prescribed.

29. Stiefel MF, Heuer GG, Smith, MJ, et al. Cerebral oxygenation following decompressive hemicraniectomy for the treatment of refractory intracranial hypertension. *J Neurosurg.* 2004;101:241–247.

Study Sample

Seven patients, 5 men and 2 women with a mean age of 30.6 ± 9.7 years were included in this study. Five experienced traumatic brain injury and 2 presented with SAH. All but 1 had an admission GCS score of 3.

Study Procedures

A Licox brain tissue oxygenation catheter (Integra NeuroSciences, Plainsboro, NJ) was placed in the frontal lobe on the side of maximal injury or edema. ICP/CPP monitoring was performed as well. CPP was maintained with vasopressors before the hemicraniectomy. For sustained increased ICP greater than 20 mm Hg and refractory to standard therapies of osmotherapy, barbiturates, and controlled hyperventilation, a decompressive hemicraniectomy was performed. The Pbto$_2$ and ICP catheters were replaced after the craniotomy on the same side as the surgery.

Key Results

Before the decompressive hemicraniectomy, the mean Pbto$_2$ was 21.2 ± 13.8 mm Hg. After the decompressive hemicraniectomy, the mean Pbto$_2$ was 45.5 ± 25.4 mm Hg, an increase of 114%. The mean ICP before the decompressive hemicraniectomy was 26 ± 4 mm Hg and after surgery 19.4 ± 11 mm Hg. The correlation between the change in ICP and Pbto$_2$ was small to moderate with an $r = 0.3$. No relationship existed between Pbto$_2$ and CPP after the hemicraniectomy.

Study Strengths and Weaknesses

Though the sample consisted of 2 patients with different diagnoses, they were similar in that none of the patients exhibited cerebral infarction, structural lesions, or vasospasm on TCD prior to the hemicraniectomy. The sample size was very small. Outcome was not noted.

Clinical Implications

Decompressive hemicraniectomy in refractory increased ICP may not only decrease the ICP but improve regional Pbto$_2$ as well.

30. Stiefel MF, Spiotta A, Gracia VH, et al. Reduced mortality rate in patients with severe traumatic brain injury treated with brain tissue oxygen monitoring. *J Neurosurg.* 2005; 103:805–81l. Comments in 105:504–506.

Study Sample

Fifty-three patients with a severe TBI, GCS score <8, were included in the study.

Study Procedures

Patients were divided into 2 groups with similar demographics, age, GCS admission score, pupillary response, pathology, initial resuscitation, and Injury Severity Score. Group A underwent routine ICP/CPP monitoring and standard severe TBI care. Group B underwent routine ICP/CPP monitoring plus continuous Pbto$_2$ monitoring with the Licox catheter (Integra NeuroSciences, Plainsboro, NJ). The Pbto$_2$ catheter was placed in healthy brain tissue on the side with the most pathology but without contusion or infarct and confirmed by CT. All patients were monitored for at least 72 hours unless they died. Patients received Pbto$_2$ based therapy in addition to ICP/CPP therapy. The Pbto$_2$ was maintained at 25 mm Hg or greater. A CPP of 60 mm Hg was maintained. Outcome at discharge from the hospital was noted as well.

Key Results

Daily ICP and CPP were similar in each group. The mortality rate in Group A using conventional ICP and CPP monitoring only was 44%. The mortality rate in Group A using Pbto$_2$ targeted therapy in addition to ICP/CPP-directed management had a reduced mortality rate of 25% (P <0.05). Pbto$_2$ targeted therapy included maintaining CPP at 60 mm Hg, increasing oxygenation, administering transfusions, aggressive management of hyperthermia and seizures, and as a last resort, decompressive hemicraniectomy. Seventeen percent of Group A required additional hospitalization or nursing home placement; none of Group B required nursing home placement. All members of Group B were discharged to home or rehabilitation.

Study Strengths and Weaknesses

This study included comparable control and treatment groups. The study size was fairly small, and historical controls were used. However, because Pbto$_2$ was not monitored in the control group, the incidence of cerebral hypoxia is not known in the control group.

Clinical Implications

The use of Pbto$_2$ targeted therapy in addition to ICP/CPP directed management may improve outcomes for severe TBI patients.

31. Stiefel MF, Spiotta AM, Udoetuk JD, et al. Intra-arterial papaverine used to treat cerebral vasospasm reduces brain oxygen. *Neurocrit Care.* 2006;4:113–118.

Study Sample

Five patients with aneurysmal SAH, poor clinical grade Hunt-Hess IV–V were included in this study. All had symptomatic vasospasm.

Study Procedures

Severe vasospasm was confirmed by angiography. A Pbto$_2$ catheter (Licox, Integra NeuroSciences, Plainsboro, NJ) was placed ipsilateral to the side with the highest MCA mean flow velocities (MFV) on TCD. ICP was monitored as well. Placement was confirmed by CT scan. All patients underwent intra-arterial papaverine 5 to 7 days after SAH. Data were collected 10 minutes before, 10 minutes during, and 10 minutes after papaverine and averaged.

Key Results

Angiographic vasospasm decreased in all 5 patients. Mean Pbto$_2$ decreased during intra-arterial papaverine in all patients from 32.99 ± 1.45 mm Hg to 22.96 ± 2.9 mm Hg (P <0.05). The Pbto$_2$ returned to the baseline 10 minutes after the injection. ICP increased from 23.04 ± 1.19 mm Hg to 29.89 ± 1.18 mm Hg. The correlation between $Pbto_2$ decrease and ICP increase was moderate ($r^2 = 0.526$).

Study Strengths and Weaknesses

The sample size was small and the study design did not include a control group. The $Pbto_2$ catheter was not necessarily in the territory that received the papaverine. MAP but not CPP results were included in the study report.

Clinical Implications

$Pbto_2$ monitoring may detect regional hypoxia associated with intra-arterial papaverine injection.

32. Stiefel MF, Udoetuk JD, Spiotta AM, et al. Conventional neurocritical care and cerebral oxygenation after traumatic brain injury. *J Neurosurg.* 2006;105:568–575.

Study Sample

Twenty-five severe traumatic brain injury patients with a mean age of 30 ± 20 years were included in the study sample. The sample consisted of 19 men and 6 women with a GCS score ≤8.

Study Procedures

A brain oxygenation catheter (Licox, Integra Neuro-Sciences, Plainsboro, NJ) was placed in the frontal lobe adjacent to the worst area of injury. The probe was allowed to stabilize over an hour and probe function was assessed with an Fio_2 challenge of 100%. CT scan was used to confirm correct placement of the catheter, adjacent but not in an area of contusion or infarct. ICP, CPP, and $Pbto_2$ were continuously monitored. Patients underwent standard traumatic brain injury care, including: intubation and mechanical ventilation; maintenance of the mean arterial blood pressure of greater than 90 mm Hg; maintenance of a pCO_2 of 30 to 40 mm Hg; head of bed elevation 15 to 30°; euvolemia, maintenance of normothermia between 35° and 37ºC; prophylactic anticonvulsants; and sedation, mannitol and CSF drainage for an ICP >20 mm Hg.

Key Results

Approximately 13 of the patients with a CPP >60 mm Hg experienced severe brain hypoxia, defined as a $Pbto_2$ value of <10 mm Hg.

Study Strengths and Weaknesses

The data were analyzed retrospectively. Traumatic brain injury patient requiring a craniotomy for the evacuation of lesions did not receive $Pbto_2$ monitoring within the first 6 hours after injury. Placement of the $Pbto_2$ probe in normal white matter rather than contused brain may have reflected global oxygenation rather than regional oxygenation.

Clinical Implications

Maintaining an ICP <20 mm Hg and a CPP >60 mm Hg alone does not protect the traumatic brain injury patient from cerebral hypoxia. The clinical parameter for monitoring secondary neuronal injury is $Pbto_2$ and not ICP and CPP.

33. Stiefel MF, Udoetuk JD, Storm PB, et al. Brain tissue oxygen monitoring in pediatric patients with severe traumatic brain injury. *J Neurosurg.* 2006;105(Suppl 4):281–286.

Study Sample

Six pediatric severe traumatic brain injury patients comprised the cohort, 4 male and 2 females with a GCS score of ≤8. Ages ranged from 6 to 16 and the GCS scores ranged from 3 to 7. Five of the 6 patients were pedestrian injuries and the other was a gunshot wound.

Study Procedures

A triple bolt ICP, $Pbto_2$, brain temperature system (Licox, Integra NeuroSciences, Plainsboro, NJ) was inserted into the noncontused tissue on the side of the lesion or cerebral edema. Placement was confirmed by CT scan. ICP, CPP, $Pbto_2$ as well as vital signs, Sao_2, end-tidal CO_2, and pH were continuously recorded. Management goals included attaining and maintaining an ICP <20 mm Hg and a CPP ≥40 mm Hg. Management of the patient included surgical evacuation of hematomas, maintaining a pCO_2 35 to 39 mm Hg and an Sao_2 >99%. Sedation, CSF drainage, neuromuscular blockade, mannitol, and 3% saline were used to maintain an ICP less than 20 mm Hg.

Key Results

A total of 346 hours of continuous monitoring of the ICP and $Pbto_2$ revealed that a higher $Pbto_2$ resulted with an ICP <20 mm Hg and a CPP >40 mm Hg. No complications from monitoring, including hemorrhage or infection, were noted. A low $Pbto_2$, defined as <10mm Hg, was associated with death. Transient decreases in $Pbto_2$ occurred despite acceptable ICP and CPP levels.

Study Strengths and Weaknesses

This study included an extremely small sample size, and data were reviewed retrospectively. However, it is one of the first studies of $Pbto_2$ in the pediatric TBI population.

Clinical Implications

Continuous $Pbto_2$ monitoring is possible in the pediatric TBI population. $Pbto_2$ values comparable to adults, <10 mm Hg, in association with ICP levels >20 mm Hg are associated with poor outcomes. Acceptable CPP values for the pediatric traumatic brain injury population are less established than for adults. Use of $Pbto_2$ monitoring with

ICP/CPP monitoring may provide additional insight into the acceptable CPP threshold for the pediatric population.

34. Stocchetti N, Paparella A, Bridelli F, Bacchi M, Piazza P, Zuccoli P. Cerebral venous oxygen saturation studied with bilateral samples in the internal jugular veins. *Neurosurgery.* 1994; 34:38–44.

Study Sample

Thirty-two severe traumatic brain injury patients with a mean age of 43.9 years were included in the study sample. All but 1 was comatose on admission.

Study Procedures

Bilateral internal jugular veins were cannulated with 20 gauge catheters; continuous recording of $Sjvo_2$ was obtained in 5. Blood was simultaneously drawn from both internal jugular veins an average of 5.34 times per patient with a total sample size of 342. Mean and standard deviation between the bilateral internal jugular samples were determined.

Key Results

Fifteen patients had greater than 15% differences in their bilateral $Sjvo_2$; 3 had greater than 10% but less than 15% differences. Only 8 patients had bilateral internal jugular $Sjvo_2$ differences of less than 5%. Ninety-five percent confidence intervals revealed that between 30% and 64% of all patients may have a bilateral $Sjvo_2$ difference of greater than 15%. Unilateral $Sjvo_2$ monitoring may not accurately reflect oxygenation in both hemispheres.

Study Strengths and Weaknesses

The correct position of the catheters in the jugular bulb was verified by x-ray. CBF to each hemisphere was not determined for comparison with the bilateral $Sjvo_2$. The rate of blood withdrawal from each catheter was not noted. Maximal rather than minimal differences between the $Sjvo_2$ of blood from both catheters was analyzed.

Clinical Implications

Because unilateral $Sjvo_2$ monitoring may not accurately reflect brain oxygenation in both hemispheres, $Sjvo_2$ data as a measure of global oxygenation must be considered in context with other data including the neurologic exam, neurodiagnostic studies, and other neurophysiologic monitoring.

35. Suazo JAC, Maas AI, van den Brink W, van Santbrink H, Steyerberg EW, Avezaat CJ. CO2 reactivity and brain oxygen pressure monitoring in severe head injury. *Crit Care Med.* 2000;28:3268–3274.

Study Sample

This study sample consisted of 90 patients with severe TBI, aged between 11 and 83 years. The mean age was 35 ± 17 years. Seventy-six percent were men. All had a GCS score ≥8. Eighty-four patients were admitted to the study within 24 hours and 6 were between 24 and 52 hours following injury; 61 had intracranial mass lesions.

Study Procedures

The minute ventilation was increased on the ventilator 20% above baseline to decrease the arterial pCO_2 for 15 minutes daily for 5 days. $Pbto_2$ was monitored with a Licox $Pbto_2$ catheter (GMS Kiel, Germany) in the frontal lobe, contralateral to the injured side. ICP, MAP, and CPP were monitored as well. The change in $Pbto_2$ to the change in pCO_2 reactivity was calculated. Hyperventilation was defined as a decrease in pCO_2 of equal to or greater than 2 mm Hg.

Key Results

Effective hyperventilation was achieved in 218 of 272 study procedures performed. Baseline pCO_2 was 32.3 ± 4.5 mm Hg. The average reduction in pCO_2 was 3.8 ± 1.7 mm Hg. The $Pbto_2/pCO_2$ reactivity was the lowest on the first study day, 0.8 ± 2.3 mm Hg, but increased on days 2 through 5, 6.1 ± 4.4 mm Hg. Hyperventilation may increase the risk of ischemia as the time since injury increases through day 5.

Study Strengths and Weaknesses

The study demonstrated decreases in $Pbto_2$ with hyperventilation in uninjured brain tissue. The injured side of the brain was not monitored. Only 272 study procedures were performed out of a possible 450.

Clinical Implications

Hyperventilation decreases $Pbto_2$ in healthy tissue following TBI. Carbon dioxide reactivity of the cerebral blood vessels increases from day 1 through day 5 of injury.

36. Torella F, Cowley RD, Thorniley MS, McCollum CN. Regional tissue oxygenation during hemorrhage: can near infrared spectroscopy be used to monitor blood loss? *Shock.* 2002; 18:440–444.

Study Sample

Forty healthy volunteers were included in this study. Ages ranged from 24 to 53 years; 27 men and 13 women participated.

Study Procedures

The rSo_2 was monitored during a 470 mL blood withdrawal. Baseline rSo_2 and the rSo_2 after each 2% of blood volume withdrawal, and 5 and 10 minutes after completion of blood withdrawal were recorded. Median blood withdrawal time was 5.4 minutes. INVOS transcranial cerebral oximeter (Somanetics) was used to monitor rSo$_2$.

Key Results

As blood loss increased, rSo$_2$ decreased ($r = -0.59$, $P < 0.001$).

Study Strengths and Weaknesses

The removal of blood occurred in a relatively short time, comparable to hemorrhage. This study was conducted in healthy volunteers, which may not reflect hemorrhage in multisystem injury nor rSo$_2$ in patients with TBI.

Clinical Implications

NIRS monitoring may be useful in the detection of systemic blood loss.

OTHER REFERENCES

1. Al-Rawi PG, Hutchinson PJ, Gupta AK, et al. Multiparameter brain tissue monitoring—correlation between parameters and identification of CPP thresholds. *Zentralbl Neurochir.* 2000;61:74–79.

2. Hoffman WE, Charbel FT, Gonzalez-Portillo G, et al. Measurement of ischemia by changes in tissue oxygen, carbon dioxide, and pH. *Surg Neurol.* 1999;51:654–658.

3. Imberti R, Bellinzona G, Riccardi F, et al. Cerebral perfusion pressure and cerebral tissue oxygen tension in a patient during cardiopulmonary resuscitation. *Intensive Care Med.* 2003;29:1016–1019.

4. Johnston AJ, Steiner LA, Coles JP, et al. Effect of cerebral perfusion pressure augmentation on regional oxygenation and metabolism after head injury. *Crit Care Med.* 2005;33:189–195.

5. Korsic M, Jugovic D, Kremzar B. Intracranial pressure and biochemical indicators of brain damage: follow-up study. *Croat Med J.* 2006;47:246–252.

6. Meixensberger J, Kunze K, Barcsay E, et al. Clinical cerebral microdialysis: brain metabolism and brain tissue oxygenation after acute brain injury. *Neurol Res.* 2001;23:801–806.

7. Menzel M, Doppenberg EM, Zauner A, et al. Cerebral oxygenation in patients after severe head injury. *J Neurosurg Anesthesiol,* 1999;11:240–251.

8. Patterson J, Bloom SA, Coyle B, et al. Successful outcome in severe traumatic brain injury: a case study. *J Neurosci Nurs.* 2005;37:236–242.

9. Rothoerl RD, Faltermeier F, Burger R, et al. Dynamic correlation between tissue pO$_2$ and near infrared spectroscopy. *Acta Neurochir Suppl.* 2002;81:311–313.

10. Soehle M, Jaeger M, Meixensberger J. Online assessment of brain tissue oxygen autoregulation in traumatic brain injury and subarachnoid hemorrhage. *Neurol Res.* 2003;25:411–417.

11. Soukup J, Zauner A, Doppenberg EMR, et al. Relationship between brain temperature, brain chemistry and oxygen delivery after severe human head injury: the effect of mild hypothermia. *Neurol Res.* 2002;24:161–168.

12. Wilensky EM, Bloom S. Brain tissue oxygen monitoring: Insertion (Assist), care and troubleshooting. In Wiegand DJL and Carlson K, eds. *AACN Procedure Manual for Critical Care,* 5th ed. St. Louis: Elsevier; 2005:712–719.

13. Charbel FT, Du X, Hoffman WE, et al. Brain tissue pO$_2$, pCO$_2$, and pH during cerebral vasospasm. *Surg Neurol.* 2000;54:432–438.

14. Hoelper BM, Hofmann E, Sporleder R, et al. Transluminal balloon angioplasty improves brain tissue oxygenation and metabolism in severe vasospasm after aneurysmal subarachnoid hemorrhage: case report. *Neurosurgery.* 2003;52:970–976.

15. Nievas MC, Toktamis S, Hollerhage HG, et al. Hyperacute measurement of brain-tissue oxygen, carbon dioxide, pH, and intracranial pressure before, during, and after cerebral angiography in patients with aneursmatic subarachnoid hemorrhage in poor condition. *Surg Neurol.* 2005;64:362–367.

16. Pennings FA, Bouma GJ, Kedaria M, et al. Intraoperative monitoring of brain tissue oxygen and carbon dioxide pressures reveals low oxygenation in peritumoral brain edema. *J Neurosurg Anesthesiol.* 2003;15:1–5.

17. Hutchinson PJ, Al-Rawi PG, O'Connell MT, et al. Monitoring of brain metabolism during aneurysm surgery using microdialysis and brain multiparameter sensors. *Neurol Res.* 1999;21:352–358.

18. Kett-White R, Hutchinson PJ, Al-Rawi PG, et al. Cerebral oxygen and microdialysis monitoring during aneurysm surgery: effects of blood pressure, cerebrospinal fluid drainage, and temporary clipping on infarction. *J Neurosurg.* 2002;96:1013–1019.

19. Littlejohns LR, Bader MK, March K. Brain tissue oxygen monitoring in severe brain injury, I. Research and usefulness in critical care. *Crit Care Nurse.* 2003;23:17–25.

20. Brain Trauma Foundation, American Association of Neurological Surgeons, Congress of Neurological Surgeons. *Management and Prognosis of Severe Traumatic Brain Injury.* 3rd ed. New York: Brain Trauma Foundation; 2007.

21. Zauner A, Doppenberg EM, Woodward JJ, et al. Continuous monitoring of cerebral substrate delivery and clearance: initial experience in 24 patients with

severe acute brain injuries. *Neurosurgery.* 1997;41:1082–1093.

22. Van den Brink WA, van Santbrink H, Avezaat C, et al. Monitoring brain oxygen tension in severe head injury: the Rotterdam experience. *Acta Neurochir.* 1998;71:190–194.

23. Van den Brink W, van Santbrink H, Steyerberg E, et al. Brain oxygen tension in severe head injury. *Neurosurgery.* 2000;46:868–878.

24. Perez A, Minces PG, Schnitzler EJ, et al. Jugular venous oxygen saturation or arteriovenous difference of lactate content and outcome in children with severe traumatic brain injury. *Pediatr Crit Care Med.* 2003;4:33–38.

25. Chan KH, Dearden NM, Miller JD. The significance of posttraumatic increase in cerebral blood flow velocity: a transcranial Doppler ultrasound study. *Neurosurgery.* 1992;30:697–700.

26. Coles JP, Fryer TD, Smielewski P, et al. Incidence and mechanisms of cerebral ischemia in early clinical head injury. *J Cereb Blood Flow Metab.* 2004: 24;202–211.

27. Latronico N, Beindorf AE, Rasulo FA, et al. Limits of intermittent jugular bulb oxygen saturation monitoring in the management of severe head trauma patients. *Neurosurgery.* 2000;46:1131–1139.

28. Mascia L, Andrews PJ, McKeating EG, et al. Cerebral blood flow and metabolism in severe brain injury: the role of pressure autoregulation during cerebral perfusion pressure management. *Intensive Care Med.* 2000;26:202–205.

29. Metz C, Holzschuh M, Bein T, et al. Jugular bulb monitoring of cerebral oxygen metabolism in severe head injury: accuracy of unilateral measurements. *Acta Neurochir Suppl.* 1998;71:324–327.

30. Moss E, Dearden NM, Berridge JC. Effects of changes in mean arterial pressure on SjO2 during cerebral aneurysm surgery. *Br J Anaesth.* 1995;75:527–530.

31. Jansen GF, van Praagh BH, Kedaria MB, et al. Jugular bulb oxygen saturation during propofol and isoflurane/nitrous oxide anesthesia in patients undergoing brain tumor surgery. *Anesth Anal.* 1999;89:358–363.

32. Diephuis JC, Moons KG, Nierich AN, et al. Jugular bulb desaturation during coronary artery surgery: a comparison of off-pump and on-pump procedures. *Br J Anesth.* 2005:94:715–720.

33. Hanel F, von Knobelsdorff G, Werner C, et al. Hypercapnia prevents jugular bulb desaturation during rewarming from hypothermic cardiopulmonary bypass. *Anesthesiology.* 1998;89:19–23.

34. Kadoi Y, Kawahara F, Saito S, et al. Effects of hypothermic and normothermic cardiopulmonary bypass on brain oxygenation. *Ann Thorac Surg.* 1999;68:34–39.

35. McCleary AJ, Gower S, McGoldrick JP, et al. Does hypothermia prevent cerebral ischaemia during cardiopulmonary bypass? *Cardiovasc Surg.* 1999;7: 425–431.

36. Millar SA, Alston RP, Souter MJ, et al. Continuous monitoring of jugular bulb oxyhaemoglobin saturation using the Edslab dual lumen oximetry catheter during and after cardiac surgery. *Br J Anaesth.* 1999;82:521–524.

37. Shaaban AM, Harmer M, Latto IP. Jugular bulb oximetry during cardiac surgery. *Anaesthesia.* 2001;56:24–37.

38. Souter MJ, Andrews PJ, Alston RP. Propofol does not ameliorate cerebral venous oxyhemoglobin desaturation during hypothermic cardiopulmonary bypass. *Anesth Analg.* 1998;86:926–931.

39. Trubiano P, Heyer EJ, Adams DC, et al. Jugular venous bulb oxyhemoglobin saturation during cardiac surgery: accuracy and reliability using a continuous monitor. *Anesth Analg.* 1996;82:964–968.

40. Takasu A, Yagi K, Ishihara S, et al. Combined continuous monitoring of systemic and cerebral oxygen metabolism after cardiac arrest. *Resuscitation.* 1995;29:189–194.

41. Kim, MB, Ward DS, Cartwright CR, et al. Estimation of jugular venous O2 saturation from cerebral oximetry or arterial O2 saturation during isocapnic hypoxia. *J Clin Monit Comput.* 2000;16:191–199.

42. Vigue B, Ract C, Benayed M, et al. Early SjvO2 monitoring in patients with severe brain trauma. *Intensive Care Med.* 1999;25:445–451.

43. Waran V, Menon DK. Mulitmodality monitoring and the diagnosis of traumatic carotid cavernous fistula following head injury. *Br J Neurosurg.* 2000; 14:469–471.

44. Sikes PJ, Segal J. Jugular bulb oxygen saturation monitoring for evaluating cerebral ischemia. *Crit Care Nurs Q.* 1994;17:9–20.

45. Sullivan J, Severance-Lossin L. Jugular venous oxygen saturation monitoring: Insertion (Assist), care, troubleshooting, and removal. In Wiegand DJL and Carlson K, eds. *AACN Procedure Manual for Critical Care,* 5th ed. St. Louis: Elsevier; 2005:738–747.

46. Bell SD, Guyer D, Snyder MA et al. Cerebral hemodynamics: monitoring arteriojugular oxygen content differences. *J Neurosci Nurs.* 1994;26:270–277.

47. Prociuk JL. Management of cerebral oxygen supply demand balance in blunt head injury. *Crit Care Nurse.* 1995;15:38–45.

48. Clay HD. Validity and reliability of the SjO2 catheter in neurologically impaired patients: a critical review of the literature. *J Neurosci Nurs.* 2000;32:194–203.

49. Buunk G, van der Hoeven JG, Meinders AE. A comparison of near-infrared spectroscopy and jugular

bulb oximetry in comatose patients resuscitated from cardiac arrest. *Anesthesia*. 1998;53:13–19.

50. Olsen KS, Svendsen LB, Larsen FS. Validation of transcranial near-infrared spectroscopy for evaluation of cerebral blood flow autoregulation. *J Neurosurg Anesthesiol*. 1996;8:280–285.

51. Madsen PL, Secher NH. Near-infrared oximetry of the brain. *Prog Neurobiol*. 1999;58:541–560.

52. Yao F-SF, Tseng CC, Ho CY, et al. Cerebral oxygen desaturation is associated with early postoperative neuropsychological dysfunction in patients undergoing cardiac surgery. *J Cardiothor Vasc Anesth*. 2004;18:562–558.

53. Samra SK, Dorje P, Zelenock GB, et al. Cerebral oximetry in patients undergoing carotid endarterectomy under regional anesthesia. *Stroke*. 1999;27:49–55.

54. Samra SK, Dy EA, Welch K, et al. Evaluation of a cerebral oximeter as a monitor of cerebral ischemia during carotid endarterectomy. *Anesthesiology*. 2000;93:964–970.

55. Newman DH, Callaway CW, Greenwald IB, et al. Cerebral oximetry in out-of-hospital cardiac arrest: standard CPR rarely provides detectable hemoglobin-oxygen saturation to the frontal cortex. *Resuscitation*. 2004;63:189–194.

56. Ejike JC, Schenkman KA, Seidel K, et al. Cerebral oxygenation in neonatal and pediatric patients during veno-arterial extracorporeal life support. *Pediatr Crit Care Med*. 2006;7:154–158.

57. Berlac PA, Rasmussen YH. Peri-operative cerebral near-infrared spectroscopy (NIRS) predicts maternal hypotension during elective caesarean delivery in spinal anaesthesia. *Int J Obstet Anesth*. 14:26–31.

58. Torella F, Haynes SL, McCollum CN. Cerebral and peripheral oxygen saturation during red cell transfusion. *J Surg Res*. 110:217–221.

59. Muellner T, Schramm W, Kwasny O, et al. Patients with increased intracranial pressure cannot be monitored using near infrared spectroscopy. *Br J Neurosurg*. 1998;12:136–139.

60. McKeating EG, Monjardino JR, Signorini DF, et al. A comparison of the INVOS 3100 and the Critikon 2020 near-infrared spectrophotometers as monitors of cerebral oxygenation. *Anaesthesia*. 1997;52:136–140.

Cerebral Blood Flow Monitoring

Catherine Kirkness, RN, PhD

CASE STUDY

Ms R.T. is a 47-year-old woman admitted to hospital following a sudden onset of dizziness, severe headache, nausea and vomiting, and a brief loss of consciousness. On admission, she was drowsy but fully oriented, photophobic, and still experiencing a severe headache. Noncontrast head computed tomography showed diffuse subarachnoid hemorrhage (SAH) with blood in the basal cisterns, along the inferior frontal lobes extending to the sylvian fissures, in the interhemispheric fissure, and a small amount of blood in the 4th and lateral ventricles. Cerebral angiography confirmed a 7-mm anterior communicating artery aneurysm. No cerebral vasospasm was seen at this time. Hunt and Hess SAH grade was III. The day after admission, Ms R.T. underwent a left craniotomy and surgical clipping of the aneurysm. Postoperatively, transcranial Doppler ultrasonography (TCD) was performed daily, and single-photon emission computed tomography (SPECT) and cerebral angiography were done intermittently. Results of these studies and a brief summary of Ms R.T.'s clinical course are presented in Table 5-1. This case illustrates the different and complementary information that different studies provide. Management decisions are based on information obtained from cerebral blood flow (CBF) studies used in conjunction with assessment of the patient's clinical status.

Highlights of the case study are as follows. Ms R.T. was admitted to the neurointensive care unit and underwent close monitoring of her neurologic status, including use of the Glasgow Coma Scale (GCS), assessment of pupillary reaction, and use of National Institutes of Health Stroke Scale (NIHSS). Daily TCD studies were initiated on the first postoperative day to monitor for increased cerebral blood flow velocities (CBFV) that could be suggestive of vasospasm. The initial TCD study was normal. A SPECT scan on the same day showed expected postoperative changes. Ms R.T. was drowsy but oriented with a GCS score of 14 and an NIHSS score of 2. On the second postoperative day increased left middle cerebral artery (MCA) flow velocities suggestive of spasm were identified via TCD and triple-H therapy was initiated. By the 5th postoperative day, TCD studies showed further increased velocities suggestive of moderate vasospasm of the left MCA and mild vasospasm of the right MCA. In an attempt to augment flow in light of evidence of increasing vasospasm, the neosynephrine dosage was increased to maintain a target systolic blood pressure of greater than 160 mm Hg. SPECT showed no new perfusion deficits and Ms R.T.'s clinical status was stable. However, on the 7th postoperative day the nurse detected deterioration in Ms R.T.'s neurologic status, with the development of increased drowsiness, confusion, and a mild right hemiparesis. Her GCS score decreased to 13 and her NIHSS score increased to 6. TCD showed moderate spasm of the left internal carotid artery (ICA). SPECT showed a new area of hypoperfusion involving the left anterior cerebral artery (ACA) territory. Given the neurologic deterioration, angiography was done on the same day and indicated moderate to severe spasm of the left ICA, MCA, and ACA. Cerebral angioplasty was therefore carried out with significant improvement of the spasm in all involved vessels. Ms R.T.'s neurologic status improved over the next 2 days and she was alert and oriented with no motor deficit. Triple-H therapy was weaned and discontinued on the postoperative day 10. TCD showed no evidence of vasospasm by postoperative day 12. She was discharged 5 days later and at 6 months following SAH was back to her previous work and recreational activities, although she was still experiencing occasional headaches and fatigue.

Table 5-1   The Case of R.T.

Postoperative Day	TCD	SPECT	Angiography	Clinical Course
1	Cerebral blood flow velocity (CBFV) of all vessels studied within normal limits.	Decreased perfusion left inferior frontal lobe. Extra-axial compression left inferior temporal lobe, probably related to post-operative swelling or hematoma, but normal perfusion as compared to right side.	No evidence of residual aneurysm or spasm	Glasgow Coma Scale (GCS) score = 14 (Eye Opening = 3, Verbal = 5, Motor = 6), motor power strong × intravenous (IV), pupils equal and reactive to light (PERL) at 3 mm. National Institutes of Health Stroke Scale (NIHSS) score = 2. 1a. Level of consciousness (LOC) = 2 (not alert, requires repeated stimulation to attend). 1b. LOC Questions: Ask patient the month and their age = 0 (answers both correctly). 1c. LOC Commands: Ask patient to open and close eyes and to grip and release hand = 0 (obeys both correctly). 2. Best Gaze = 0 (normal). 3. Visual = 0 (no visual field loss). 4. Facial Palsy = 0 (normal symmetrical movement). 5. Motor Arm = 0 (right and left arm) (normal). 6. Motor Leg = 0 (right and left leg) (normal). 7. Limb Ataxia = 0 (no ataxia). 8. Sensory = 0 (normal). 9. Best Language = 0 (no aphasia). 10. Dysarthria = 0 (normal articulation). 11. Extinction and Inattention = 0 (normal).
2	Increased flow velocity of the left middle cerebral artery (MCA) suggestive of mild spasm.			GCS score = 14 (Eye Opening = 3, Verbal = 5, Motor = 6), motor power strong × IV, PERL at 3 mm. NIHSS score = 2 (no change). Hypervolemic, hemodilution therapy was started using alternating normal saline and 5% albumin boluses to keep central venous pressure greater than 12 mm Hg. A neosynephrine drip was started to maintain systolic blood pressure greater than 140 mm Hg.
4	Elevated left MCA flow velocity suggestive of mild spasm			GCS score = 14 (Eye Opening = 3, Verbal = 5, Motor = 6), motor power strong in all extremities, PERL at 3 mm. NIHSS score = 2 (no change). Triple-H therapy continued.
5	Further elevation of left MCA flow velocity suggestive of moderate spasm; elevated right MCA flow velocity suggestive of mild spasm.	Left frontal perfusion deficit remains, no new perfusion deficits.		GCS score = 14 (Eye Opening = 3, Verbal = 5, Motor = 6), motor power strong in all extremities, PERL at 3 mm. NIHSS score = 2 (no change). Triple-H therapy continued, with neosynephrine drip now to keep systolic blood pressure greater than 160 mm Hg.

Table 5-1   The Case of R.T., continued

Postoperative Day	TCD	SPECT	Angiography	Clinical Course
6	Mild left internal carotid artery (ICA) spasm, global hyperdynamic flow.			GCS score = 14 (Eye Opening = 3, Verbal = 5, Motor = 6), motor power strong in all extremities, PERL at 3 mm.
				NIHSS score = 2 (no change).
				Triple-H therapy continued.
7	Further elevation of left ICA flow velocity suggestive of moderate spasm, global hyperdynamic flow.	Stable left frontal perfusion deficit, new area of mild hypoperfusion left anterior cerebral artery (ACA) territory	Moderate to severe spasm left ICA, MCA, and ACA. Cerebral angioplasty done with significant improvement of the ICA, MCA, and ACA spasm.	In early AM, the nurse noted that R.T. was confused and had developed mild right hemiparesis, leg : arm. GCS score = 13 (Eye Opening = 3, Verbal = 4, Motor = 6), PERL at 3 mm.
				Pre-angioplasty NIHSS score = 6.
				1a. Level of consciousness = 2 (not alert, requires repeated stimulation to attend).
				1b. LOC Questions: Ask patient the month and their age = 1 (answers 1 correctly).
				1c. LOC Commands: Ask patient to open and close eyes and to grip and release hand = 0 (obeys both correctly).
				2. Best Gaze = 0 (normal).
				3. Visual = 0 (no visual field loss).
				4. Facial palsy = 0 (normal symmetrical movement).
				5. Motor Arm = 1 (right and left arm; right drift).
				6. Motor Leg = 2 (right and left leg; some effort against gravity).
				7. Limb Ataxia = 0 (no ataxia).
				8. Sensory = 0 (normal).
				9. Best Language = 0 (no aphasia).
				10. Dysarthria = 0 (normal articulation).
				11. Extinction and Inattention = 0 (normal).
8	Elevated flow velocities suggestive of mild left ICA and MCA spasm.			GCS score = 14 (Eye Opening = 3, Verbal = 5, Motor = 6), motor power strong in all extremities, PERL at 3 mm.
				NIHSS score = 2 (not alert, requires repeated stimulation to attend).
				Triple-H therapy continued.
9	Elevated flow velocities suggestive of mild left ICA and MCA spasm.			GCS score = 15 (Eye Opening = 4, Verbal = 5, Motor = 6), motor power strong in all extremities, PERL at 3 mm.
				NIHSS score = 0.
				Triple-H therapy continued.
10	Elevated flow velocities suggestive of mild left ICA and MCA spasm.			GCS score = 15 (Eye Opening = 4, Verbal = 5, Motor = 6), motor power strong in all extremities, PERL at 3 mm.
				NIHSS score = 0.
				Triple-H therapy weaned and discontinued.
12	CBFV within normal limits in all vessels examined.			GCS score = 15 (Eye Opening = 4, Verbal = 5, Motor = 6), motor power strong in all extremities, PERL at 3 mm.
				NIHSS score = 0.

GENERAL DESCRIPTION

Measurement of CBF is relevant in a number of acute and chronic conditions where individuals are at risk for alterations in CBF that may lead to cerebral ischemia and infarction. The use of CBF studies in acute and critical care is the emphasis of this chapter. Examples of such conditions include ischemic stroke, aneurysmal SAH, and traumatic brain injury (TBI).

Early techniques of measuring CBF using nitrous oxide provided for measurement of global CBF. However, CBF is not homogenous throughout the brain and cerebral ischemia may be present within a particular region of the brain despite normal global CBF. More recent techniques of measuring CBF allow for measurement of regional or local CBF. These measures have the advantage of being able to identify localized areas of decreased CBF, such as the area supplied by an occluded artery or around a cerebral contusion. These are likely to represent areas at greatest risk for ischemia and infarction, and therefore are the most relevant targets of intervention strategies. For techniques to assess regional or local CBF, placement of the monitoring devices is critical to the usefulness of the information obtained in clinical decision-making.

CBF can be assessed using a number of techniques that measure CBF either directly or indirectly. Those that provide direct measures of CBF include xenon-computed tomography (Xe-CT), perfusion computed tomography (perfusion CT), positron emission tomography (PET), SPECT, and perfusion-weighted magnetic resonance imaging (MRI). Although there is considerable literature on the use of Xe-CT and the technique is well validated, currently it is used infrequently in the United States and its discussion is limited.

All of these techniques require transport of the individual to the site of the scanning equipment. However, because CT scanners have become more portable, some institutions are able to bring these techniques to the bedside. Transcranial Doppler ultrasonography (TCD) provides an indirect measure of CBF in that it measures CBFV and is a technique that currently can be carried out at the bedside. Other techniques, such as brain tissue oxygenation, are associated with CBF but are impacted by other factors and so are not strict measures of CBF alone. Cerebral angiography, which provides information about cerebral vessel patency, is also not strictly a measure of CBF.

CBF measurement techniques can provide quantitative or qualitative measures of CBF. Xe-CT provides a quantitative measure of CBF that is standardized over time and between different scanners. SPECT can provide a semi-quantitative measure of CBF, with the flow compared to a control region that is assumed to be normal. Perfusion CT and perfusion MRI can provide quantitative measures of CBF, but these are relative measures rather than absolute quantification. For studies using diffusible tracers (that pass the blood-brain barrier and go into the brain tissue), such as SPECT, Xe-CT, or PET, the concentration of the tracer in the feeding artery must be known in order to quantify CBF.

Most CBF measurement techniques do not allow for continuous measurement. TCD can allow for extended monitoring but the difficulty in maintaining the ultrasound probe in position to obtain an adequate signal limits its use for extended continuous monitoring. Continuous CBF measurement can be achieved using laser Doppler flowmetry (LDF) or thermal diffusion flowmetry (TDF), which involves insertion of probes on or near the surface of the brain and provides information regarding regional or local CBF.

Other, less used measurements of CBF, such as continuous jugular thermodilution, double-indicator dilution techniques, or near infrared spectroscopy, are not addressed in this chapter, nor is intraoperative monitoring.

Although CBF studies can identify changes in CBF, this information alone does not indicate whether the change is associated with ischemia or infarction. It is also difficult to define an absolute level of CBF that results in cerebral ischemia in TBI, given that a decrease in CBF may be coupled with a decrease in cerebral metabolism and may not reflect ischemia. Therefore, combining CBF studies with measures of cerebral oxygenation and metabolism will provide greater information to guide interventions directed at restoring adequate CBF and preventing ischemia or infarction.

There is considerable overlap as to which CBF study is appropriate for a particular clinical situation and different CBF studies may provide complementary information. The decision as to which CBF study to use is based on a number of factors such as patient acuity, equipment availability, expense, ease of carrying out the study, invasiveness, resolution, and whether the study provides a quantitative or qualitative measure of CBF. General information about different CBF techniques that influence decisions for use is included under the first listed clinical application for which the study was performed, but this information may be relevant to the other clinical situations.

This chapter presents information about the most common uses of CBF measurement, primarily in acute and critical care. Use of CBF study techniques varies by institution and region, and despite the considerable literature documenting the use of various CBF measurement techniques in a variety of clinical situations, as yet there is a lack of well-designed studies to provide strong evidence as to the value of CBF measurement in clinical decision-making, determining prognosis, and improving outcome. There continues to be a lack of standardization and quantification of findings, and a need for further definition of normal and abnormal values and their meanings. Thus, findings are often interpreted in light of both the expertise of practitioners and other clinical results. Levels of recommendation for use are based on the degree to which there is evidence to support the ability of the studies to be informative in terms of CBF in general and the degree to which each study has been used in a particular condition.

ACCURACY

Technical considerations continue to affect the accuracy of CBF studies. Patient movement affects the accuracy of many of the study results. Different CBF measurement techniques allow for different resolution of findings, with SPECT providing lower resolution and CT, PET, and MRI allowing higher resolution. More subtle areas of decreased CBF may be missed by techniques with lower resolution.

CBF studies that provide qualitative measures of CBF lack standardization of findings across patients and differing equipment, and between studies of the same patient carried out at different times. Except for Xe-CT, techniques that provide quantitative measures of CBF also lack standardization of results over time with the same scanner and between different scanners. With perfusion CT, quantification of CBF requires the selection of an input artery to provide information about the concentration of tracer in the feeding artery; thus, the choice of input artery affects results. Although a quantitative measure of CBF can be obtained using perfusion CT, the accuracy of this has not yet been fully validated and requires further comparison with other established methods of CBF measurement. Perfusion-weighted MRI also allows for quantification of CBF but values are relative values and not absolute, and parameters are not comparable between MRI units. PET also permits only relative quantification of CBF. TCDs are used to measure CBFV at intermittent intervals, usually daily. Accuracy of the test is dependent on the skill level of the technician performing the TCD measurement. Accuracy of bedside TDF or LDF (regionally parenchymal placed) probes is dependent on correct placement of the probe into the white matter of the cerebral hemisphere. There are different CBF rates for gray matter versus white matter. The neurosurgeon must ensure the appropriate placement of the probe. Also, regional measurements of CBF reflect a local area and significant differences occur in varying locations in 1 hemisphere as well as between hemispheres. Thus this type of CBF monitoring is helpful in trending CBF rates.

COMPETENCY

Nurses typically do not actually perform CBF studies, although they may be involved in patient preparation, patient and family education, patient monitoring, and in the interventions initiated as a result of findings. Patient and family preparation requires knowledge of contraindications and precautions for specific studies (eg, risk for adverse reactions to contrast media or risk related to the presence of devices that will be affected by the magnet during MRI)

and of study procedures. Nursing care may include monitoring of patients during CBF studies (eg, during MRI), where the individual is in an enclosed scanner, may require sedation, and may be critically ill, and during the study's aftercare, including monitoring for adverse effects and ongoing monitoring of neurologic status. Given that individuals undergo CBF studies because of conditions that put them at increased risk for cerebral ischemia and infarction, nurses have an important role in monitoring patients for signs and symptoms of cerebral ischemia. Providing this care requires knowledge of principles of cerebrovascular hemodynamics, cerebrovascular anatomy and physiology, and neurologic assessment. In addition, knowledge of interventions targeted at altering CBF is necessary, for example, thrombolytic administration or manipulation of blood pressure (BP). The interpretation of CBF studies typically involves individuals with specialized knowledge in relation to the particular study and may include neuroradiologists and nuclear medicine personnel. Nurses have an important role in helping patients and families understand the meaning of CBF study results that are presented to them.

FUTURE RESEARCH

Although numerous articles describe the use of CBF studies in a variety of conditions, further study is needed to establish the clinical usefulness of information obtained and its impact on management and outcome in the different clinical situations where these studies may be used. As technology for the measurement of CBF continues to advance and provide better quantification, better resolution, and greater standardization of CBF data, research will need to continue to incorporate this new information.

Further research is needed to better understand the meaning of alterations of CBF in different conditions and in different areas of the brain, both in relation to directing management and to outcome. In addition to testing the ability of interventions to alter CBF, research also must focus on defining the optimal CBF in various conditions, and on examining whether therapies to alter CBF do or do not translate into improved patient outcome. Particular areas of interest include determining the value of CBF information in TBI and using CBF studies to define ischemic tissue and predict response to treatment and outcome in ischemic stroke. There is a lack of nursing research in this area. Nursing research will be needed to further examine the impact on both short- and longer-term outcomes of independent and collaborative nursing interventions directed at altering CBF and to further develop and validate protocols for such interventions.

CLINICAL RECOMMENDATIONS

The rating scale for the Level of Recommendation ranges from I to VI, with levels indicated as follows: I, manufacturer's recommendations only; II, theory based, no research data to support recommendations; recommendations from expert consensus group may exist; III, laboratory data only, no clinical data to support recommendations; IV, limited clinical studies to support recommendations; V, clinical studies in more than 1 or 2 different populations and situations to support recommendations; VI, clinical studies in a variety of patient populations and situations to support recommendations.

Period of Use	Recommendation	Rationale for Recommendation	Level of Recommendation	Supporting References	Comments
Selection of Patients	CBF studies may be used in the following circumstances. Most current evidence supports only possible or probable value in clinical management decision-making and impact on outcome. Further study is required to fully establish its value.				
	After aneurysmal SAH The technique most commonly used is TCD, followed by SPECT. PET, perfusion-weighted MRI, Xe-CT, perfusion CT. TDF and LDF may also be used.	Allows for detection and monitoring of decreases in CBF due to cerebral vasospasm that may lead to ischemia and/or infarction. Provides a guide for management decisions (eg, triple-H therapy or angioplasty) and monitoring of the response to management of cerebral vasospasm.		See Other References: 1–4 (Management of SAH)	The effect on outcome of the use of CBF studies in the management of cerebral vasospasm remains to be fully determined. Angiography has been the gold standard to which other methods of measuring cerebral vasospasm have been compared. However, the presence of angiographic vasospasm may or may not be accompanied by clinical signs and symptoms of cerebral ischemia (clinical vasospasm). Angiography is invasive, has associated risks, is expensive, and cannot be repeated frequently.
	• TCD	TCD has particular value in that it can be performed at the bedside and used for serial monitoring (repeated daily). TCD is most useful for monitoring vasospasm in the basal intracranial arteries, particularly the middle cerebral artery (MCA) and basilar artery. It is less effective for detecting changes in distal arteries. TCD measures cerebral blood flow velocity (CBFV) rather than CBF. Cerebral blood vessel narrowing as a result of vasospasm is associated with increased CBFV. However, increased CBFV can also be associated with other states, such as hyperemia, so it is not specific to vasospasm.	VI	See Annotated Bibliography: 4	

Period of Use	Recommendation	Rationale for Recommendation	Level of Recommendation	Supporting References	Comments
Selection of Patients (*cont.*)		There is evidence for the usefulness of TCD in monitoring vasospasm. However, there is variability in the correlation between TCD findings, CBF measures, and delayed neurologic deficits. Thus TCD is best used in conjunction with other parameters, such as CBF measures and the neurologic exam, in making decisions regarding therapies.		See Other References: 5–15 (TCD, angiography)	
	• SPECT	Provides information about regional CBF and gives a semiquantitative relative measure of CBF by comparing an area on 1 side of the brain with a comparable area on the other side, with the assumption that flow on the other side is normal. Absolute CBF quantification can be obtained by determining arterial input using arterial blood samples but this is infrequently done. SPECT can detect perfusion deficits related to spasm of more distal cerebral vessels, but it is not as easily repeated as TCD. SPECT has relatively low resolution compared to CT, MRI, and PET. In addition, SPECT does not provide the anatomic information provided by CT or MRI.	VI	See Other References: 7 See Annotated Bibliography: 1	Although it is recommended that SPECT be combined with TCD for the detection of vasospasm and delayed ischemic deficits, its usefulness and predictive ability are not strongly established.
	• PET	PET is related to SPECT but the radioisotope that is used has a much shorter half-life (minutes to hours), requiring that the cyclotron where it is produced is very close to where the scan will be done. PET has better resolution than SPECT and can show more rapid changes (seconds) with good resolution. PET can also provide metabolic information. CT scans may be used along with PET to provide anatomic information. However, the use of PET is limited by its expense and lack of widespread availability.	VI	See Other References: 9	PET studies have shown a range of CBF patterns from reduced to hyperemic flow in patients with delayed neurologic deficit following SAH, suggesting factors other than large vessel spasm may contribute to these delayed deficits.

Period of Use	Recommendation	Rationale for Recommendation	Level of Recommendation	Supporting References	Comments
Selection of Patients (*cont.*)	• Perfusion-weighted MRI	A relatively new technique that provides a measure of relative CBF of the entire brain. It is being examined as a means of detecting tissue at risk for infarction in patients with cerebral vasospasm. Perfusion-weighted MRI can be carried out relatively quickly and can be used emergently in cases of neurologic deterioration. It can be combined with other MRI studies such as MR angiography and diffusion-weighted MRI to provide anatomic information and detect infarcted tissue. A number of limitations remain, including analysis techniques, lack of absolute quantification of CBF, lack of standardization of MRI units, and expense. In addition, monitoring of patients while inside the scanner may be challenging.	VI	See Other References: 15, 16	Further study is needed to determine the role of perfusion-weighted MRI in the management of cerebral vasospasm. Although there are many reports of the use of perfusion MRI, there is yet a lack of adequate well-designed studies to establish its usefulness in relation to clinical decision-making, predictive ability, and effect on outcome.
	• Xe-CT	Although Xe-CT has the advantage of giving an absolute value of CBF in mL/100 g/min and being well validated, it is currently used infrequently in the United States. With Xe-CT, quantitative CBF data can be superimposed on an anatomic image in gray or color scale. Xe-CT can provide information about regions of low blood flow associated with cerebral vasospasm that may be used to monitor vasospasm and its management (e.g., the effect of triple-H therapy on CBF).	VI	See Other References: 11 See Annotated Bibliography: 6	There is currently limited use of Xe-CT in the United States.
	• Perfusion CT	The area of the brain that is imaged and the quantification of CBF depend on the specific technique used. Quantitative CBF information can be obtained for an area of interest (not the entire brain). Accuracy of CBF quantification and technical issues related to perfusion	VI	See Other References: 17–20	Further study is needed to determine the ability of perfusion CT to predict delayed cerebral ischemia following SAH and its use to guide management.

Period of Use	Recommendation	Rationale for Recommendation	Level of Recommendation	Supporting References	Comments
Selection of Patients (*cont.*)		CT require further attention. It is being examined for its ability to predict the development of delayed cerebral ischemia following SAH and to identify cerebral ischemia and guide medical and endovascular management.			
	• TDF	Allows for continuous quantitative measurement of cortical blood flow at the patients' bedside. Probes are located on the cortical surface or in the brain parenchyma. TDF provides absolute values of CBF in mL/100 g/min. TDF measurement of CBF has high temporal resolution and sensitivity to even small flow changes, making it useful to monitor response to interventions to alter flow. TDF has been validated by comparing it with Xe-CT.	IV	See Other References: 21–23	Further study is needed to establish the value of TDF following SAH.
	• LDF	An invasive technique that allows for continuous real-time measure of local cortical CBF by measuring the velocity of red blood cells within the microcirculation (capillaries). LDF has been used to monitor CBF intraoperatively and in the intensive care unit. LDF only allows for measurement of CBF over a very small area (1–2 mm^3), is prone to artifact, does not provide absolute quantification of CBF (units are arbitrary), and its reliability depends on probe positioning (determination of the most clinically relevant site and avoidance of placement near larger vessels). LDF can be used to assess CBF changes in response to physiologic and pathophysiologic stimuli.	V	See Other References: 24	Further study is needed to establish the value of LDF following SAH.

Period of Use	Recommendation	Rationale for Recommendation	Level of Recommendation	Supporting References	Comments
Selection of Patients *(cont.)*	**After traumatic brain injury, during the acute phase**				
	TCD, perfusion CT, PET, LDF, TDF, or Xe-CT may be used.	Can detect areas of low CBF that may represent brain tissue at risk for ischemic injury. Low CBF is associated with poor outcome.		See Annotated Bibliography: 5	Because CBF studies provide information about decreased CBF but not whether the decrease is associated with ischemia, combining CBF studies with measures of cerebral oxygenation and metabolism will yield greater information regarding the therapeutic use of hyperventilation and interventions to alter CBF in TBI.
		Information regarding areas of inadequate CBF may be used to direct interventions to improve CBF and prevent or minimize secondary ischemic injury.			
		Therapies include maintenance of adequate oxygenation, maintenance of adequate cerebral perfusion pressure (CPP), and prevention of increased intracranial pressure (ICP).		See Other References: 25–27	
		Provides a guide to the degree of hyperventilation that can safely be used to decrease ICP through cerebral vasoconstriction without causing a potentially detrimental decrease in CBF to ischemic levels.			
		Used to assess cerebral autoregulation, which is the ability to maintain a relatively constant CBF despite changes in ABP and CPP. Impaired autoregulation seen after brain injury may make the brain more vulnerable to increased ICP with hypertension and to secondary ischemic injury, and has been associated with poorer outcome.		See Other References: 28–33	
		Interest has grown in using a measure of autoregulation to determine optimal CPP level on an individual basis.			
	• TCD	Commonly used to assess cerebral autoregulation. Relative MCA flow velocity changes are measured in response to rapid or steady-state changes in BP (dynamic or static autoregulation, respectively). BP changes may be spontaneous or induced (eg, pharmacologically)	V		

Period of Use	Recommendation	Rationale for Recommendation	Level of Recommendation	Supporting References	Comments
Selection of Patients *(cont.)*		following rapid release of bilateral thigh cuffs. An index of autoregulation may be calculated based on: 1) The rate of return of CBFV in relation to return of BP or CPP. 2) A moving correlation coefficient between CPP and MCA flow velocity.			
	• Xe-CT	Evidence indicates that Xe-CT with testing of cerebral autoregulation and response to physiologic challenges can probably be used to predict outcome following TBI, but this requires further validation.	V	See Other References: 34, 35 See Annotated Bibliography: 2, 6	
	• SPECT	Although there is some evidence that SPECT shows greater perfusion abnormalities than changes seen on CT, the significance is not clear and the value of SPECT in patients with TBI is not yet established.	IV	See Other References: 36 See Annotated Bibliography: 1, 2	
	• Perfusion CT	Perfusion CT has recently been examined for its ability to assess autoregulation, but there are inadequate data to establish its value.	IV	See Other References: 19, 37, 38 See Annotated Bibliography: 2	
	• TDF	TDF may be useful following TBI to detect changes in regional CBF and monitor response to therapy.	IV	See Other References: 39	
	• LDF	The clinical value of LDF monitoring following TBI is not yet established.	IV	See Other References: 40, 41	
	• PET	PET has been used in a small sample to examine the effect of augmentation of CPP. PET is less commonly used to assess autoregulation.	IV	See Other References: 31, 42, 43 See Annotated Bibliography: 3	

Period of Use	Recommendation	Rationale for Recommendation	Level of Recommendation	Supporting References	Comments
Selection of Patients (*cont.*)	**Acute ischemic stroke** Perfusion CT technology is advancing and its availability and use in acute ischemic stroke is increasing. Other techniques that may be used include SPECT, perfusion MRI, PET, and Xe-CT.	To allow for differentiation of areas of reversible and nonreversible ischemia; evaluate whether the tissue is salvageable, evaluate the risk of bleeding from thrombolytic administration, and contribute to prognostic information. While tissue at the core of an ischemic area may be infarcted, nearby tissue may be salvageable if flow can quickly be restored. However, restoring flow to areas with severe ischemia or infarction may increase the risk of edema and hemorrhage, resulting in greater mortality and morbidity. Therefore, the benefits of interventions to restore flow must be carefully weighed against the risks. Information from perfusion imaging studies may be of significant value in determining relative benefits versus risks.		See Other References: 1, 44, 45	Further study is needed to determine the role of different techniques of CBF measurement in treatment decisions and ability to predict outcome in acute ischemic stroke.
	• Perfusion CT	Can be carried out rapidly and done in conjunction with unenhanced CT (the current standard to rule out hemorrhage in suspected acute stroke), or CT angiography. Perfusion CT is being examined for its ability to differentiate reversible from nonreversible ischemia and identify salvageable tissue, thereby providing information related to risk and benefits of interventions to restore flow, such as thrombolytic administration.	V	See Other References: 46–48 See Annotated Bibliography: 2, 7	Evidence suggests that perfusion CT may be useful to differentiate between reversible and irreversible ischemia but its ability to predict hemorrhage following thrombolytic administration is yet unknown.
	• SPECT	Strong evidence exists for its ability to detect hypoperfusion following acute stroke, and to predict reversibility of ischemia and threshold for hemorrhage with the use of thrombolytics. SPECT also has been shown to be useful in correlating hypoperfusion with neurologic deficit severity, infarct size, and clinical outcome in cases where reperfusion does not occur.	VI	See Other References: 46–49 See Annotated Bibliography: 1, 2, 7	

Period of Use	Recommendation	Rationale for Recommendation	Level of Recommendation	Supporting References	Comments
Selection of Patients (*cont.*)	• Perfusion-weighted MRI	Evidence suggests that MRI techniques are probably useful in differentiating reversible and irreversible ischemia. However, the predictive ability and value of perfusion-weighted MRI (often combined with diffusion-weighted MRI, which provides information on the extent of infarcted tissue) to guide management decisions (eg, thrombolysis) or to predict complications is not yet clear.	V	See Other References: 50 See Annotated Bibliography: 2, 7	
	• Xe-CT	Studies indicate that Xe-CT provides accurate CBF values, allowing identification of areas that are nonischemic, and those with reversible and irreversible ischemia. Xe-CT provides predictive information regarding risk of edema, hemorrhage, and herniation related to reperfusion.	VI	See Other References: 46–48 See Annotated Bibliography: 2, 7	
	• PET	Can be used in acute stroke to define the penumbra and has been compared with other methods but is used less frequently.	IV	See Other References: 51, 52	
	Assessment of vasomotor reactivity in patients at risk for decreased cerebrovascular reserve/ autoregulation (eg, with symptomatic or asymptomatic extracranial ICA stenosis or occlusion, or MCA occlusive disease) TCD, SPECT, perfusion CT, perfusion MRI, PET, or Xe-CT may be used.	Allows for identification of individuals who are at increased risk for stroke because of the inability of cerebral blood vessels to further dilate to maintain CBF in the face of a drop in BP. Acetazolamide is commonly administered as a vasodilator to test vasomotor reactivity.			
	• TCD	Studies indicate that TCD is probably useful in assessing cerebrovascular reserve.	IV	See Other References: 53	
	• SPECT	SPECT carried out before and after acetazolamide administration allows identification of impaired cerebrovascular reserve. Further validation and study to define stroke risk in relation to CBF measures obtained by SPECT are needed.	IV	See Other References: 54	

Period of Use	Recommendation	Rationale for Recommendation	Level of Recommendation	Supporting References	Comments
Selection of Patients (*cont.*)	• Perfusion CT and perfusion-weighted MRI	There are inadequate data to determine the usefulness and predictive ability of perfusion CT and perfusion MRI in relation to cerebrovascular reserve.	IV	See Other References: 48	
	• PET	PET has been used in carotid stenosis to evaluate altered hemodynamics by assessing CBF before and after acetazolamide administration.	V	See Other References: 53–55	
	• Xe-CT	Has been shown to be of value in identifying a subgroup at high risk for infarction that has a decrease in CBF in response to acetazolamide administration.	VI	See Other References: 56 See Annotated Bibliography: 6	
	Assessment of collateral circulation with temporary artery occlusion SPECT, perfusion CT, perfusion-weighted MRI, TDF, or Xe-CT may be used.	Used to assess the adequacy of collateral blood flow during a period of temporary occlusion of an artery (eg, ICA) when prolonged or permanent occlusion is considered (eg, for management of a cerebral aneurysm that cannot be clipped or appropriately managed otherwise). CBF information from SPECT, perfusion CT, perfusion MRI, or Xe-CT during temporary arterial occlusion may provide information beyond neurologic assessment but further study is needed to establish the usefulness in determining risk of arterial sacrifice.	V	See Other References: 47, 57–62 See Annotated Bibliography: 6	
	To confirm a clinical diagnosis of brain death, in conjunction with other criteria				
	TCD or SPECT may be used. • TCD	An absence of CBF is associated with brain death. TCD shows small early systolic peaks with no diastolic flow or reverberating flow.	VI	See Other References: 63	Approximately 10% of patients may not have a temporal window so CBFV signals must have been previously present to use TCD in the confirmation of brain death.
	• SPECT	SPECT will show no radioisotope uptake in the brain parenchyma.	VI	See Other References: 63, 64 See Annotated Bibliography: 1	

Period of Use	Recommendation	Rationale for Recommendation	Level of Recommendation	Supporting References	Comments
Application of Device and Initial Use	• Nurses may or may not be involved in the actual performance of CBF studies. However, nurses have an important role in patient preparation, patient and family education, patient monitoring (eg, for adverse effects, of neurologic status), and in interventions initiated as a result of findings.				
	• Nurses must be prepared to institute interventions directed at altering CBF, such as BP manipulation, based on an understanding of cerebral hemodynamics.			See Other References: 65	
	• Particularly in the case of acute ischemic stroke when administration of IV thrombolytic agents must be carried out within 3 hours of symptom onset, nurses must be aware of specific screening, monitoring, and management protocols related to thrombolytic administration.			See Other References: 45	
	• A normal CBF value is approximately 50 mL/100 g tissue/min, although flow varies to some degree in different areas of the brain (higher in gray matter than white matter).			See Other References: 48	
	• Failure of electrical activity and neurologic dysfunction occur when CBF falls to 18 to 20 mL/100 g/min. While CBF between 10 and 20 mL/100 g/min may be tolerated for minutes to hours before infarction, CBF of less than 10 mL/100 g/min leads rapidly to neuronal death. At low CBF states, the clinical exam is not useful in determining the level of perfusion present.				

Period of Use	Recommendation	Rationale for Recommendation	Level of Recommendation	Supporting References	Comments
Application of Device and Initial Use *(cont.)*	• Most CBF studies do not involve the direct application of a device; rather external devices that emit and/or detect signals are used.				
	• Most CBF studies (Xe-CT, perfusion CT, PET, SPECT, MRI) generally require that the patient be transferred to the site of the scanner. Depending on patient acuity, nursing accompaniment and continuous monitoring may be required.				
	• Patients may be positioned within closed or open scanning devices. Particularly when closed scanning devices are involved, teaching should be done to prepare patients for the experience of being in an enclosed space during the study. They should be informed that they will be able to communicate if they need something.	Movement affects the validity of data obtained during CBF studies, particularly MRI, PET, and Xe-CT.			
	• For CT, PET, and MRI studies, patients move/are moved to the scanner table, which is then moved inside the doughnut-shaped scanner.				
	• Ensure that patients are positioned comfortably with the head stabilized (eg, supports around the head, pillows under the knees, arms in a comfortable position, and with appropriate covers/blankets).				
	• Administer analgesics prior to the study as needed.				
	• Administer sedation as needed during the study.				
	• The contrast agent or radioisotope is generally injected intravenously. For CT perfusion study techniques requiring a rapid bolus injection of contrast, a large bore	Use of a larger IV injection site will minimize potential extravasation of contrast.			

Period of Use	Recommendation	Rationale for Recommendation	Level of Recommendation	Supporting References	Comments
Application of Device and Initial Use *(cont.)*	antecubital IV site is preferable. The IV site should be monitored for extravasation. • Food and fluid intake are not generally restricted prior to CBF studies (although may be restricted for 4 to 6 hours prior to PET if 18-fluorodeoxyglucose is used). **TCD** • Onset of cerebral vasospasm can occur as early as 3 days post-SAH, typically peaking on days 4 to 12, and resolving after about 2 weeks. Close nursing monitoring of the patient's neurological condition, in conjunction with TCD findings, can allow for early diagnosis of vasospasm, initiation of treatment, and monitoring of treatment response. • There is considerable variation in normal CBFV, so relative changes may be of greater value than absolute numbers. An increase of greater than 50% over baseline is consistent with vasospasm. • Despite variation in normal CBFV, a mean MCA flow velocity greater than 120 cm/sec is generally considered suggestive of vasospasm. A velocity greater than 200 cm/sec is suggestive of severe vasospasm. Calculation of the ratio of flow velocities in the MCA and the ICA (Lindegaard or Hemispheric ratio) can help to differentiate whether increased MCA flow velocity is due to vasospasm or to increased flow. This			See Other References: 2–4, 8, 66	

Period of Use	Recommendation	Rationale for Recommendation	Level of Recommendation	Supporting References	Comments
Application of Device and Initial Use (*cont.*)	ratio is independent of flow. A ratio of 3 suggests MCA spasm and a ratio of greater than 6 suggests severe vasospasm.				
	• For the basilar artery, vasospasm is suggested by a flow velocity of greater than 70 cm/sec and a ratio of the basilar artery and extracranial vertebral artery flow velocities (Soustiel ratio) of greater than 2. Severe spasm is suggested by a basilar artery flow velocity of greater than 85 cm/sec and a Soustiel ratio of greater than 3.				
	• TCD requires careful positioning and application of the ultrasound device and adjustment of ultrasound parameters, including angle of insonation and depth of ultrasound signal, to obtain valid and reliable information.				
	• Areas of the skull that allow penetration of the ultrasound signal, termed *windows*, are the temporal bone, the orbit, and the foramen magnum.				
	• CBFV can be obtained for the ICA, carotid siphon, anterior, middle and posterior cerebral arteries, as well as the ophthalmic, vertebral, and basilar arteries.				
	• Gel is placed on the ultrasound transducer, which is then placed over the appropriate cranial window, and parameters are adjusted until an adequate signal is obtained. Use of a headband device helps to secure the placement of the ultrasound transducer.				
	• Systolic, diastolic, and mean blood flow velocities are calculated as cm/sec.				

Period of Use	Recommendation	Rationale for Recommendation	Level of Recommendation	Supporting References	Comments
Application of Device and Initial Use (*cont.*)	**SPECT** • Involves the IV injection of a radioisotope, followed by a scan that is carried out in the nuclear medicine area within a period of a few hours after the injection. The procedure takes approximately 15 minutes. **PET** • Involves the IV injection of a radioisotope, followed by a scan within a period of 30 to 90 minutes that takes approximately 30 to 45 minutes. **Perfusion-weighted MRI** • Perfusion-weighted MRI typically involves the injection of a gadolinium contrast medium followed by the scan. **Perfusion CT** • An initial unenhanced CT is done followed by a second scan obtained quickly after intravascular injection of an iodinated contrast agent. **Xe-CT** • Involves obtaining a baseline CT scan. A mixture of xenon and oxygen is administered by inhalation, followed by a repeat scan. • For individuals who are not intubated, an occlusive mask that covers the nose and mouth is used for inhalation of the xenon-oxygen mixture. The mask should be adjusted to ensure proper fit and comfort. • For individuals who are intubated, the gas mixture is administered via the endotracheal tube. • Patients may experience sedation when inhaling the gas and for a short period afterwards.			See Other References: 67 See Other References: 68	

Period of Use	Recommendation	Rationale for Recommendation	Level of Recommendation	Supporting References	Comments
Application of Device and Initial Use *(cont.)*	• Patients should be aware that they may experience headache or extremity tingling.				
	• Because xenon increases CBF, there is a potential risk of increased ICP in those at risk. This has not been associated with cerebral ischemia and appears to be related to $Paco_2$ levels. However, the nurse should be aware of this potential complication and monitor respiratory status and for signs of increased ICP.				
	• Patients with high oxygen demands may be unable to tolerate Xe-CT.				
	TDF • Using sterile technique, the thermal diffusion microprobe is inserted into brain parenchyma through a burr hole or at the time of craniotomy. Earlier probes were placed on the cortical surface. Current intraparenchymal probes allow for monitoring of a larger area around the probe. The probe is generally inserted into normal tissue of a vascular territory at risk for ischemia (eg, due to vasospasm) but avoiding major blood vessels. Probe placement is dependent on practitioner skill.				
	• Probe position is confirmed by a CT scan.				
	• The probe consists of a thermistor at the tip and a temperature sensor located slightly proximally. The thermistor is heated to a constant temperature and the proximal sensor monitors tissue temperature. Mathematical calculations using the amount of power dissipated by the				

Period of Use	Recommendation	Rationale for Recommendation	Level of Recommendation	Supporting References	Comments
Application of Device and Initial Use *(cont.)*	thermistor, which reflects the tissue's ability to transport heat and depends on tissue perfusion, provide absolute values of CBF in mL/100 g/min. • Tissue perfusion and temperature can be displayed graphically. • The monitor can perform in situ calibration followed by a short delay for stabilization of measurements. **LDF** • Probes are typically placed in the operating room under sterile technique on the cortical surface or a few mms below.				
Ongoing Monitoring	• The majority of CBF studies does not allow for continuous monitoring and provides only a snapshot of CBF at the particular time of the study. • Serial monitoring, however, may be used and involves repeated administration of the study methods at discrete times. • Although TCD may be used for extended periods of monitoring, the technical difficulty of maintaining the ultrasound probe placement and an adequate signal limits its continuous use. • TDF and LDF, however, can allow for continuous bedside monitoring of CBF. Both of these techniques are invasive and require insertion of probes on the cortical surface or into the parenchyma under sterile technique, with ongoing maintenance of the site with a sterile dressing. The insertion site should be observed for drainage, redness, or swelling.				

Period of Use	Recommendation	Rationale for Recommendation	Level of Recommendation	Supporting References	Comments
	• Trends in CBF measures and response to care should be monitored.				
Prevention of Complications	For studies involving the injection of contrast media, particularly iodinated contrast (eg, that used in perfusion CT), determine whether the patient has had an adverse reaction to a contrast in the past. Reactions may be immediate (occurring within 1 hour of contrast administration; approximately 70% occurring within the first 5 minutes) or nonimmediate (occurring from 1 hour to 1 week after contrast administration). Symptoms of immediate reactions to monitor for include flushing, urticaria, pruritus, angioedema, nausea, vomiting, diarrhea, hoarseness, cough, rhinorrhea, bronchospasm, dyspnea, laryngeal edema, tachycardia or bradycardia, hypotension or hypertension, and rarely shock, respiratory arrest, or cardiac arrest. Symptoms of nonimmediate reactions may include headache, urticaria, pruritus, angioedema, skin reactions such as a maculopapular rash, erythema, which are generally of mild-to-moderate severity and are self-limiting, although severe skin reactions such as Stevens-Johnson may occur. Although the incidence of immediate anaphylactic-like reactions to contrast media is low (0.02%–0.04% with nonionic contrast media), with a mortality rate of 1 in 100 000, an appropriate immediate response is critical. Resuscitation equipment always should be immediately available and checked regularly, and guidelines for management of acute reactions should be established.	A patient who has had a prior reaction to a contrast is more likely to have a reaction to subsequent contrast administration.	VI	See Other References: 69–71	Use of nonionic agents significantly decreases the incidence of immediate reactions. About 90% of iodinated contrast media currently used clinically is nonionic. Most adverse reactions are mild or moderate.

Period of Use	Recommendation	Rationale for Recommendation	Level of Recommendation	Supporting References	Comments
Prevention of Complications (*cont.*)	For studies involving the injection of contrast media, determine whether the patient:		VI		
	• Has allergies, asthma, heart disease, or is taking a beta-blocker.	Associated with a higher risk of an immediate reaction.			
	• Is being treated with interleukin-2 and has a history of drug and contact allergy.	Associated with a higher risk of a nonimmediate reaction.			
	Patients at risk for an adverse reaction to contrast media may be pretreated with corticosteroids or antihistamines.	Some studies have shown that pretreatment can reduce adverse reactions, but this is primarily related to minor reactions. However, repeat nonimmediate reactions and severe anaphylactic-like reactions may still occur despite pretreatment with corticosteroids.	IV		The role of premedication to prevent severe contrast media reactions has yet to be established.
	For studies involving the injection of contrast media, determine whether the patient has decreased renal function. Obtain serum creatinine, and preferably calculate creatinine clearance, in patients with abnormal renal function.	Decreased renal function is associated with a higher risk of nephrotoxicity related to contrast administration. Serum creatinine may be used for screening but normal levels do not exclude renal dysfunction, so creatinine clearance is a more useful measure.	VI		
	Ensure that patients at risk for nephrotoxicity are adequately hydrated (IV fluid administration if unable to take orally).	Contrast induced nephrotoxicity is thought to be related to decreased glomerular flow, so ensuring good flow may be renoprotective.	VI		Nephrotoxicity has not been associated with IV administration of gadolinium chelates, used as contrast agents with MRI.
	Be aware that adverse reactions, such as nausea and hives, can occur with gadolinium chelates used as contrast agents with MRI but are uncommon. Anaphylactoid reactions are rare. Patients should be screened for asthma, allergies, and drug sensitivities.		VI		

Period of Use	Recommendation	Rationale for Recommendation	Level of Recommendation	Supporting References	Comments
Prevention of Complications (*cont.*)	Patients undergoing MRI must be screened for ferromagnetic objects such as metal implants, foreign objects, or other devices that will be affected by the magnet or cause damage to the area of the body being affected by the magnet; examples include pacemakers, some aneurysm clips, metallic bone or joint pins, and everyday items such as metallic jewelry.	The magnet could damage such objects, leading to their malfunction, or could cause movement of the objects and damage to the body.			
	Provide earplugs or other appropriate ear protection for patients undergoing MRI.	The MRI scanner makes very loud noises during the scan that may temporarily affect hearing if ears are unprotected.			
	SPECT and PET are contraindicated during pregnancy.	Avoid exposure of the fetus to ionizing radiation.			
Quality Control Issues	Accurate calculation of CBF using nondiffusible tracer techniques (tracer remains within the vasculature) requires an intact blood-brain barrier.	CBF calculations are based on the concentration of the tracer (contrast) in the feeding arteries and draining veins.			
	Metallic objects, even though not magnetic, may cause artifact in MRI data.				
	Movement causes artifact in MRI, PET, and Xe-CT data.				
	Accuracy of TCD study findings is dependent on operator technique and requires a skilled operator.				

ANNOTATED BIBLIOGRAPHY

Given the number of CBF measurement techniques and clinical situations in which each CBF study may be used, guidelines and articles summarizing the use of various techniques are presented rather than a multitude of individual articles focused on validation of each technique in a particular clinical situation.

1. **Atrocchi PH, Brin M, Fergusion JH, Goldstein ML, Gorelick PB, Hanley DF, Lange DJ, Nuwer MR, van den Noort S. Assessment of brain SPECT: Report of the Therapeutics and Technology Assessment Subcommittee of the American Academy of Neurology.** *Neurology.* **1996;46:278–285.**

Description

This report presents the history and technique of SPECT and summarizes its use in specific clinical situations.

Key Results

The efficacy of SPECT was rated as *established* for the detection of acute ischemia, and *promising* in the determination of stroke subtypes, vasospasm following SAH, and the determination of brain death. The efficacy of SPECT was rated *investigational* in the determination of prognosis/recovery following stroke, monitoring therapies in stroke, diagnosis and prognosis of transient ischemic attack, and traumatic brain injury.

Strengths and Limitations

This report by a panel of experts on the clinical utility of brain SPECT was based on a review of the literature and expert opinion. Thus, it presents the best evidence currently available. However, based on the limitations of the evidence to support the use of the CBF measures discussed, the panel rates their use only as investigational.

2. **Latchaw RE, Yonas H, Hunter GJ, et al. Guidelines and recommendations for perfusion imaging in cerebral ischemia: a scientific statement for healthcare providers by the writing group on perfusion imaging, from the Council on Cardiovascular Radiology of the American Heart Association.** *Stroke.* **2003;34;1084–1104.**

Description

This scientific statement examines the quality of research involving a number of CBF studies, including Xe-CT, perfusion CT, SPECT, and perfusion and diffusion MRI, provides graded recommendations for their clinical use, and identifies for areas of further study. The rationale of each technique, method of carrying out the technique, and infor-

mation related to quantification, accuracy, and reproducibility are presented. Clinical situations in which the techniques are used are described, as are the advantages and disadvantages relative to other techniques. The strengths of recommendation as to usefulness are graded as established, probable, possible, or having inadequate data.

Key Results

The report acknowledges that the accuracy and reliability of data from these techniques is generally high but their ability to predict outcome with or without treatment and their influence on treatment decisions is less well studied. Although the main focus is the use of CBF studies in ischemic stroke, use in traumatic brain injury is also addressed because of the common denominator of ischemic brain injury.

Strengths and Limitations

The article provides recommendations for clinical use of CBF studies based on a comprehensive assessment by experts of the quality of research examining their use. The conclusions reflect the limited evidence currently available to validate the effect of use of these studies on treatment and outcome.

3. **Menon DK. Brain ischemia after traumatic brain injury: lessons from $^{15}O_2$ positron emission tomography.** *Curr Opin Crit Care.* **2006; 12:85–89.**

Description

This article reviews the use of $^{15}O_2$ PET in studying cerebral ischemia following traumatic brain injury. Interesting points regarding the role and definition of ischemia following traumatic brain injury are discussed as well as implications for further research.

Key Results

Given the heterogeneity of pathophysiology in the injured brain, PET has an advantage in better identifying pathophysiology that may be masked when global CBF measures are used or missed by measures in a very focal area. PET also has the benefit of providing measures of cerebral metabolism. Its combined use with other imaging and monitoring modalities is recommended to better define cerebral ischemia in traumatic brain injury and assess the effect of interventions.

Strengths and Limitations

The article identifies how challenges in measuring cerebral ischemia due to the pathophysiologic heterogeneity of brain injury limit current ability to fully characterize the pathophysiology. Limitations in current knowledge and technology necessitate further study, particularly related to the use of complementary physiologic monitoring techniques to increase understanding of the pathophysiology following brain injury and to guide treatment.

4. **Sloan MA, Alexandrov AV, Tegeler CH, Spencer MP, Caplan LR, Feldmann E, Wechsler LR, Newell DW, Gomez CR, Babikian VL, Lefkowitz D, Goldman RS, Armon C, Hsu CY, Goodin DS. Assessment: Transcranial Doppler ultrasonography: Report of the Therapeutics and Technology Assessment Subcommittee of the American Academy of Neurology. *Neurology*. 2004;62:1468–1481.**

Description

This report reviews the evidence in the literature relating to the usefulness of TCD in specific clinical situations, whether TCD information improves clinical decision making, and if TCD is the preferred diagnostic test in a particular clinical situation.

Key Results

It was concluded that the clinical utility of TCD is established in the detection and monitoring of cerebral vasospasm following aneurysmal SAH, although the effect on clinical outcome is yet to be determined. TCD was concluded to be informative but its clinical utility compared to other diagnostic studies yet to be determined in intracranial steno-occlusive disease and cerebral circulatory arrest. Clinical utility of TCD in a number of other clinical situations, including cerebral thrombolysis and vasomotor reactivity testing was rated as undetermined.

Strengths and Limitations

A strength of this report is that it has been prepared by a committee of experts who have examined the current literature on the use of TCD. A limitation of the report is that the authors were unable to determine the impact of the use of TCD on outcome because of a lack of studies addressing this issue.

5. **Steiner LA, Czosnyka M. Should we measure cerebral blood flow in head-injured patients? *Br J Neurosurg*. 2002;16:429–439.**

Description

This article addresses 3 fundamental issues in relation to CBF measurement in traumatic brain injury: 1) which method to use, 2) how to manipulate CBF, and 3) does manipulating CBF improve outcome.

Key Results

The importance of spatial resolution of CBF techniques is an issue in traumatic brain injury, given the heterogeneity of lesions. In addition, adequate detection of short episodes

that may contribute to ischemic brain injury requires high temporal resolution, versus snapshot measurement of CBF provided by many measures. The authors conclude that CBF techniques do not yet provide quantitative data with reliable spatial and temporal resolution, so there is no gold standard for CBF measurement in head injury. Multimodality monitoring may improve ability to identify relevant episodes of inadequate perfusion. The limited methods of manipulating CBF are identified, such as changing CPP or partial pressure of carbon dioxide ($Paco_2$) levels, as is the importance of cerebral autoregulatory status in the response to therapies targeted at altering CBF. Further study is recommended to examine the use of treatment strategies to optimize CPP based on cerebral autoregulation. The authors cite 2 contradictory studies using CBF management strategies and conclude there is no adequate evidence that manipulating CBF is better than using ICP or CPP to guide treatment, thus making the benefit of CBF monitoring unclear. However, indices of vascular reactivity derived from CBF studies may provide prognostic information. The need to be able to define thresholds of ischemia and hyperemia in traumatic brain injury is raised, recognizing that there will be interindividual and temporal variability, and CBF may not be the best parameter to use.

Strengths and Limitations

One strength of this article is that it provides a general review by the authors of CBF measurement in patients with head injury. Limitations are that the references are primarily related to the measurement techniques and the clinical application of findings from CBF studies are addressed only in general terms. Conclusions that CBF monitoring is an option for which a clear clinical benefit has not been established, reflect current limitations of CBF measures and a lack of research in the area.

6. **Yonas H, Pindzola RR, Johnson DW. Xenon/computed tomography cerebral blood flow and its use in clinical management. *Neurosurg Clin N Am*. 1996;7:605–616.**

Description

Although Xe-CT is currently used only on a very limited basis in the United States, there are many reports in the literature of its use and it has been used to validate many other CBF studies. This article provides a review of the technique and its application in various clinical situations, including assessing cerebrovascular reserve, response to temporary artery occlusion, traumatic brain injury, and SAH.

Strengths and Limitations

The authors have published extensively on this topic and trace the development of Xe-CT measurement of CBF. However, more recent issues cannot be addressed given the date of the publication. Clinical use of the CBF techniques is described, with some supporting references included. Although the authors support the use of Xe-CT further study is needed to determine its ultimate value.

7. Latchaw RE. Cerebral perfusion imaging in acute stroke. *J Vasc Interv Radiol.* 2004; 15:S29–S46.

Description

This article summarizes 4 CBF measurement techniques (Xe-CT, SPECT, perfusion CT, and perfusion MR), focusing on their application in acute stroke. The study methods, important issues in carrying out the studies, accuracy, and advantages and disadvantages of each are presented. The article identifies the need for further study in relation to the relative value of quantifying perfusion data versus identifying of patterns of mismatch between irreversible and potentially reversible (penumbral) ischemic tissue in guiding decision-making regarding the administration of thrombolytics. A key general summary point is that the value of CBF data in decision-making, predicting outcome, and establishing risks and benefits associated with a particular treatment, such as thrombolytic therapy, have not yet been established with certainty. Once these are established, decisions as to which technique to use can be based on relative advantages and disadvantages, ease of performing the study, and accuracy of study results.

Strengths and Limitations

The author has a number of other publications in this area and summarizes complex information in an understandable way. Highlighting the advantages and disadvantages of the different techniques is useful to provide clinicians with an understanding of when and why a particular study would be used. References provided are mainly related to study technique. The author identifies the potential importance of CBF studies in acute stroke but also clearly identifies the limitations of current knowledge in relation to the value of these studies and the need for further study.

OTHER REFERENCES

1. Hinkle JL, Guanci MM, Bowman L, Hermann l, McGinty LB, Rose J. Cerebrovascular events of the nervous system. In: Hinkle JLC, Bader MK, Little-johns LR, eds. *AANN Core Curriculum for Neuroscience Nursing,* 4th ed. St. Louis, MO: Elsevier Inc.; 2004:536–585.

2. Kosty T. Cerebral vasospasm after subarachnoid hemorrhage: an update. *Crit Care Nurs Q.* 2005;28:122–134.

3. Oyama K, Criddle L. Vasospasm after aneurysmal subarachnoid hemorrhage. *Crit Care Nurse.* 2004; 24:58–67.

4. Treggiari MM, Walder B, Suter PM, Romand JA. Systematic review of the prevention of delayed ischemic neurological deficits with hypertension, hypervolemia, and hemodilution therapy following subarachnoid hemorrhage. *J Neurosurg.* 2003;98: 978–984.

5. Lysakowski C, Walder B, Costanza MC, Tramer MR. Transcranial Doppler versus angiography in patients with vasospasm due to a ruptured cerebral aneurysm: a systematic review. *Stroke.* 2001;32:2292–2298.

6. Wardlaw JM, Offin R, Teasdale GM, Teasdale EM. Is routine transcranial Doppler ultrasound monitoring useful in the management of subarachnoid hemorrhage? *J Neurosurg.* 1998;88:272–276.

7. Rajendran JG, Lewis DH, Newell DW, Winn HR. Brain SPECT used to evaluate vasospasm after subarachnoid hemorrhage: correlation with angiography and transcranial Doppler. *Clin Nucl Med.* 2001;26:125–130.

8. Sloan MA, Alexandrov AV, Tegeler CH, et al. Assessment: transcranial Doppler ultrasonography: report of the Therapeutics and Technology Assessment Subcommittee of the American Academy of Neurology. *Neurology.* 2004;62:1468–1481.

9. Minhas PS, Menon DK, Smielewski P, et al. Positron emission tomographic cerebral perfusion disturbances and transcranial Doppler findings among patients with neurological deterioration after subarachnoid hemorrhage. *Neurosurgery.* 2003;52:1017–1024.

10. Newell DW, Aaslid R, Lam A, Mayberg TS, Winn HR. Comparison of flow and velocity during dynamic autoregulation testing in humans. *Stroke.* 1994;25:793–797.

11. Clyde BL, Resnick DK, Yonas H, Smith HA, Kaufmann AM. The relationship of blood velocity as measured by transcranial Doppler ultrasonography to cerebral blood flow as determined by stable xenon computed tomographic studies after aneurysmal subarachnoid hemorrhage. *Neurosurgery.* 1996;38: 896–905.

12. Lindegaard KF, Nornes H, Bakke SJ, Sorteberg W, Nakstad P. Cerebral vasospasm diagnosis by means of angiography and blood velocity measurements. *Acta Neurochir (Wein).* 1989;100:12–24.

13. Sviri GE, Ghodke B, Britz GW, et al. Transcranial Doppler grading criteria for basilar artery vasospasm. *Neurosurgery.* 2006;59:360–366; discussion 360–366.

14. Soustiel JF, Shik V, Shreiber R, Tavor Y, Goldsher D. Basilar vasospasm diagnosis: investigation of a modified "Lindegaard Index" based on imaging studies and blood velocity measurements of the basilar artery. *Stroke.* 2002;33:72–77.

15. Griffiths PD, Wilkinson ID, Mitchell P, et al. Multi-modality MR imaging depiction of hemodynamic

changes and cerebral ischemia in subarachnoid hemorrhage. *AJNR Am J Neuroradiol.* 2001;22:1690–1697.

16. Hertel F, Walter C, Bettag M, Morsdorf M. Perfusion-weighted magnetic resonance imaging in patients with vasospasm: a useful new tool in the management of patients with subarachnoid hemorrhage. *Neurosurgery.* 2005;56:28–35; discussion 35.

17. Harrigan MR, Magnano CR, Guterman LR, Hopkins LN. Computed tomographic perfusion in the management of aneurysmal subarachnoid hemorrhage: new application of an existent technique. *Neurosurgery.* 2005;56:304–317.

18. Moftakhar R, Rowley HA, Turk A, et al. Utility of computed tomography perfusion in detection of cerebral vasospasm in patients with subarachnoid hemorrhage. *Neurosurg Focus.* 2006;21:E6.

19. Wintermark M, Ko NU, Smith WS, Liu S, Higashida RT, Dillon WP. Vasospasm after subarachnoid hemorrhage: utility of perfusion CT and CT angiography on diagnosis and management. *AJNR Am J Neuroradiol.* 2006;27:26–34.

20. van der Schaaf I, Wermer MJ, van der Graaf Y, Velthuis BK, van de Kraats CIB, Rinkel GJE. Prognostic value of cerebral perfusion-computed tomography in the acute stage after subarachnoid hemorrhage for the development of delayed cerebral ischemia. *Stroke.* 2006;37:409–413.

21. Carter LP. Thermal diffusion flowmetry. *Neurosurg Clin N Am.* 1996;7:749–754.

22. Vajkoczy P, Horn P, Thome C, Munch E, Schmiedek P. Regional cerebral blood flow monitoring in the diagnosis of delayed ischemia following aneurysmal subarachnoid hemorrhage. *J Neurosurg.* 2003;98:1227–1234.

23. Vajkoczy P, Horn P, Bauhuf C, et al. Effect of intra-arterial papaverine on regional cerebral blood flow in hemodynamically relevant cerebral vasospasm. *Stroke.* 2001;32:498–505.

24. Johnson WD, Bolognese P, Miller JI, Heger IM, Liker MA, Milhorat TH. Continuous postoperative lCBF monitoring in aneurysmal SAH patients using a combined ICP-laser Doppler fiberoptic probe. *J Neurosurg Anesthesiol.* 1996;8:199–207.

25. The Brain Trauma Foundation. The American Association of Neurological Surgeons. The Joint Section on Neurotrauma and Critical Care. Hyperventilation. *J Neurotrauma.* 2000;17:513–520.

26. Kirkness CJ, March K. Intracranial Pressure Management. In: Mitchell PHCE, Bader MK, Littlejohns LR, eds. *AANN Core Curriculum for Neuroscience Nursing,* 4th ed. St. Louis, MO: Elsevier Inc.; 2004:249–267.

27. Stocchetti N, Maas AI, Chieregato A, van der Plas AA. Hyperventilation in head injury: a review. *Chest.* 2005;127:1812–1827.

28. Steiger HJ, Aaslid R, Stooss R, Seiler RW. Transcranial Doppler monitoring in head injury: relations between type of injury, flow velocities, vasoreactivity, and outcome. *Neurosurgery.* 1994;34:79–85; discussion 85–76.

29. Tiecks FP, Lam AM, Aaslid R, Newell DW. Comparison of static and dynamic cerebral autoregulation measurements. *Stroke.* 1995;26:1014–1019.

30. Czosnyka M, Smielewski P, Kirkpatrick P, Menon DK, Pickard JD. Monitoring of cerebral autoregulation in head-injured patients. *Stroke.* 1996;27:1829–1834.

31. Steiner LA, Coles JP, Johnston AJ, et al. Assessment of cerebrovascular autoregulation in head-injured patients: a validation study. *Stroke.* 2003;34:2404–2409.

32. Lang EW, Lagopoulos J, Griffith J, et al. Noninvasive cerebrovascular autoregulation assessment in traumatic brain injury: validation and utility. *J Neurotrauma.* 2003;20:69–75.

33. Howells T, Elf K, Jones PA, et al. Pressure reactivity as a guide in the treatment of cerebral perfusion pressure in patients with brain trauma. *J Neurosurg.* 2005;102:311–317.

34. Marion DW, Bouma GJ. The use of stable xenon-enhanced computed tomographic studies of cerebral blood flow to define changes in cerebral carbon dioxide vasoresponsivity caused by a severe head injury. *Neurosurgery.* 1991;29:869–873.

35. Bouma GJ, Muizelaar JP. Evaluation of regional cerebral blood flow in acute head injury by stable xenon-enhanced computerized tomography. *Acta Neurochir (Wein).* 1993;59:34–40.

36. Assessment of brain SPECT. Report of the Therapeutics and Technology Assessment Subcommittee of the American Academy of Neurology. *Neurology.* 1996;46:278–285.

37. Wintermark M, Chiolero R, van Melle G, et al. Relationship between brain perfusion computed tomography variables and cerebral perfusion pressure in severe head trauma patients. *Crit Care Med.* 2004;32:1579–1587.

38. Wintermark M, Chiolero R, Van Melle G, et al. Cerebral vascular autoregulation assessed by perfusion-CT in severe head trauma patients. *J Neuroradiol.* 2006;33:27–37.

39. Sioutos PJ, Orozco JA, Carter LP, Weinand ME, Hamilton AJ, Williams FC. Continuous regional cerebral cortical blood flow monitoring in head-injured patients. *Neurosurgery.* 1995;36:943–949; discussion 949–950.

40. Arbit E, DiResta GR. Application of laser Doppler flowmetry in neurosurgery. *Neurosurg Clin N Am.* 1996;7:741–748.

41. Lam JM, Hsiang JN, Poon WS. Monitoring of autoregulation using laser Doppler flowmetry in patients with head injury. *J Neurosurg.* 1997; 86:438–445.

42. Johnston AJ, Steiner LA, Coles JP, et al. Effect of cerebral perfusion pressure augmentation on regional oxygenation and metabolism after head injury. *Crit Care Med.* 2005;33:189–195.

43. Menon DK. Brain ischaemia after traumatic brain injury: lessons from $^{15}O_2$ positron emission tomography. *Curr Opin Crit Care.* 2006;12:85–89.

44. NINDS. NIH Stroke Scale. Available at: http://www.ninds.nih.gov/doctors/NIH_Stroke_Scale _Booklet.pdf. Accessed August 14, 2007.

45. Adams H, Adams R, Del Zoppo G, Goldstein LB. Guidelines for the early management of patients with ischemic stroke: 2005 guidelines update a scientific statement from the Stroke Council of the American Heart Association/American Stroke Association. *Stroke.* 2005;36:916–923.

46. Latchaw RE. Cerebral perfusion imaging in acute stroke. *J Vasc Interv Radiol.* 2004;15:S29–S46.

47. Hoeffner EG, Case I, Jain R, et al. Cerebral perfusion CT: technique and clinical applications. *Radiology.* 2004;231:632–644.

48. Latchaw RE, Yonas H, Hunter GJ, et al. Guidelines and recommendations for perfusion imaging in cerebral ischemia: a scientific statement for healthcare professionals by the writing group on perfusion imaging, from the Council on Cardiovascular Radiology of the American Heart Association. *Stroke.* 2003;34:1084–1104.

49. Ueda T, Sakaki S, Yuh WT, Nochide I, Ohta S. Outcome in acute stroke with successful intra-arterial thrombolysis and predictive value of initial single-photon emission-computed tomography. *J Cereb Blood Flow Metab.* 1999;19:99–108.

50. Keir SL, Wardlaw JM. Systematic review of diffusion and perfusion imaging in acute ischemic stroke. *Stroke.* 2000;31:2723–2731.

51. Sobesky J, Zaro Weber O, Lehnhardt FG, et al. Does the mismatch match the penumbra? Magnetic resonance imaging and positron emission tomography in early ischemic stroke. *Stroke.* 2005;36:980–985.

52. Sobesky J, von Kummer R, Frackowiak M, et al. Early ischemic edema on cerebral computed tomography: its relation to diffusion changes and hypoperfusion within 6 h after human ischemic stroke. A comparison of CT, MRI and PET. *Cerebrovasc Dis.* 2006;21:336–339.

53. Minhas PS, Smielewski P, Kirkpatrick PJ, Pickard JD, Czosnyka M. Pressure autoregulation and positron emission tomography-derived cerebral blood flow acetazolamide reactivity in patients with carotid artery stenosis. *Neurosurgery.* 2004;55:63–67; discussion 67–68.

54. Ogasawara K, Ito H, Sasoh M, et al. Quantitative measurement of regional cerebrovascular reactivity to acetazolamide using 123I-N-isopropyl-p-iodoamphetamine autoradiography with SPECT: validation study using $H_2^{15}O$ with PET. *J Nucl Med.* 2003;44: 520–525.

55. Bisdas S, Nemitz O, Berding G, et al. Correlative assessment of cerebral blood flow obtained with perfusion CT and positron emission tomography in symptomatic stenotic carotid disease. *Eur Radiol.* 2006;16:2220–2228.

56. Yonas H, Smith HA, Durham SR, Pentheny SL, Johnson DW. Increased stroke risk predicted by compromised cerebral blood flow reactivity. *J Neurosurg.* 1993;79:483–489.

57. Guckel FJ, Brix G, Schmiedek P, et al. Cerebrovascular reserve capacity in patients with occlusive cerebrovascular disease: assessment with dynamic susceptibility contrast-enhanced MR imaging and the acetazolamide stimulation test. *Radiology.* 1996;201:405–412.

58. Eastwood JD, Alexander MJ, Petrella JR, Provenzale JM. Dynamic CT perfusion imaging with acetazolamide challenge for the preprocedural evaluation of a patient with symptomatic middle cerebral artery occlusive disease. *AJNR Am J Neuroradiol.* 2002;23:285–287.

59. Michel E, Liu H, Remley KB, et al. Perfusion MR neuroimaging in patients undergoing balloon test occlusion of the internal carotid artery. *AJNR Am J Neuroradiol.* 2001;22:1590–1596.

60. Mathis JM, Barr JD, Jungreis CA, et al. Temporary balloon test occlusion of the internal carotid artery: experience in 500 cases. *AJNR Am J Neuroradiol.* 1995;16:749–754.

61. Sugawara Y, Kikuchi T, Ueda T, et al. Usefulness of brain SPECT to evaluate brain tolerance and hemodynamic changes during temporary balloon occlusion test and after permanent carotid occlusion. *J Nucl Med.* 2002;43:1616–1623.

62. Thome C, Vajkoczy P, Horn P, Bauhuf C, Hubner U, Schmiedek P. Continuous monitoring of regional cerebral blood flow during temporary arterial occlusion in aneurysm surgery. *J Neurosurg.* 2001;95:402–411.

63. Practice parameters for determining brain death in adults (summary statement). The Quality Standards Subcommittee of the American Academy of Neurology. *Neurology.* 1995;45:1012–1014.

64. Munari M, Zucchetta P, Carollo C, et al. Confirmatory tests in the diagnosis of brain death: comparison between SPECT and contrast angiography. *Crit Care Med.* 2005;33:2068–2073.

65. Kirkness CJ. Cerebral blood flow monitoring in clinical practice. *AACN Clin Issues.* 2005;16:476–487.

66. Aaslid R. *Transcranial Doppler Sonography.* NY: Springer-Verlag Wien; 1986.

67. Hinkle JL. SPECT: A powerful imaging tool. *Am J Nurs.* 2002;102:24A–24G.

68. Plougmann J, Astrup J, Pedersen J, Gyldensted C. Effect of stable xenon inhalation on intracranial pressure during measurement of cerebral blood flow in head injury. *J Neurosurg.* 1994;81:822–828.

69. Idee JM, Pines E, Prigent P, Corot C. Allergy-like reactions to iodinated contrast agents. A critical analysis. *Fundam Clin Pharmacol.* 2005;19:263–281.

70. Costa N. Understanding contrast media. *J Infus Nurs.* 2004;27:302–312.

71. Bettmann MA. Frequently asked questions: iodinated contrast agents. *Radiographics.* 2004;24(Suppl 1): S3–10.

Electroencephalograph-Derived Monitoring

Richard Arbour, RN, MSN, CCRN, CNRN, FAAN

CASE STUDY

R.B., a 74-year-old man, presented to the emergency department with productive cough, shortness of breath, and poor activity tolerance. His past medical history consisted of chronic obstructive pulmonary disease (COPD) and hypertension. He reported living with his wife and that he no longer smoked.

Examination revealed R.B. with generalized weakness and shortness of breath that was exacerbated with activity. Lung sounds were generally diminished with a few rhonchi. More significant decrease in lung sounds was noted over the right middle and lower lobes. He required supplemental oxygen at a fraction of inspired oxygen (FIO_2) of 0.5 to maintain an oxygen saturation of >93% as measured by pulse oximetry.

R.B. was admitted to the medical intensive care unit (ICU) for monitoring and supportive care as well as treatment of COPD exacerbation and presumed community-acquired pneumonia. His medication regimen included furosemide, captopril, moxifloxacin, and ranitidine. Sequential compression stockings were utilized for prevention of deep vein thrombosis. His condition remained stable for the initial 36 hours following ICU admission. At the end of ICU day 2, his condition deteriorated. R.B. became increasingly restless, anxious, and hypoxemic despite an increase in supplemental oxygen to 100% delivered by nonrebreather facemask. After failure of a trial of noninvasive positive-pressure ventilation, he was electively intubated and placed on controlled ventilation. With controlled ventilation, FIO_2 was titrated down to 0.6. Initially, assist/control ventilation was utilized. His condition continued to deteriorate as evidenced by increasing oxygen requirements (FIO_2 increased to 0.8 to maintain oxygen saturation of 90% to

92%), increased ventilation requirements, and poor synchrony with controlled ventilation. For these reasons, R.B. received aggressive sedation and analgesia using a balanced technique with midazolam and fentanyl, respectively. This therapy was titrated to endpoints of synchrony with ventilation, adequate sedation and analgesia while maintaining ability to assess neurologic status.

Over the ensuing 24 hours following intubation and controlled ventilation, there was further decline in R.B.'s clinical status as evidenced by increased oxygen requirements to FIO_2 of 1.0, poor interface with controlled ventilation, significant decrease in lung compliance, and refractory hypoxemia. In addition to "white-out" on chest radiograph, these clinical findings indicated progression to acute respiratory distress syndrome. Assist/control ventilation was now inadequate for oxygenation and ventilation needs. Anticipating the need for nonphysiologic ventilation modes, R.B. received additional sedation/analgesia to produce a marked decrease in responsiveness followed by neuromuscular blockade (NMB) with cis-atracurium.

With onset of skeletal muscle relaxation, ventilator support was changed to pressure control/inverse ratio ventilation with permissive hypercapnia. Following stabilization, maintaining serum pH ≥ 7.20 was accomplished using sodium bicarbonate. The goal for pH support was a pH 7.20 to 7.30. In the event pH exceeded 7.30, the sodium bicarbonate dosing would be titrated down.

Thirty-six hours following utilization of NMB, R.B.'s family was approached for participation in a study evaluating the bispectral index (BIS) in the ICU. After informed consent was obtained, BIS monitoring was initiated. Monitoring of the clinical effects of NMB was done by means of clinical assessment of meeting goals/endpoints of therapy that included synchrony with controlled ventilation and resolution of excessive muscle movement. NMB also was monitored by peripheral nerve stimulation and assessment of the evoked response. In R.B.'s case, 2 evoked responses from a series of 4 stimulations (the train-of-four) yielded a train-of-four of 2/4, which correlated with R.B. meeting therapeutic goals. Initial BIS monitoring revealed a value of 20 to 25, a low BIS value that generally corresponds with a burst suppression electroencephalogram (EEG) pattern. This EEG state was not easily explained by current sedation/analgesia therapy. The BIS did not increase in response to vigorous endotracheal suctioning and primarily electrocardiographic (ECG) artifact was the only activity noted in the EEG channel of the monitoring system. Initial BIS trend, EEG channel, and comparable ECG rhythm are illustrated in Figure 6-1.

Aggressive weaning of NMB followed and when recovery of neuromuscular function was documented, R.B. was weaned off sedative/analgesic agents. Recovery of neuromuscular function following withdrawal of NMB therapy was determined by clinical assessment and peripheral nerve stimulation with assessment of the evoked response. Clinical assessment of recovery was indicated by recovery of cough, gag, and corneal reflexes as well as recovery of residual respiratory drive/ventilator triggering. Electrophysiologic recovery of neuromuscular function was documented by a train-of-four of 4/4. Stat neurology consult and comprehensive neurologic examination revealed minimal responsiveness. Bedside diagnostic EEG evaluation was completed and showed minimal brain activity and significant suppression of EEG activity indicating global brain injury. The formal EEG

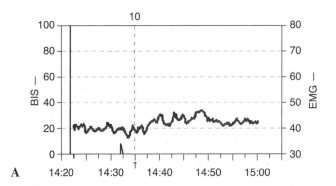

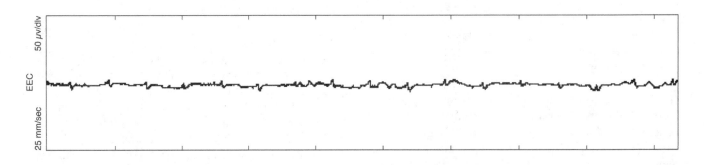

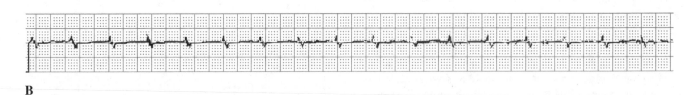

Figure 6-1   (A) Initial BIS trend. (B) EEG channel and ECG rhythm for comparison and illustration of degree of EEG suppression.

Source: Figure appeared previously in: Arbour R. Continuous nervous system monitoring: EEG, the bispectral index and neuromuscular transmission. *AACN Clin Iss/AACN Adv Crit Care*. 2003;14:185–207. Used with permission.

interpretation was: severely suppressed EEG, excessive ECG artifact, and rare periods of theta activity suggesting severe anoxic event. Normal EEG tracing consistent with awake and interactive patient is illustrated in Figure 6-2 as a basis for comparison. EEG tracing from R.B. illustrating severe global brain injury as evidenced by significant suppression and rare theta activity with significant ECG artifact is illustrated in Figure 6-3.

Case Discussion

Given this information, the family was called back to the hospital and all findings were explained to them. This led to their decision to elect a "do not resuscitate" status and subsequent withdrawal of ventilation and extubation with appropriate palliative care for R.B. He died peacefully the following day. This case study effectively illustrates use of EEG and EEG-derived monitoring techniques that provide real-time feedback on brain state as affected by drug therapy or severe injury. In this case, EEG-based information as an adjunct to clinical evaluation gave information to clinicians as well as family and enabled further, more informed decisions to be made on the patient's behalf.

GENERAL DESCRIPTION

Monitoring EEG and EEG-derived data in the critical care setting is an effective means to obtain real-time feedback regarding cerebral stability in response to global physiologic states as well as drug therapy. Specifically, EEG data may be used to guide sedative/analgesic therapy, drug-induced coma, anticonvulsant therapy as well as identify evolving brain injury at a potentially reversible stage.[1–5] It also may enable dramatic changes in therapy in response to a potentially treatable condition. A key application of EEG and EEG-derived technology is that it can provide additional information on global physiologic changes affecting brain physiology and localized changes in brain state that may not be available on clinical examination. EEG/EEG-derived monitoring may be cost-effective when collected data are utilized to navigate between extremes of over- versus undersedation and limit increases in ICU length of stay due to prolonged effects of sedative/analgesic agents. Examples include patients with depressed consciousness/coma states, NMB/sedation/analgesia management as well as brain trauma, metabolic encephalopathies and clinical versus subclinical seizure activity.[1,2]

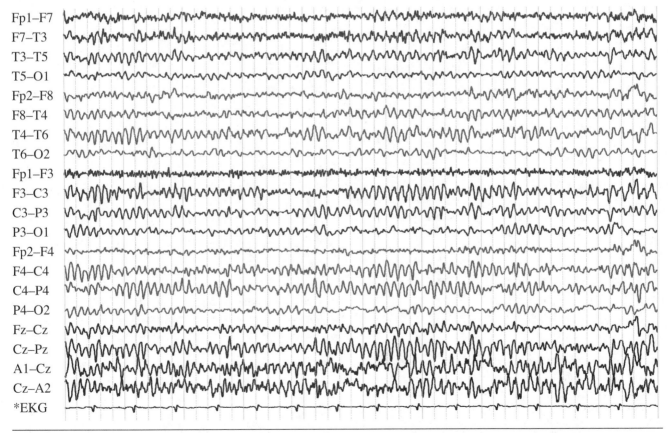

Figure 6-2   Normal EEG tracing consistent with awake and interactive patient illustrated as a basis for comparison with EEG trace of global brain injury. Tracing illustrates high-frequency, low amplitude EEG activity. Sensitivity: 7 uV/mm; data interval 10 seconds.

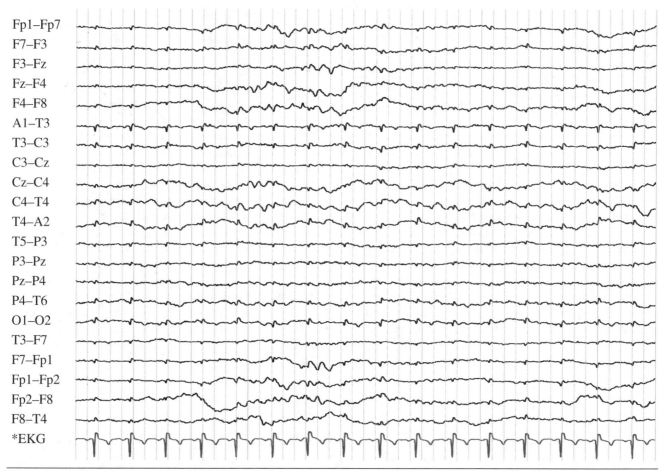

Figure 6-3   EEG tracing from R.B. in the case study, illustrating severe global brain injury as evidenced by **significant suppression and rare theta activity with significant ECG artifact.** Sensitivity 3 uV/mm, data interval 10 sec.

THE TECHNOLOGY

Electroencephalogram Data Collection

EEG and EEG-derived data, waveforms, and waveform analysis are utilized with increasing frequency in clinical practice. EEG activity is intimately linked with cerebral metabolic state. Diagnostic EEG tracings and waveforms as well as data from EEG-derived technology are typically obtained by application of electrodes to the scalp and head. Neuronal electrical activity is detected and recorded.[1,2,6] Data obtained in this manner from diagnostic EEG technology or EEG-derived technology, such as the BIS or patient state analyzer, potentially can be utilized to guide drug therapy or provide early warning of central nervous system (CNS) dysfunction.

On the most basic level, EEG waveforms reflect summation of electrical impulses generated at the cerebral cortex, which in turn reflects electrical discharges in other areas of the brain such as the thalamus. EEG activity also reflects the interaction between and among excitatory and inhibitory electrical discharges and presynaptic neurotrans-

mitter release. Postsynaptic alterations in membrane permeability allow for the controlled membrane instability and ion exchange ultimately responsible for conduction of electrical impulses.[1,4,6–8]

Diagnostic EEG electrodes are placed on areas of the scalp including the frontal, temporal, parietal, and occipital areas. As such, information about global brain physiologic stability and response to drug therapy is obtained. Diagnostic EEG can be used to identify a seizure focus within a discrete brain area or demonstrate global EEG abnormalities consequent to an encephalopathic state. BIS electrodes are placed in a frontal-temporal configuration and reflect the response to drug therapy as it affects the underlying brain tissue. A brain lesion in the occipital lobe, for example, may not immediately cause a change in BIS value. Over time however, an expanding mass lesion such as brain hemorrhage or brain ischemia can produce global effects such as severe ICP elevations and loss of consciousness (LOC). At this stage, BIS monitoring in the frontal-temporal montage electrode placement can reflect these changes.

Physiologic events responsible for generation and conduction of neuronal electrical activity as reflected in EEG waveforms are multiple and energy-requiring steps. Given this physiologic basis, EEG waveforms intimately reflect the underlying cerebral metabolic state and, as such, any physiologic state such as hypothermia, cerebral ischemia, or brain state after cardiac arrest can be reflected in EEG data.[1,3,5,7] In addition, multiple drug therapies such as sedative/hypnotics including benzodiazepines, propofol, and barbiturates can alter and suppress cerebral metabolic activity; their effects can be reflected in EEG data. For a more comprehensive discussion of brain physiology and drug effects as related to an EEG state, the reader is referred to any of the superb references available on this topic.[1,2,8,9] Comparison of normal EEG versus EEG consistent with severe encephalopathy is seen in Figures 6-2 and 6-3. As stated, EEG reflects global physiologic stability as well as brain activity within specific areas. Severe global encephalopathy (ie, stage 4 hepatic encephalopathy with LOC) may produce significant slowing of EEG waveform frequencies as well as potentially significant EEG suppression. Cerebral ischemia in early stages may change EEG waveforms from high-frequency, low amplitude to lower frequencies and higher amplitude and, in either event, reflect compromised brain physiology.

In an evaluation of EEG data, waveform frequency, amplitude, morphology, and degree of EEG suppression are primary factors. Waveform frequency and amplitude generally correspond with clinical states. Alpha waves (8–12/second) are seen primarily in awake, relaxed individuals. Beta waves (>13/second) may indicate initial levels of sedation such as amnesia/anxiolysis. Theta waves (4–7/second) are normally seen in sleep states. Delta waves (≤3/second) are seen normally in deep sleep.[1,9–11] Typically with onset of sleep or a state of depressed consciousness following administration of sedative/hypnotic or anesthetic agents in a dose-related manner, the EEG waveform changes from a low amplitude/higher frequency state to a high amplitude/lower frequency state.[1,9]

Degree of responsiveness of EEG waveform/amplitude to external stimulation is also evaluated as a means to determine integrity of CNS/peripheral nervous system pathways. Under normal circumstances, the EEG should change in response to stimulation such as visual or auditory evoked potentials. Noxious stimulation, particularly in the absence of significant analgesia, typically produces an arousal response at the cerebral cortex and alters EEG data. An absolutely invariant EEG absent any potentially reversible causes usually carries a grim prognosis. For these reasons, the reactivity of EEG and response of EEG-derived data to stimulation gives additional, vital data on CNS integrity and function.[1,12–15] Also, given the risk of increased morbidity related to seizure activity following brain trauma or intracerebral hemorrhage, EEG monitoring should be initiated and maintained as clinically indicated as part of aggressive treatment early in the ICU course.

Additional information regarding the corresponding clinical state is obtained from the degree of EEG suppression.[1,3,5] A completely suppressed and nonreactive EEG state not accounted for by drug therapy (ie, excessive barbiturate dosing) or a reversible clinical state (eg, severe hypothermia), in context with clinical evaluation showing complete unresponsiveness to stimulation, dilated, fixed, and nonreactive pupils, and total unresponsiveness to brainstem reflex evaluation concurrent with a nonreversible brain lesion such as devastating intracerebral hemorrhage, is confirmatory for brain death.[1,16–20] A state of burst suppression, for example, in response to appropriate barbiturate dosing to control ICP elevations indicates a near maximal reduction in cerebral metabolic rate. Metabolic suppression therapy is typically titrated to 3 to 5 bursts per minute. Burst-suppression EEG patterns are characterized by occasional bursts or short intervals of higher amplitude activity over a background of a predominately suppressed EEG. Significant EEG suppression also can occur in response to reversible encephalopathic states such as high-grade hepatic encephalopathy. In such cases, a deeply unconscious patient having a significantly suppressed EEG may not have a grave prognosis. Aggressive management and physiologic support may lead to recovery of consciousness/responsiveness concurrent with recovery of EEG activity.

Alterations in EEG waveform morphology such as spike and wave activity indicate seizure activity. Increased spike/wave activity indicates electrical instability within the cerebral cortex, which potentially can increase the cerebral metabolic rate and exhaust available fuel substrates (oxygen/glucose). Seizure activity (clinical or subclinical) can occur from electrolyte imbalance, drug toxicity, and space-occupying cerebral tumors as well as occur consequent to brain trauma among many other causes. For these reasons, early recognition and intervention are paramount and vital to provide the best opportunity for optimal clinical/neurologic outcome. The resulting mismatch between cerebral oxygen supply and demand may result in ischemia and possible permanent brain dysfunction. In select centers, concurrent EEG and video monitoring are available for seizure monitoring, diagnosis, and correlation of physical symptoms of seizure symptoms with corresponding EEG waveforms.

Select EEG-Derived Parameters: The Bispectral Index and Patient State Analyzer

Bispectral Index

Initial clinical applications of the BIS began in the operating room (OR) setting. The BIS is a processed EEG parameter utilized to monitor responses to sedative/hypnotic and anesthetic agents. Clinical applications of BIS technology have been investigated beyond the OR setting to include sedation assessment in the ICU.[1] The gold standard for assessing brain function, arousal, cognition level of sedation, and neurologic stability will always remain the clinical neurologic examination.[1,21,22] There are situations

Table 6-1   BIS Values and Corresponding Level of Sedation and EEG State

BIS Value	Corresponding Level of Sedation	Corresponding EEG State/Descriptors
100	Awake state; patient is able to respond appropriately to verbal stimulation.	Baseline state before sedation.
80	Patient is able to respond to loud verbal and limited tactile stimulation such as mild prodding or shaking.	Anxiolysis/high-frequency EEG activity (beta augmentation). Moderate sedation.
60	Low probability of explicit recall; patient is unresponsive to verbal stimulation.	Low frequency EEG activity (theta/delta activity). Deep sedation.
40	Patient is unresponsive to verbal stimulation and less responsive to physical stimulation.	Low frequency EEG activity. Deep hypnotic state.
20	Minimal responsiveness.	Drug-induced coma. Burst suppression EEG pattern.
0	No responses are mediated by brain function; spinal reflexes may be present.	Isoelectric or completely suppressed EEG.

Data are from References.[1,9,21–23,24]

where the ability to assess neurologic status or level of sedation may be severely limited or equivocal. Under these circumstances, use of EEG-based technology as an adjunct to clinical evaluation may provide useful information not available on clinical assessment. Examples of these clinical situations include patients receiving NMB, drug-induced coma for ICP management following brain injury, or deep-sedation/analgesia in management of severe respiratory failure.[1,21,22] When BIS is utilized in brain-injured patients, the electrodes are typically placed over the uninjured area of the brain.

BIS is derived from EEG data; therefore, changes in EEG waveform frequency, amplitude, and level of EEG suppression whether drug-induced (as with sedative/hypnotic administration) or induced by physiologic changes (eg, moderate to severe hypothermia) may be reflected in BIS values. BIS determination begins with EEG data acquisition obtained from a single electrode strip across the patient's forehead placed in a frontal-temporal montage. Brain activity within this localized area will be reflected in the BIS value. If the brain injury involves the monitored area, this may affect BIS value. A single channel of EEG data is obtained and digitized prior to being channeled through multiple processing steps. Each processing step evaluates a specific EEG feature such as degree of suppression or synchrony of fast versus slow wave activity.[1,9,21–23] The resulting EEG-derived parameter—the BIS value—is on a linear scale (0 to 100). A BIS value of "0" indicates no brain activity and a BIS value at or near "100" generally corresponds with an awake/interactive patient. Correlation between EEG state, BIS value, and corresponding clinical state is found in Table 6-1. A comprehensive discussion of BIS derivation from EEG data is beyond the scope of this chapter. The reader is referred to any of the superb references available on this topic.[1,9,21–24]

BIS monitoring, as based on the EEG, has been demonstrated to show varying degrees of positive correlation with clinical assessment.[1,22–28] In addition, BIS demonstrates sensitivity to altered cerebral physiology independent of sedative/hypnotic administration.[1,22,29–31] Given the correlation between BIS and clinical assessment of sedation and sensitivities of BIS to altered brain physiology, BIS monitoring can have an adjunctive role complementing clinical evaluation of brain function, particularly in sedation assessment. Data available from BIS monitoring include EMG activity generated from the muscles of the face/forehead, BIS value (0 to 100 on a linear scale), suppression ratio (SR; a measure of the percentage of EEG suppression in the previous 63 seconds of collected data), and signal quality index (SQI). BIS values may be tracked over time and in response to stimulation as well as drug therapy, providing real-time feedback with which to make therapeutic decisions. An example of a BIS trend over time in response to drug therapy is in Figure 6-4. In patient care situations where clinical assessment is equivocal or not available, such as deep sedation/analgesia or NMB, BIS monitoring may help identify patients at risk of under- or oversedation. If clinical assessment provides all necessary information with which to guide therapy and BIS monitoring adds nothing to guide therapeutic decisions, it becomes unnecessary. BIS utilization may be emerging as an alternative to diagnostic EEG monitoring in determining depth of barbiturate-induced coma in ICP management following traumatic brain injury.[1,21,32] It also needs to be determined whether BIS changes sedation practice if the clinician is a novice versus an experienced/expert in critical care practice.

Patient State Analyzer

As with the BIS, the patient state analyzer (PSA) is derived from the EEG. The specific value, the patient state index (PSI), was developed as an objective electrophysiologic measure of hypnosis during anesthesia. In contrast with BIS monitoring, the PSA utilizes anterior/posterior placement of scalp electrodes for EEG data acquisition. EEG data

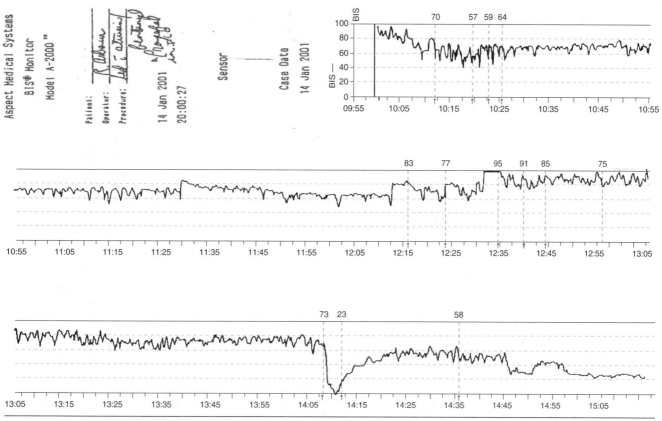

Figure 6-4   BIS trend recording of sedation/analgesia management in a critically ill patient.

BIS monitoring was initiated at approximately 10:00 AM. Sedation was managed initially with fentanyl and lorazepam. Decline in BIS from the 90–97 range to 55–65 range occurred over 25 to 30 minutes in response to therapy. Decline in BIS value matched clinical assessment of increased level of sedation. The patient had periods of breakthrough agitation and ventilator dys-synchrony at 12:15 and 12:35 PM. Agitation was refractory to current therapy despite an upward titration of sedative/analgesic agents. The sedation management was changed to propofol at approximately 14:05 PM. The precipitous drop in BIS value indicated increased sedation. Propofol was titrated back in a controlled, incremental manner. Sedation was more closely and optimally managed with application of EEG-based monitoring adjunctive with clinical evaluation. In a controlled manner, extremes of excessive versus inadequate sedation were avoided.

Source: This figure appeared originally in: Arbour R. Chapter 86; Bispectral index monitoring. In *AACN Procedure Manual for Critical Care*, 5th Edition; Wiegand DL, and Carlson KK, editors. Elsevier Inc. 2005. Used with permission. This tracing has been utilized by Aspect Medical Systems in electronic format.

obtained are then subjected to processing through a multivariate algorithm that quantifies the most probable hypnotic state.[33–35] The resulting parameter, the PSI, is a value on a linear scale (0 to 100) with a deeper hypnotic state generally corresponding with a lower number of the continuum.[33–35] Research is ongoing to determine to what degree the PSI may be useful in ICU practice for sedation assessment. Available but limited research shows a positive correlation between PSI and clinical assessment of sedation.[36,37]

Continued clinical experience and research ultimately will determine best practices regarding patient selection, length of monitoring, and clinical applications in critically ill patients. In selected circumstances, EEG-derived monitoring technology can offer additional information about the depth of sedation/hypnosis that may not be available on clinical assessment alone. Thus, it can assist clinicians in

navigating therapeutic choices between extremes of under- versus oversedation. Each sedation extreme carries risks including prolonged physiologic stress, prolonged recovery, and increased ICU length of stay. Additional ventilator days add significantly to both human and financial costs associated with critical illness.[38] With experienced clinicians and optimal patient selection, cost-avoidance related to best practice in sedation management may be enabled with the integration of EEG-based monitoring into practice.[22,23]

ACCURACY

Whether obtained from an integrated system within a bedside monitoring system or from a full diagnostic EEG machine, EEG data may be continuously displayed and recorded. Generally, diagnostic EEG data are stored

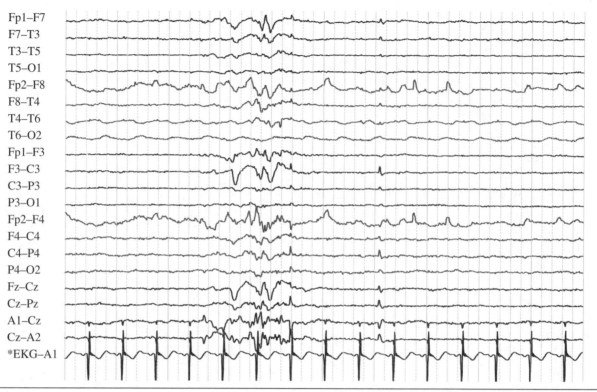

Figure 6-5   Diagnostic EEG tracing illustrating characteristic burst suppression pattern in a patient receiving barbiturate-induced coma for control of ICP elevation. Sensitivity 5 uV/mm 10 sec of EEG data.

digitally and may be recorded on a disc for teaching /research purposes or later review. Review of diagnostic EEG data may be correlated with clinical assessment of the patient's neurologic stability and be useful in helping to determine prognosis and the most appropriate direction of clinical management. Diagnostic EEG consistent with an awake, interactive patient as basis for comparison is found in Figure 6-2. Diagnostic EEG consistent with severe, catastrophic global brain injury is found in Figure 6-3. Real-time monitoring of diagnostic EEG data is also well utilized in titration of drug-induced coma. For example, 3 to 5 bursts per minute is considered at or near maximal therapeutic reduction of brain metabolism during drug-induced coma.[21] Periods of relative electrocerebral silence interspersed with higher frequency/higher amplitude activity is an EEG pattern characteristic of burst suppression. Figure 6-5 shows a diagnostic EEG tracing illustrating burst suppression pattern in a patient receiving barbiturate-induced coma to control ICP elevation. In coordination with a clinical evaluation of grade IV hepatic encephalopathy, diagnostic EEG can directly assess and record the degree of EEG suppression consequent to hepatic dysfunction and elevated serum ammonia levels in hepatic encephalopathy and serve as a baseline to determine effectiveness of aggressive supportive care. A diagnostic EEG tracing consistent with grade IV

hepatic encephalopathy and showing significant EEG suppression is illustrated in Figure 6-6. Following extensive and aggressive supportive care with recovery of responsiveness, diagnostic EEG may be utilized adjunctively to assess recovery of cerebral function and complement the neurologic examination. Figure 6-7 is a diagnostic EEG tracing of grade I–II hepatic encephalopathy from the same patient as in Figure 6-6, and shows the resolution of EEG suppression. In patients with depressed consciousness, cerebral function must be evaluated to rule out subclinical seizure activity and guide anticonvulsant therapy in a controlled monitored setting. A diagnostic EEG illustrating subclinical seizure activity is shown in Figure 6-8. This patient has a depressed consciousness but was arousable to tactile and loud verbal stimulation. EEG-derived parameters such as the BIS can display BIS trend, EMG, SR, and 1 channel of raw EEG (Figures 6-1 and 6-4).

Electrical interference such as that produced by bedside monitoring or other technology as well as patient movement may interfere with data acquisition from EEG and EEG-derived technology. Patient movement and EMG activity may cause a spurious increase in the BIS value independent of hypnotic state. For these reasons, data must be interpreted within the context of clinical assessment as well as overall goal of therapy.

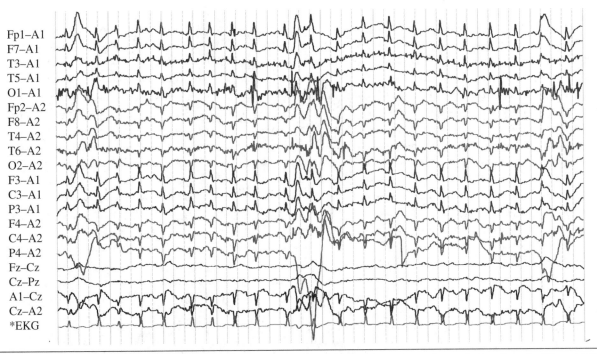

Figure 6-6   Diagnostic EEG tracing consistent with grade IV hepatic encephalopathy and showing significant EEG suppression. Significant EEG suppression is seen as prominent ECG artifact with low-frequency background activity and occasional spike/wave activity. Sensitivity 5 uV/mm and 10 seconds of EEG data are shown.

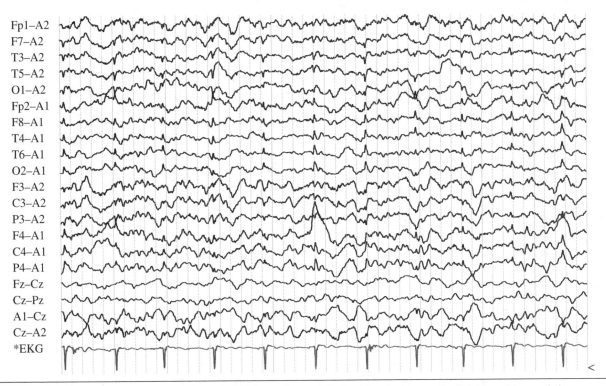

Figure 6-7   Diagnostic EEG tracing of grade I-II hepatic encephalopathy in the same patient as Figure 6-6, showing resolution of EEG suppression, illustrating effect of aggressive supportive care/management for hepatic encephalopathy. Clinical examination shows grade I–II hepatic (ie, confused but arousable and responsive to commands) encephalopathy. EEG shows lower frequency activity but significantly less EEG suppression. Sensitivity at 10 uV/mm and 10 seconds of EEG data are shown.

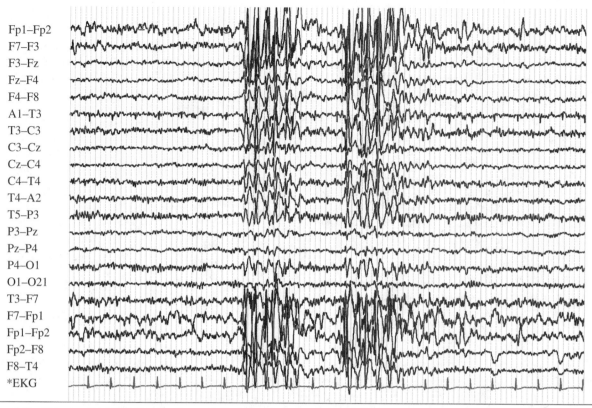

Figure 6-8   Diagnostic EEG illustrating subclinical seizure activity with characteristic spike/wave pattern and abrupt beginning from background activity. Sensitivity at 5 uV/mm/20 seconds of EEG data are illustrated.

COMPETENCY

Competency requirements and prerequisite knowledge related to the use of EEG and EEG-derived technology for patient monitoring of critically ill adults include the ability to:

- Describe the interrelationships between EEG activity, EEG-derived processed parameters, and cerebral physiology as related to sedative/hypnotic administration and metabolic versus structural brain injury.
- Identify the close relationship between EEG and BIS as well as between EEG and the PSI.
- Analyze factors affecting brain metabolism, responsiveness, and EEG activity. These factors include CNS depressant administration as well as brain injury, hypoxemia, and other factors.
- State the indications for EEG and EEG-derived technology for evaluation of clinical states such as depressed consciousness, NMB, deep sedation/analgesia, and procedural sedation as well as in select circumstances, including monitoring level of burst suppression in drug-induced coma.
- Identify the factors affecting data obtained through EEG and EEG-derived technology. Such factors may include sedative/analgesic administration, NMB use (decreases

EMG activity and may decrease BIS value), painful stimuli, sleep states, hypothermia, brain ischemia, encephalopathies, and electrical interference. During NMB use, peripheral nerve stimulation and assessment of the evoked response potentially increases the BIS value consequent to high-frequency electrical activity generated by the pulse generator. To assure accurate measurements, BIS should be allowed to return to baseline following peripheral nerve stimulation for consistency.

- Describe the monitor display and specific data obtained from specific monitoring parameters such as EEG waveform recognition (seizure activity, burst suppression pattern/level of overall EEG suppression, and basic waveform recognition).
- Interpret data as related to therapeutic decision-making.
- Assess when there is a need to obtain baseline data (when possible) and use as a basis for comparison in response to therapy and pathophysiological changes such as hypoxemia and/or hemodynamic instability. As clinically indicated and when possible, BIS monitoring may be initiated prior to initiation of aggressive sedation/analgesia.
- Relate the knowledge of clinical assessment parameters to the specific drug therapies utilized for CNS depression.

- Facilitate and maintain optimal electrode placement for EEG and EEG-derived data acquisition.
- Prepare the patient and provide patient and family education for EEG and EEG-derived data acquisition.

The above list of competency points were adapted with permission from, Bispectral index monitoring, Chapter 86 in the *AACN Procedure Manual for Critical Care*.[39]

Competency verification may be accomplished by a combination of pretest/posttest as well as the return demonstration, and also may be dictated by institutional policy.

FUTURE RESEARCH

There is significant potential benefit in EEG and EEG-derived monitoring in critical care practice. The benefits of diagnostic EEG data acquisition and use of derived EEG parameters include monitoring level of burst suppression, seizure activity, degree of encephalopathy, and extension or evolution of ischemia or other CNS dysfunction as well as monitoring the level of sedation. Additional applications of diagnostic EEG, such as identifying patients at risk for delirium, offer significant opportunities for well-constructed studies and great possible benefit given the risks associated with delirium in practice.

Additional avenues for research in EEG-derived parameters include determining whether and to what degree EEG-derived monitoring improves clinical outcomes. Currently, studies examining clinical outcomes in the critical care setting with parameters such as BIS are limited. Additional research focusing on outcomes such as number of ventilator days, cost avoidance, drug utilization, and ICU length of stay will further determine the role of this technology in patient monitoring and therapeutic decision-making. Efficacy of specific monitoring technologies can and should be determined also as related to specific drug therapies and combinations. Additionally, because there are multiple EEG-derived technologies available, research evaluating degree of correlation between individual parameters and clinical evaluation of sedation is necessary and should be ongoing. Evaluating and determining best patient selection criteria for using EEG-derived technology in practice are important as well. Because most EEG technologies store data/waveforms electronically, research pursuits and later clinical review are facilitated.

REFERENCES

1. Arbour R. Continuous nervous system monitoring: EEG, the bispectral index and neuromuscular transmission. *AACN Clin Issues*. 2003;14:185–207.
2. Markland ON. Pearls, perils and pitfalls in the use of the electroencephalogram. *Semin Neurol*. 2003;23:7–46.
3. Stewart-Amidei C. Neurologic monitoring in the ICU. *Crit Care Nurs Q*. 1998;21:47–60.
4. Grissom TE, Grissom J. *Neurologic Monitoring in the ICU*. Anesthesiology Online 2000. San Antonio, TX: Dannemiller Memorial Educational Foundation.
5. Jordan KG. Continuous EEG monitoring in the neuroscience intensive care unit and emergency department. *J Clin Neurophysiol*. 1999;16:14–39.
6. Misulis KE, Head T. *Essentials of Clinical Neurophysiology,* 3rd Edition. Newton, MA: Butterworth-Heinemann; 2003.
7. Guerit JM. Medical technology assessment: EEG and evoked potentials in the intensive care unit. *Neurophysiol Clin*. 1999;29:301–317.
8. Wallace BE, Wagner AK, Wagner EP, McDeavitt JT. A history and review of quantitative electroencephalography in traumatic brain injury. *J Head Trauma Rehabil*. 2001;16:165–190.
9. Rampil IJ. A primer for EEG signal processing in anesthesia. *Anesthesiology*. 1998;89:980–1002.
10. Luders HO, Noachtar S. *Atlas and Classification of Electroencephalography*. Philadelphia, PA: Saunders; 2000.
11. Louis S. Normal EEG waveform from Neurology/electroencephalography and evoked potentials. New York: E-Medicine; first accessed in 2001, updated 11/2006. Available at: http://emedicine.com/neuro/topic275.htm. Accessed August 26, 2007.
12. Huszar L. Clinical utility of evoked potentials. New York: E-Medicine; first accessed in 2001, updated 4/2006. Available at: http://www.emedicine.com/neuro/topic69.htm. Accessed August 26, 2007.
13. Leim LK. Intraoperative neurophysiological monitoring from neurology/encephalography and evoked potentials. New York: E-Medicine; first accessed in 2001, updated 4/2006. Available at: http://www.emedicine.com/neuro/topic102.htm. Accessed August 26, 2007.
14. Schwartz G. Evoked potentials for coma diagnosis and prognosis. Brussels, Belgium: European Society of Anesthesia. http://www.euroanesthesia.org/education/rc_vienna/07rc3.HTM. Accessed September 24, 2007.
15. Young GB. The EEG in coma. *J Clin Neurophysiol*. 2000;17:473–485.
16. Arbour R. Clinical management of the organ donor. *AACN Clin Issues*. 2005;16:551–580.
17. Henneman EA, Karras GE. Determining brain death in adults: a guideline for use in critical care. *Crit Care Nurse*. 2004;24:50–56.
18. Sullivan J, Seem DL, Chabalewski F. Determining brain death. *Crit Care Nurse*. 1999;19:37–46.
19. Lovasik D. Brain death and organ donation. *Crit Care Nurs Clin North Am*. 2000;12:531–538.

20. Morenski JD, Oro JJ, Tobias JD, Singh A. Determination of death by neurological criteria. *J Intensive Care Med*. 2003;18:211–221.

21. Bader MK, Arbour R, Palmer S. Refractory increased intracranial pressure in severe traumatic brain injury: Barbiturate coma and bispectral index monitoring. *AACN Clin Issues*. 2005;16:526–541.

22. Arbour R. Impact of bispectral index monitoring on sedation and outcomes in critically ill adults: a case series. *Crit Care Nurs Clin North Am*. 2006;18:227–241.

23. Arbour R. Using bispectral index monitoring to detect potential breakthrough awareness and limit duration of neuromuscular blockade. *Am J Crit Care*. 2004;13:66–73.

24. Rosow C, Manberg PJ. Bispectral index monitoring. *Anesthesiol Clin North America* 1998;2:89–107.

25. Deogaonkar A, Gupta R, DeGeorgia M, Sabharwal V, Gopakumaran B, Schubert A, Provencio JJ. Bispectral index monitoring correlates with sedation scales in brain-injured patients. *Crit Care Med*. 2004;32:2403–2406.

26. Mondello E, Siliotti R, Noto G, et al. Bispectral index in ICU: Correlation with Ramsay Score on assessment of sedation level. *J Clin Monit Comput*. 2002;17:271–277.

27. Courtman SP, Wardburgh A, Petros AJ. Comparison of the bispectral index monitor with the Comfort score in assessing level of sedation of critically ill children. *Intensive Care Med*. 2003;29:2239–2246.

28. Simmonds LE, Riker RR, Prato BS, Fraser GL. Assessing sedation during intensive care unit mechanical ventilation with the bispectral index and the sedation-agitation scale. *Crit Care Med*. 1999;27:1499–1504.

29. Mourisse J, Booij L. Bispectral index detects period of cerebral hypoperfusion during cardiopulmonary bypass. *J Cardiothorac Vasc Anesth*. 2003;17:76–78.

30. Azim N, Wang CY. Case report: the use of bispectral index during a cardiopulmonary arrest: a potential indicator of cerebral perfusion. *Anesthesia*. 2004;59:610–612.

31. Vivien B, Langeron O, Riou B. Increase in bispectral index (BIS) while correcting a severe hypoglycemia. *Anesth Analg*. 2002;95:824–825.

32. Riker RR, Fraser GL, Wilkins ML. Comparing the bispectral index and suppression ratio with burst suppression of the electroencephalogram during pentobarbital infusions in adult intensive care patients. *Pharmacotherapy*. 2003;23:1087–1093.

33. Drover DR, Lemmens HJ, Pierce ET, Plourde G, Loyd G. Titration of delivery and recovery from propofol, alfentanyl, and nitrous oxide anesthesia. *Anesthesiology*. 2002;97:82–89.

34. White PF, Tang J, Ma H, et al. Is the patient state analyzer with the PSA2 array a cost-effective alternative to the bispectral index monitor during the perioperative period? *Anesth Analg*. 2004; 99:1429–1435.

35. Prichep LS, Gugino LD, John ER, et al. The patient state index as an indicator of the level of hypnosis under general anesthesia. *Br J Anaesth*. 2004;92:393–399.

36. Shah N, Quijano A. Is patient state index of EEG better than bispectral index of EEG in assessing different levels of sedation as judged by Ramsay Sedation Score in ICU patients? *Anesthesiology*. 2004;101:A293. Abstract.

37. Chisholm CJ, Zurica J, Mironov D, Sciacca RR, Ornstein E, Heyer EJ. Comparison of electrophysiologic monitors with clinical assessment of level of sedation. *Mayo Clin Proc*. 2006;81:46–52.

38. Dasta JF, McLaughlin TP, Mody SH, Piech CT. Daily cost of an intensive care unit day: the contribution of mechanical ventilation. *Crit Care Med*. 2005;33:1266–1271.

39. Arbour R. Bispectral Index Monitoring. In Weigand DLM, Carlson KK, eds. *AACN Procedure Manual for Critical Care Nursing*, 5th ed. Philadelphia: Elsevier; 2005:699–711.

CLINICAL RECOMMENDATIONS

The rating scale for the Level of Recommendation ranges from I to VI, with levels indicated as follows: I, manufacturer's recommendations only; II, theory based, no research data to support recommendations; recommendations from expert consensus group may exist; III, laboratory data only, no clinical data to support recommendations; IV, limited clinical studies to support recommendations; V, clinical studies in more than 1 or 2 different populations and situations to support recommendations; VI, clinical studies in a variety of patient populations and situations to support recommendations.

Period of Use	Recommendation	Rationale for Recommendation	Level of Recommendation	Supporting References	Comments
Patient Selection Neurologic examination indicates depressed consciousness without a readily apparent cause.	Electrodiagnostic evaluation should be performed to evaluate subclinical seizure activity, extension of injury, or differentiate type(s) of encephalopathy. EEG monitoring would be most appropriate here.	During periods where the ability to perform an adequate clinical neurologic examination is compromised, patients are at risk for extension of injury, subclinical seizure activity, and brain injury consequent to global cardiopulmonary instability. EEG data to complement the neurologic assessment may identify evolving CNS dysfunction at a potentially reversible stage. Real-time EEG data facilitate appropriate drug titration during drug-induced coma and sedation/analgesia during NMB.	VI	See Annotated Bibliography: 1–4, 5–10 See References: 1, 2, 4, 5, 7, 9, 10, 14, 15 See Other References: 4, 8, 9, 11–15, 18, 20, 21, 23, 25–28, 31–35, 41–46, 48, 51, 52, 54	A variety of patients may benefit from EEG and EEG-derived monitoring. Key point is that EEG data are complementary or adjunctive to the clinical neurologic assessment. The clinical examination remains the gold standard for assessing CNS stability. For example, in sedation assessment in the ICU, if able to clinically evaluate sedation level and EEG-derived parameters add nothing to change direction of care, they probably should not be used. Also, education with personnel remains paramount in order to avoid "monitoring the machine" rather than monitoring the patient. During NMB, effects of paralyzing agents should be monitored by clinical assessment and peripheral nerve stimulation/ assessment of the evoked response (train-of-four). Metabolic suppression therapy (propofol or barbiturate therapy) should be titrated to achieve 3–5 bursts per minute.
Equivocal or severely compromised ability for thorough clinical neurologic examination.	As clinically appropriate, EEG evaluation should be utilized for determining prognosis and direction of clinical management.		VI		
When receiving NMB, having declined LOC following head trauma, seizure history, or deep sedation/analgesia in ventilator management.	Should be evaluated with EEG or EEG-derived monitoring to assess level of sedation/arousal. The gold standard for electrophysiologic monitoring for seizure activity, extension of injury, or ischemia is EEG. More data are needed before BIS is recommended for routine use in sedation assessment.		IV		
Drug-induced coma with/without therapeutic hypothermia.	Should receive continuous EEG monitoring to determine therapeutic endpoints and facilitate real-time drug titration.		VI		
Application of Device and Initial Monitoring Skin integrity should be assessed in areas of proposed electrode placement for EEG or EEG-derived monitoring.	EEG electrodes should not be placed over areas of skin breakdown. Skin prep (cleaning) is done using soap and water or alcohol pads. The area should be thoroughly dried prior to electrode placement.	Infection risk is associated with skin breakdown.	II	See Annotated Bibliography: 1–3, 5–7. References: 1–3, 15, 21–23, 32, 39. See Other References: 2–4, 10, 12, 15, 30, 32, 35, 37–39, 47, 50, 51, 54, 55.	Skin integrity should be carefully assessed in all patients. Skin breakdown may occur over pressure points such as the occipital area. If this occurs, electrode placement may prove problematic. Obtaining baseline data from clinical and EEG-based evaluation remains paramount to assess

Period of Use	Recommendation	Rationale for Recommendation	Level of Recommendation	Supporting References	Comments
At risk for skin breakdown.	If skin irritation occurs following placement of BIS electrodes (eg,, electrodes should be removed or repositioned if possible.	Infection risk, electrodes may potentially loosen, depending on severity and thus limit data obtained.	I		changes in response to drug therapy, induction of hypothermia or evolution/extension of injury, seizure activity over time.
Determining baseline neurologic assessment concurrent with EEG data is appropriate.	Baseline neurologic assessment data should be compared/correlated with EEG or EEG-derived data.	Obtaining baseline clinical and EEG-based data serves as a basis for comparison and identifying evolution/extension of injury, progression to deeper hypnotic state or drug overdosing during hypothermia/drug-induced coma.	VI		Continuous EEG monitoring is most appropriate for diagnosis of seizure waveform morphology, location, and responsiveness to drug therapy. Concurrent clinical evaluation is optimal. In select centers, video/EEG monitoring is available to aid diagnosis/management.
Ongoing Monitoring Patients requiring EEG/EEG-derived data for clinical management of short-term versus long-term therapy.	All patients receiving drug-induced coma with/without induced hypothermia benefit from EEG/EEG-derived monitoring.	In drug-induced coma with/without hypothermia, drug kinetics may change, predisposing to deeper or lighter coma state than indicated. After head trauma, seizures may occur in up to 1/5 of patients and morbidity/mortality may be dramatically increased. Evolution of injury may occur and early identification of injury, seizures, and extension of injury enables a longer treatment window before neurologic changes become permanent.	VI	See Annotated Bibliography: 2, 5, 6, 8, 9 See References: 1, 3, 5, 7, 8, 13–15, 16, 22, 23, 29, 31, 32, 39 See Other References: 2–4, 12–15, 19, 20, 22, 23, 28, 30–32, 35, 48, 51, 52, 54	In the absence of a reliable neurologic examination, EEG data extend clinicians' ability to objectively measure CNS stability. Where the neurologic examination is equivocal or masked by decreased LOC, deep sedation/analgesia, or NMB, EEG data can provide real-time data and enable more timely therapeutic decisions. Ongoing or surveillance monitoring can detect changes in clinical state as well as altered drug kinetics as reflected in EEG activity.
	Ongoing seizure management; decreased LOC requires EEG-based evaluation.	Patients receiving NMB benefit due to drug tolerances altered over time, risking pain and awareness.	VI		
	Patients receiving NMB potentially benefit from EEG/EEG-derived monitoring.		IV		
Device Removal and Prevention of Complications Patients receiving NMB, drug-induced coma with/without induced hypothermia need EEG-derived	EEG technology and electrodes as well as those used for EEG-derived monitoring should be utilized as indicated and removed when: 1. EEG data are no longer necessary or will not impact therapeutic decisions. If coma/decreased LOC state is prolonged,	Compromised skin integrity can occur in clinical practice or be related to electrode placement. Infection risk increases with compromised skin integrity. EEG technology is effective at extending clinical observations to the level of brain	VI	See Annotated Bibliography: 1, 2, 7, 9 See References: 1, 39 See Other References: 2–4, 17, 27, 30, 52, 53	EEG/EEG-derived technology adds a great deal to the clinicians' ability to assess CNS stability. This technology is best utilized when information obtained does not increase risk (eg, compromise skin integrity) and when data obtained facilitate clinical decision-

Period of Use	Recommendation	Rationale for Recommendation	Level of Recommendation	Supporting References	Comments
monitoring as clinically indicated and as long as no complications occur as related to device or electrode placement.	recovery is not anticipated and EEG does not impact therapeutic decisions, so it may be discontinued. 2. Skin breakdown occurs in area of electrode placement.	electrophysiology. It generates significant amounts of data that, if no longer "actionable," in therapeutic decisions becomes unnecessary.	II		making. When EEG-derived data do not facilitate therapeutic decision-making, a cost-benefit analysis must be done as to how appropriate it is in patient management at a given point in time. Generally speaking, there are virtually no complications associated with EEG/ EEG-derived data acquisition beyond issues related to skin integrity.
Quality Control Issues During patient monitoring, quality control issues related to technology, utilization, and clinician education need to be addressed.	EEG technology, software, processor, and data storage must be fully operational and undergo self-test at start of monitoring and periodic review by biomedical engineering.	Ensures monitoring/ diagnostic system is fully operational, data storage is appropriate.	III	See Annotated Bibliography: 1 See References: 1, 2, 3, 5, 7, 9, 22–24, 39 See Other References: 5–7, 24, 27, 30, 36, 40, 49, 56.	Equipment quality control is managed by institutional biomedical engineering departments. Quality control in EEG/EEG-based monitoring is also multidisciplinary, often involving neurology and neurodiagnostic technologist personnel. Appropriate education and continued competency in multiple areas must be determined and main-
	For derived EEG technology such as BIS, monitor self-testing at start-up/activation is necessary and automatic.	Ensures system is fully operational.	III		
Optimal patient outcomes depend on most appropriate utilization of available technology and appropriate skill mix/education for clinicians.	Quality of electrical contact between scalp and monitoring device should be assessed at the start of monitoring and throughout.	Ensures quality of EEG data acquisition, integrity of electrical contact, and reliability.	IV		tained. This should include data acquisition and interpretation based on clinician education, training and experience as well as institutional policy and procedure. Research-based practice in data interpretation, technology utilization, and patient care should be done. Documentation of EEG-acquired data, particularly as related to therapeutic decisions, should be documented at baseline and with any changes. Reportable conditions include EEG-derived data that are unexpected given clinical goals and endpoints for the patient. For additional documentation, quality guidelines see Reference 39 and Other Reference 30.
	Thorough cleaning of scalp and facial area prior to electrode placement should be done prior to electrode application. Monitor EMG as secondary parameter during BIS monitoring.	Ensures optimal electrical contact between monitoring system and patient. Removes skin oils and residue. High EMG can cause spurious elevation in BIS value.	VI		
	Electrodes should be placed specific to appropriate anatomic landmarks.	Ensures consistency of anatomic location for sensor placement.	IV		
	EEG/EEG-derived monitor settings and sensitivities should be patient-specific and determined by goals of therapy and purpose of monitoring. This may be determined by neurology consultation and is not always a nursing responsibility.	Ensures optimal data utilization and display.	III		

ANNOTATED BIBLIOGRAPHY

1. **Arbour R. Impact of bispectral index monitoring on sedation and outcomes in critically ill adults: a case series. *Crit Care Nurs Clin North Am* 2006;18:227–241.**

Study Sample

Fifteen heterogeneous patients with no CNS pathology at the start of data collection were monitored with clinical assessment and BIS to determine level of sedation/arousal in the ICU. Outcomes related to ventilator days, time to attain recovery of baseline level of consciousness, drug utilization, and length of NMB as well as awareness during NMB were measured. In addition, degree of correlation between clinical assessment using the Sedation-Agitation-Scale (SAS) and BIS for level of sedation was determined for the patients in this series.

Comparison Studied

These outcomes were compared with data collected from a heterogeneous sample of patients monitored with standard clinical assessment techniques.

Study Procedure

Families of patients meeting inclusion criteria were approached by the investigator for study enrollment. BIS monitoring was initiated and data obtained was utilized in therapeutic decision-making for sedation/hypnotic/analgesic dosing. Drug therapies and related outcomes were compared between control (clinical assessment alone) and study enrollees (clinical assessment and BIS) to determine whether and to what degree BIS monitoring made a difference in clinical outcomes. In addition, correlation between clinical and EEG-based monitoring was determined.

Key Results

Moderate positive correlation between BIS and clinical assessment of sedation was found. BIS A-2000/SAS with 134 paired observations: Pearson's coefficient = 0.8072; Spearman rank coefficient = 0.8240. BIS A-2000XP with 52 paired observations: Pearson's coefficient = 0.7271; Spearman coefficient = 0.7348. In select patients in this series, NMB withdrawal was facilitated by a closer objective assessment of sedation. Following withdrawal of NMB, recovery of baseline level of consciousness occurred more quickly. Patients in the control group (clinical assessment) experienced increased ICU length of stay related to prolonged recovery from sedation following NMB. In patients receiving NMB, easier navigation between risk of awareness and excessive sedation was possible. The most significant difference was in patients receiving NMB.

Study Strengths and Weaknesses

This is among the first publications to directly examine clinical outcomes as well as correlation between clinical and EEG-derived sedation assessment. However, the small sample size in the clinical assessment group and the clinical assessment/BIS group limited statistical viability specific to comparing outcomes between groups, and limits the study's generalizability.

Clinical Implications

Results from this series support BIS utilization in the ICU. There is moderate correlation between clinical and BIS sedation assessment that validates BIS when used to assess sedation in patients using NMB as well as determining when patients are progressing to a deeper level of sedation that may not be immediately apparent on clinical evaluation.

2. **Riker RR, Fraser GL, Wilkins ML. Comparing the bispectral index and suppression ratio with burst suppression of the electroencephalogram during pentobarbital infusions in adult intensive care patients. *Pharmacotherapy.* 2003;23:1087–1093.**

Study Sample

Twelve consecutive patients during 62 patient-days who were treated with pentobarbital infusions for elevated intracranial pressure.

Comparison Studied

Comparison and correlation were made between BIS and raw EEG specific to level of burst suppression/EEG suppression between both EEG measures.

Study Procedure

All research subjects were monitored continuously with Aspect A-1050 BIS/EEG monitor using a bilateral referential montage. Pentobarbital dosing was titrated based on raw EEG to attain burst suppression of 3 to 5 bursts/min. Barbiturate dosing, ICP, CPP, bursts/minute, BIS value and SR were recorded.

Key Results

BIS correlated well with SR (r = .99, P <.001). During intervals of burst-suppression BIS value (version 3.2; r = .90, P <.001) and SR (r = .89, P <.001) strongly correlated with number of bursts/minute. Mean BIS value corresponding to 3 to 5 bursts/minute was 15 (95% CI, 10–20); SR value was 71 (95% CI, 61–80).

Study Strengths and Weaknesses

Study strengths include demonstrable direct correlation between raw EEG and parameters derived from the EEG

(BIS value and SR). If further validated, using EEG derived parameters may facilitate more widespread monitoring of burst suppression during drug-induced coma. Weaknesses include small sample size and limited number of patient days, potentially limiting large-scale generalizations when compared to the vastly larger number of patients receiving drug-induced coma. The larger question remains: Is this a representative enough sample to generalize to a vastly larger population? This study identifies intriguing avenues for further research.

Clinical Implications

Potentially, with good patient selection, these findings may support BIS technology utilization in monitoring drug induced coma.

3. **Deogaonkar A, Gupta R, DeGeorgia M, Sabharwal V, Gopakumaran B, Schubert A, Provencio JJ. Bispectral index monitoring correlates with sedation scales in brain-injured patients.** *Crit Care Med* **2004;32:2403–2406.**

Study Sample

Thirty critically ill patients were admitted to the neurointensive care unit with brain injury/decreased LOC.

Comparison Studied

Comparison/correlation between clinical assessment (sedation scales) and EEG-derived data (BIS) was determined for BIS-XP and BIS 2.1.1.

Study Procedures

Patients were prospectively evaluated for level of consciousness with the Richmond Agitation-Sedation Scale (RASS), the Sedation-Agitation Scale (SAS), and Glasgow Coma Scale (GCS) simultaneously with BIS. Spearman's coefficient was utilized to correlate BIS/clinical assessment.

Key Results

With the newer BIS technology (n-15, BIS-XP), significant correlation was found with clinical evaluation tools: BIS/RASS (R^2 = .810; P <.0001); BIS/SAS (R^2 = .725; P <.0001); BIS/GCS (R^2 = .655; P <.0001). With the older technology (version 2.1.1): BIS/RASS (R^2 = .30; P <.008); BIS/SAS (R^2 = .376; P <.001); BIS/GCS (R^2 = .274; P <.015). During sedation therapy, these correlations remained consistent.

Study Strengths and Weaknesses

Strengths were the assessment of the correlation between BIS and clinical assessment in patients with brain injury and potentially validating BIS utilization in patients having brain pathology. Within the context of this study, BIS was

shown to provide useful data beyond sedation assessment to include quantification of level of consciousness. Weaknesses included the small sample size and narrow range of diagnoses. The results from this study may not be applicable to patients following head trauma, delirium, or other CNS pathologies.

Clinical Implications

Implications of this study are multiple. One is identifying the potential for BIS utilization for sedation assessment in the setting of brain pathology. This represents a promising application of BIS technology given the challenges in clinical evaluation of sedation in neurologic critical care.

4. **Chisholm CJ, Zurica J, Mironov D, Sciacca RR, Ornstein E, Heyer EJ. Comparison of electrophysiologic monitors with clinical assessment of level of sedation.** *Mayo Clin Proc.* **2006;81:46–52.**

Study Sample

Fifty patients who were scheduled for elective surgery were included: 24 patients were monitored with the patient state analyzer (PSA) 4000 and 26 patients were monitored with the BIS A-2000XP system.

Comparison Studied

The correlation between 2 clinical assessment tools for sedation level (Ramsay Sedation Scale and the Observer's Assessment of Alertness/Sedation (OAA/S) scale) and 2 EEG-derived tools for assessing level of sedation (BIS A-2000 XP and PSA 4000) were evaluated.

Study Procedure

Level of sedation in patients scheduled for elective surgery was determined clinically with 2 sedation scales (Ramsay and OAA/S) and using 2 derived EEG measures (BIS A-2000XP and PSA 4000 monitoring systems). Correlation between these measures (clinical and EEG-based) was tested using nonparametric statistical tests (partial Mann-Kendall statistical tests). The resulting correlation coefficient was subjected to Fisher transformation and group comparisons of BIS XP and PSA 4000 were performed using unpaired *t* tests or analysis of variance.

Key Results

Ramsay and OAAS scores correlated strongly with one another (r = −.96; P <.001) and with the BIS-XP (r = −.89 and −.91, P <.001). Ramsay and OAAS scores correlated with the PSA 4000 (r = −.80 and −.80; P <.001). This correlation was strongest only at extremes of sedation (light vs. excessive depth). Intermediate levels of sedation are not easily distinguished by the derived EEG parameters from the results in this study.

Study Strengths and Weaknesses

Strengths included the large numbers of data points for assessing correlation among both clinical and both EEG-derived monitoring tools. Patients enrolled in this study had no CNS pathology and as such, clinical effects of sedative/hypnotic agents were reflected in assessment findings and monitor data. Also, this study focused on intermediate levels of sedation such as might be utilized for outpatient procedures such as endoscopies. Given the increasing numbers of such procedures being performed, validating monitoring guidelines and technology potentially have widespread benefit. Weaknesses include the homogenous patient population (elective surgical procedures) and short-term use of the technology (duration of procedure) limits the potential applicability of these data to a larger population such as that encountered in the ICU setting. In addition, critically ill patients at times are sedated for several days rather than hours. Given the differences in population, it may be problematic to generalize results from this study to a larger ICU population. It does heighten awareness of potential avenues for research on these technologies in the ICU population. In addition, it assesses correlation and as presented, does not necessarily highlight improved outcomes.

Clinical Implications

Clinical implications of this study include renewed focus on reliance on clinical evaluation of sedative/hypnotic state. Perhaps more so for less experienced nurses and physicians there may be a temptation to "nurse the machine" and not as readily notice indications of the patient progressing to a more deeply sedated state. It cannot be overemphasized that when clinical assessment data are available for sedation assessment, that should be the primary determinant of therapeutic decisions.

5. **Jordan KG. Continuous EEG monitoring in the neuroscience intensive care unit and emergency department. *J Clin Neurophysiol.* 1999;16:14–39.**

Multiple case series of patients encompassing populations from the emergency department (ED) and neuroscience ICU were studied. The first case series consisted of 200 patients monitored with continuous EEG. Of the 200 patients in this series, EEG monitoring was decisive in 54% (n = 109) in determining a direction of clinical management. In an additional 32% (n = 64), EEG data was a contributing factor in therapeutic decision-making. The second case series consisted of 518 patients having risk factors for seizure activity. Of the 518 patients in this series, 25.9% of patients (n = 134) were identified as having only subtle indications of seizure activity. Both clinical areas highlighted by Jordan (emergency department and neuroscience critical care unit) have a high incidence of patients at high risk of neurologic dysfunction or extension of an existing neurologic injury. The multiple case series examined in this article included

cerebral ischemia and hemorrhage, seizure activity (nonclinical episodic or nonclinical status epilepticus), brain tumor, brain trauma, and intracranial infection. Benefits of continuous EEG availability include earlier detection of seizure activity or brain dysfunction at a potentially reversible stage and, in monitored patients, shortening the interval between occurrence of seizure activity/further neurologic dysfunction and aggressive clinical management. Jordan further identifies that longer intervals between onset of seizure activity, particularly subclinical status epilepticus, can lead to higher morbidity, mortality, and resistance to treatment.

This article reviews the literature on applications of EEG technology and their efficacy at complementing the neurologic examination in identifying CNS dysfunction not immediately available on clinical assessment. Clinical areas highlighted include the emergency department and neuroscience critical care unit. Both clinical areas have a high incidence of patients at high risk of having neurologic dysfunction or an extension of an existing neurologic injury. Benefits of a continuous availability of EEG monitoring technology are highlighted in multiple situations. The multiple case series highlighted in this article include patients following acute cerebral ischemia and hemorrhage, seizure activity (nonclinical episodic or nonclinical status epilepticus), brain tumor, intracranial infection, and brain trauma. Early aggressive clinical management of these patient populations is vital to optimal clinical outcomes. Early data indicating brain dysfunction at a potentially reversible stage can be decisive in determining direction of clinical management. Of the 200 patients in this series, EEG monitoring was decisive in 54% (n = 109) with regard to changing the direction of management because it yielded information not clearly evident from clinical examination. In an additional 32% (n = 64), it was a contributing factor in changing direction of care. Jordan noted the significant benefit in availability of EEG technology toward optimal patient outcomes. A second patient series was documented. Of all of the patients (n = 518) with risk factors for seizure activity, a significant number (n = 134) were described as having only "subtle" indications of seizure activity. Jordan further identifies the time to treatment following onset of seizure activity, particularly subclinical status epilepticus. A longer time elapsed from seizure onset can lead to higher morbidity, mortality, and resistance to treatment.

Clinical Implications

Implication are twofold: a compelling case for increased availability (24/7) of EEG monitoring and appropriate training of nursing and physician staff for optimal use/clinical benefit from the technology.

6. **Stecker MM, Cheung AT, Pochettino A, Kent GP, Patterson T, Weiss SJ, Bavaria JE. Deep hypothermic circulatory arrest: I. Effects of cooling on electroencephalogram and evoked potentials. *Ann Thorac Surg.* 2001;71:14–21.**

Study Sample

One hundred nine patients underwent surgical procedures requiring circulatory arrest.

Comparison Studied

This investigation focused on 5 electrophysiologic events indicating significant reduction in cerebral metabolism at various stages of cooling as reflected in the EEG. These events were periodic complexes ($26.9° ± 3°C$), burst suppression ($24.4° ± 4°C$), electrocerebral silence ($17.8° ± 4°C$), and 2-phase ablation of somatosensory evoked responses ($21.4° ± 4°C$ and $17.3 ± 4°C$, respectively).

Study Procedures

EEG and somatosensory evoked potential (SSEP) recordings using a 16-channel EEG machine were initiated at baseline (prior to hypothermia induction) and EEG/SSEP changes at varying stages of cooling were correlated with specific temperature ranges. Analysis of variance was used to test for differences between variables across 3 groups of patients (neurologically normal, preoperative CVA, postoperative neurologic impairment).

Key Results

The main results of the study were close evaluation of EEG changes (decreasing frequency and increased suppression) in association with significant decreases in core body temperature. With regards to predictive value of a given body temperature on EEG state, Stecker et al. found the only absolute predictor of an isoelectric EEG was a core body temperature below $12.5°C$ for longer than 50 minutes.

Study Strengths and Weaknesses

Study strengths include close electrophysiologic monitoring with 16-channel EEG hardware as well as a heterogenous patient population (with/without CNS disease). Additionally, induced hypothermia was done on a patient-specific basis rather than choosing an arbitrary temperature endpoint for all patients. This took into account individualized neurophysiologic effects of hypothermia. As such, using isoelectric EEG is a more reproducible endpoint for monitoring. It also tracked electrophysiologic changes to temperature in a clinical setting. Weaknesses included the fact that this was done on a surgical setting rather than an adult critical care setting. Also, the only drug therapy utilized in this study was isoflurane and no other CNS depressants were documented. These factors make generalizability problematic to other populations and clinical settings.

Clinical Implications

Clinical implications are multiple. One is that during induced hypothermia concurrent with drug-induced coma, EEG monitoring is necessary. There may be wide differences in patient responses to hypothermic states as well as clinical effects of barbiturate therapy, for example. Burst

suppression or isoelectric EEG may occur at a much higher temperature when barbiturate therapy is utilized. In addition, with known pharmacokinetic changes consequent to hypothermic states, a more profound CNS depressant effect and duration of action may be associated with a given drug dosage at lower body temperatures, mandating continuous EEG monitoring and drug/temperature titration to specific endpoints to protect patients from dangerous side effects and prolonged/profound CNS depression.

7. Mathew JP, Weatherwax KJ, East CJ, White WD, Reves JG. Bispectral analysis during cardiopulmonary bypass: the effect of hypothermia on the hypnotic state. *J Clin Anesth.* 2001;13:301–305.

Study Sample

One hundred patients with no CNS dysfunction undergoing cardiothoracic surgery required cardiopulmonary bypass.

Comparison Studied

The study objective was to evaluate the relationship between data obtained from BIS monitoring and therapeutic hypothermia such as that utilized during surgical procedures requiring cardiopulmonary bypass.

Study Procedures

BIS monitoring was initiated using the A-1050 monitoring system. Induction and maintenance of anesthesia were accomplished with bolus followed by infusion dosing of midazolam (targeted to effect site concentration of 150 ng/mL) and fentanyl (targeted to effect site concentration of 2.2 ng/mL). NMB was provided using pancuronium bromide, and isoflurane was administered by the anesthesia provider as clinically indicated. BIS values, drug dosing, and related predicted brain concentrations as well as temperature were monitored before cardiopulmonary bypass and throughout. Arterial $Paco_2$ was maintained between 35 and 40 mm Hg, and arterial $Paco_2$ was maintained between 150 and 250 mm Hg. A repeated-measures, mixed-effects statistical method was used to analyze effects of all variables (age, drug dosing, and temperature) on BIS values.

Key Results

A relationship was found between BIS and body temperature, specifically, a decrease in BIS value of 1.12 for each degree centigrade decrease in body temperature.

Study Strengths and Weaknesses

Strengths included large sample size (100 patients) analysis and accounting for multiple factors (ie, administration of CNS depressants) that may impact BIS values. Hypothermia and advanced age are known to decrease anesthetic requirements and this investigation identified the specific relationship between hypothermia, EEG-derived brain evaluation and drug dosing. Weaknesses include a homogenous patient population and serum concentrations of fentanyl and midazolam that were not measured. If higher than expected, then the association between BIS and body temperature was less defined. Given the population studied and drug therapy regimens during anesthesia, ability to generalize this study to patients in the ICU is limited. Matthew et al. rightly point out that with profound hypothermia, exogenous CNS depressant dosing requirements were dramatically reduced.

Clinical Implications

This investigation has potential implications for monitoring patients receiving drug-induced (barbiturate) coma during therapeutic hypothermia. Real-time EEG and EEG-derived brain monitoring can assist in identifying patients at risk for excessive CNS depression and facilitate downward dose titration of barbiturate therapy as dictated by objective data. It is well known that EEG and induced hypothermia are closely related. This study begins to potentially validate the relationship between BIS (as an EEG-derived parameter) and hypothermia.

8. Markland ON. Pearls, perils and pitfalls in the use of the electroencephalogram. *Semin Neurol* 2003;23:7–46.

Markland initially discusses baseline or normal EEG activity as a basis of comparison and follows with correlation between multiple pathologic states with corresponding EEG states through use of multiple detailed examples of specific brain pathologies, clinical findings, and corresponding EEG states. The correlation between EEG state, clinical findings, and optimal clinical management is illustrated. One example is the specific EEG state with triphasic waves that differentiate specific neurologic pathologic states such as subclinical status epilepticus and metabolic encephalopathy. A second example is the identification of specific EEG seizure waveform morphologies that help to determine optimal drug therapies. Markland provides guidance on optimal use of diagnostic EEG data to determine brain pathology, direction of therapeutic interventions, as well as prognosis. EEG provides data that may not be evident on clinical evaluation but may complement clinical and neuroimaging evaluation.

This article reviews literature, applications of EEG technology, and its efficacy at complementing the neurologic examination in identifying CNS dysfunction not immediately available on clinical assessment. The correlation between degree of cerebral dysfunction, clinical evaluation, and corresponding EEG state is extensively reviewed. Specific EEG states such as triphasic waves are highlighted as differentiating between specific neurologic pathologic states such as subclinical status epilepticus and metabolic encephalopathy. Multiple detailed examples are given of specific pathologic states, clinical findings, and correspond-

ing EEG state(s). This correlation between characteristic EEG state and specific brain pathology is paramount not only in differentiating brain disease or injury but also in determining the direction of therapeutic intervention(s) as well as prognosis. Markland first discusses baseline or normal EEG activity and then uses this as a basis to compare additional pathologic states for EEG patterns, pathophysiology, and corresponding clinical examination findings. Specific aspects of EEG utilization and findings are illustrated as determining drug therapies for various types of seizure waveform morphologies. Ultimately, Markland provides guidance on the optimal use of diagnostic EEG data to determine brain pathology not immediately evident, and posits that it is complementary to both the clinical examination and neuroimaging studies.

9. Claassen J, Mayer SA, Kowalski RG, Emerson RG, Hirsch LJ. Detection of electrographic seizures with continuous EEG monitoring in critically ill patients. *Neurology.* 2004;62: 1743–1748.

Study Sample

Five hundred seventy consecutive critically ill patients underwent continuous EEG monitoring.

Comparison Studied

EEG data were evaluated from the patient sampling in order to detect seizure activity not evident on clinical examination. Patients who had an otherwise unexplained decrease in level of consciousness were included in the sample. The duration of the study/data collection was 6.5 years.

Study Procedure

Following patient enrollment, baseline demographics and clinical and EEG data were recorded; multivariate logistic regression analysis was performed to identify factors associated with electrographic seizure activity as well as onset of seizure activity greater than 24 hours following the start of EEG monitoring.

Key Results

In 19% of the sample (n = 110 patients), seizure activity was detected. In 92% of this subset (n = 101), the seizure activity was not evident on clinical examination. Of the patients in whom seizure activity was identified, 89% (n = 98) were in critical care units. Subclinical seizure was associated with coma (odds ratio [OR] 7.7; 95% CI 4.2–14.2), age <18 years (OR 6.7; 95% CI 2.8–16.2), history of seizure disorder (OR 2.7; 95% CI 1.3–5.5) and clinically evident seizure activity during the current illness (OR 2.4; 95% CI 1.4–4.3). In 88% of patients who had subclinical seizure activity, it was detected within the first 24 hours of EEG monitoring.

Study Strengths and Weaknesses

Strengths are the large sample size and variety of admitting diagnoses. The investigation also identified specific subgroups of the patient demographic who were more at risk for seizure activity such as depressed consciousness, and it further supports more widespread use of EEG monitoring in clinical practice within critical care settings. Weaknesses include the narrow applicability of the results. It was done at only 1 institution, which limits the ability to generalize the data to other clinical settings and patient diagnoses.

Clinical Implications

This study supports more widespread use of continuous EEG monitoring in clinical practice. Roughly 1 in 5 patients with depressed consciousness over a 5-year period were identified as having seizure activity. This represents a significant proportion of patients being admitted to critical care units. Also, it highlights early detection and intervention, and illustrates the effiacy of EEG technology in identifying seizure activity early at a more treatable stage that will contribute to more favorable clinical and neurologic outcomes.

10. Vespa PM, Boscardin WJ, Hovda DA, et al. Early and persistent impaired alpha variability on continuous electroencephalography monitoring as predictive of poor outcome after traumatic brain injury. *J Neurosurg.* **2002;97:84–92.**

Study Sample

Eighty-nine consecutive patients with moderate to severe traumatic brain injury (TBI) as defined by GCS scores between 3 and 12 comprised this cohort.

Comparison Studied

Vespa et al. hypothesized that a reduced percentage of alpha variability (PAV) on diagnostic EEG recording indicates a poor prognosis as measured by clinical and neurologic outcome.

Study Procedures

Continuous EEG was prospectively monitored on 89 consecutive patients. The PAV was calculated daily and the evolution in trends in PAV was analyzed in comparison with the patient's Glasgow Outcome Scale score at discharge.

Key Results

In patients with a GCS of ≤ 8, a PAV of 0.1 or lower was predictive of poor outcome or death (positive predictive value, 86%). The determining PAV was obtained by day 3 postinjury. Persistent PAV values ≤ 0.1 or a PAV that declined within 3 days postinjury indicated a high likelihood of poor outcome. Early PAV during initial 3 days postinjury improved prognostic ability ($P < .001$).

Study Strengths and Weaknesses

Strengths include a priori hypothesis testing, large sample size, and use of objective information readily available from EEG data. Conduct of the study is also consistent with recognizing value in reactivity of EEG. Under normal circumstances, EEG waveforms should be responsive to brain arousal or stimulation. A less responsive EEG state is already recognized as a poor prognostic sign. Weaknesses include narrow patient sampling focusing only on patients following TBI. The sample size of 89 patients in this single study when compared with the vastly larger number of patients who suffer a TBI limits generalizability. Thus, generalization of the results to other neurologic disorders such as cerebral infarction or subarachnoid hemorrhage is limited. Vespa et al. also didn't differentiate between global and focal brain injury in terms of correlating injury type with reduced PAV.

Clinical Implications

This study supports early use of EEG monitoring following brain injury. If replicated, this may greatly help in determining prognosis early in clinical management, which would provide more data for clinicians and families to use in making more appropriate decisions about the direction of care (palliative vs. aggressive curative care).

OTHER REFERENCES

1. Arbour R. Aggressive management of intracranial dynamics. *Crit Care Nurse.* 1998;18:30–40.
2. Arbour R. Mastering neuromuscular blockade. *Dimens Crit Care Nurse.* 2000;19:4–20.
3. Arbour RB. Sedation and pain management in critically ill adults. *Crit Care Nurse.* 2000;20:39–56.
4. Arbour RB. Using the bispectral index to assess arousal response in a patient with neuromuscular blockade. *Am J Crit Care.* 2000;9;383–387.
5. Aspect Medical Systems. *A-2000™ Operating Manual.* Norwood, MA: Aspect Medical Systems, Inc.; 2001.
6. Aspect Medical Systems. *Technology overview: Bispectral Index* (White Paper). Norwood, MA: Aspect Medical Systems Inc.; 1997.
7. Aspect Medical Systems. *Overview: The Effects of Electromyography (EMG) and Other High-Frequency Signals on the Bispectral Index (BIS)* (White Paper). Norwood, MA: Aspect Medical Systems Inc.; 2000.
8. Barbato M. (2001). Bispectral index monitoring in unconscious palliative care patients. *J Palliat Care.* 2001;17:102–108.
9. Benbadis SR, Rielo D. *EEG atlas: Normal sleep EEG-Stage III and IV.* E-Medicine 2001 (updated 9/2006). Available at: http://www.emedicine.com/neuro/topic689.htm. Accessed August 24, 2007.

10. Brandl KM, Langley KA, Dork LA, Levy H. Conforming the reliability of the Sedation-Agitation Scale administered by ICU nurses without experience in its use. *Pharmacotherapy*. 2001;21:431–436.

11. Brunh J, Myles PS, Sneyd R, Struys MMRF. Depth of anaesthesia monitoring: what's available, what's validated, and what's next? *Br J Anaesth*. 2006; 97:85–94.

12. Censullo JL, Sebastian S. Pentobarb sodium coma for refractory intracranial hypertension. *J Neurosci Nurs*. 2003;35:252–262.

13. Chonj DJ, Hirsch LJ. Which EEG patterns warrant treatment in the critically ill? Reviewing the evidence for treatment of periodic epileptiform discharges and related patterns. *J Clin Neurophysiol*. 2005;22:79–91.

14. DeDeyne C, Struys M, Decruyenaere J, Creupelandt J, Hoste E, Colardyn F. Use of continuous bispectral EEG monitoring to assess depth of sedation in ICU patients. *Intensive Care Med*. 1998;24:1294–1298.

15. Del Castillo MA.. Monitoring neurologic patients in intensive care. *Curr Opin Crit Care*. 2001;7:49–60.

16. Dereeper E, Berré J, Vandesteene A, LeFranc F, Vincent JL. Barbiturate coma for intracranial hypertension: clinical observations. *J Crit Care*. 2002;17: 58–62.

17. Doi M, Morita K, Mantzaridis M, Sato S, Kenny GN. Prediction of responses to various stimuli during sedation: a comparison of three EEG variables. *Intensive Care Med*. 2005;31:41–47.

18. Ely EW, Siegel MD, Inouye SK. Delirium in the intensive care unit: an under-recognized syndrome of organ dysfunction. *Semin Respir Crit Care Med*. 2001;22:115–126.

19. Epstein J, Breslow MJ. The stress response of critical illness. *Crit Care Clin*. 1999;15:17–34.

20. Frenzel D, Griem CA, Sommer C, Bauerle K, Roewer N. Is the bispectral index appropriate for monitoring the sedation level of mechanically ventilated surgical ICU patients? *Intensive Care Med*. 2002;28:178–183.

21. Gilbert TT, Wagner MR, Halukurike V, Paz HL, Garland A. Use of bispectral electroencephalogram monitoring to assess neurologic status in unsedated, critically ill patients. *Crit Care Med*, 2001; 29:1996–2000. Comment in 29:2036–2037.

22. Halliburton JR, McCarthy EJ. Perioperative monitoring with the electroencephalogram and bispectral index monitor. *AANA J*. 2000;68:333–340.

23. Hilbish C. Bispectral Index monitoring in the neurointensive care unit. *J Neurosci Nurs*. 2003;35: 336–338.

24. Honan DM, Breen PJ, Boylan JF, McDonald NJ, Egan TD. Decrease in bispectral index preceding intraoperative hemodynamic crisis: evidence of acute alteration of propofol pharmacokinetics. *Anesthesiology*. 2002;97:1303–1305.

25. Huff JS. *Status epilepticus*. Emedicine 2001. Available at: http://www.emedicine.com/emerg /topic554.htm. Accessed August 24, 2007.

26. Inoue S, Kawaguchi M, Sasaoka N, Hirai K, Furuya H. Effects of neuromuscular block on systemic and cerebral hemodynamics and bispectral index during moderate or deep sedation in critically ill patients. *Intensive Care Med*. 2006;32:391–397.

27. Jacobi J, Fraser GL, Coursin DB, et al. Clinical practice guidelines for the sustained use of sedatives and analgesics in the critically ill adult. *Crit Care Med*, 2002;30:119–141. Comments in 2002;30:2609–2610, 2613–2614; 2003;31:664–665, 2417–2418; 2004;32: 1435–1436.

28. Kelly SD. *Monitoring Level of Consciousness During Anesthesia and Sedation. A Clinician's Guide to the Bispectral Index*. Norwood, MA: Aspect Medical Systems; 2003. Available at: http://www.aspectmed ical.com/resources/handbook/default.mspx.

29. Kin N, Konstadt SN, Sato K, Hanaoka K. Reduction of bispectral index value associated with clinically significant cerebral air embolism. *J Cardiothorac Vasc Anesth*. 2004;18:82–84.

30. Luginbuhl M, Schnider TW. Detection of awareness with the bispectral index: two case reports. *Anesthesiology*. 2002;96:241–243.

31. March K, Wellwood J, Arbour, R. Technology, chapt 7. In: *AANN Core Curriculum for Neuroscience Nursing*, 4th ed. St. Louis: W. B. Saunders Co.; 2004.

32. Mathew JP, Weatherwax KJ, East CJ, White WD, Reves JG, Bispectral analysis during cardiopulmonary bypass: the effect of hypothermia on the hypnotic state. *J Clin Anesth*. 2001;13:301–305.

33. Merat S, Levecque JP, Gulluche YL, Diraison Y, Brinquin L, Hoffmann JJ. BIS monitoring may allow detection of severe cerebral ischemia. *Can J Anesth*. 2001;48:1066–1069.

34. Misulis KE. *Essentials of Clinical Neurophysiology*. Newton, MA: Butterworth-Heinemann; 1997.

35. Mondello E, Siliotti R, Noto G, Cuzzocrea E, Scollo G, Trimarchi G, Venuti FS. Bispectral index in ICU: correlation with Ramsay Score on assessment of sedation level. *J Clin Monit Comput*. 2002;17: 271–277.

36. Mourisse J, Booij L. Bispectral index detects period of cerebral hypoperfusion during cardiopulmonary bypass. *J Cardiothor Vasc Anesth*. 2003;17:76–78.

37. Nasraway SA. The bispectral index: expanded performance for everyday use in the intensive care unit? *Crit Care Med*. 2005;33:685–687.

38. Nasraway SA. Use of sedative medications in the intensive care unit. *Semin Resp Crit Care Med*. 2001;22:165–174.

39. Nasraway SA, Wu EC, Kelleher RM, Yasuda CM, Donnelly AM. How reliable is the bispectral index in critically ill patients? A prospective, comparative,

single-blinded observer study. *Crit Care Med.* 2002;30:1483–1487.

40. Parker BM. Anesthetics and anesthesia techniques: impacts on perioperative management and postoperative outcomes. *Clev Clin J Med.* 2006;73(Suppl 1): S13–S17.

41. Prielipp RC, Coursin DB, Wood KE, Murray MJ. Complications associated with sedative and neuromuscular blocking drugs in critically ill patients. *Crit Care Clin.* 1995;11:983–1002.

42. Primak LK, Lowrie L. Paralyzation and sedation of the ventilated trauma patient. *Respir Care Clin N Am.* 2001;7:97–126.

43. Rhoney DH, Parker D. Use of sedative and analgesic agents in neurotrauma patients: effects on cerebral physiology. *Neurol Res.* 2001;23:237–259.

44. Riker RR, Fraser GL, Simmons LE, Wilkins ML. Validating the sedation-agitation scale with the bispectral index and visual analog scale in adult ICU patients after cardiac surgery. *Intensive Care Med.* 2001;27:853–858.

45. Riker RR, Fraser GL. Sedation in the intensive care unit: refining the models and defining the questions. *Crit Care Med.* 2002;30:1661–1663.

46. Rutkove SB. Effects of temperature on neuromuscular electrophysiology. *Muscle Nerve.* 2001;24: 867–882.

47. Simmons LE, Riker RR, Prato BS, Fraser GL. Assessing sedation during intensive care unit mechanical ventilation with the bispectral index and the sedation-agitation scale. *Crit Care Med.* 1999;27:1499–1504.

48. Sleigh JW, Andrezejowski J, Steyn-Ross M. The Bispectral Index: a measure of depth of sleep. *Anesth Analg.* 1999;88:659–661.

49. Stecker MM, Cheung AT, Pochettino A, Kent GP, Patterson T, Weiss SJ, Bavaria JE. Deep hypothermic circulatory arrest: I. Effects of cooling on electroencephalogram and evoked potentials. *Ann Thorac Surg.* 2001;71:14–21.

50. Tonner PH, Wei C, Bein B, Weiler N, Paris A, Scholz J. Comparison of two bispectral index algorithms in monitoring sedation in postoperative intensive care patients. *Crit Care Med.* 2005;33:580–584. Comment in 33:685–687.

51. Vanluchene ALG, Vereecke H, Thas O, Mortier EP, Shafer SL, Struys MM. Spectral entropy as an electroencephalographic measure of anesthetic drug effect. *Anesthesiology.* 2004;101:34–42.

52. Vespa, P. Continuous EEG monitoring for the detection of seizures in traumatic brain injury, infarction and intracerebral hemorrhage: "To detect and protect." *J Clin Neurophysiol.* 2005;22:99–106.

53. Vivien B, Paqueron Z, Le Cosquer P, Langeron O, Coriat P, Riou B. Detection of brain death onset using the bispectral index in severely comatose patients. *Intensive Care Med.* 2002;28:419–425.

54. Wagner BK, Zavotsky KE, Sweeney JB, Palmeri BA, Hammond JS. Patient recall of therapeutic paralysis in a surgical critical care unit. *Pharmacotherapy.* 1998;18:358–363.

55. Watson BD, Kane-Gill SL. Sedation assessment in critically ill adults: 2001–2004 update. *Ann Pharmacother.* 2004;38:1898–1906.

56. Welsby IJ, Ryan M, Booth JV, et al. The bispectral index in the diagnosis of perioperative stroke: A case report and discussion. *Anesth Analg.* 2003;96: 435–437.